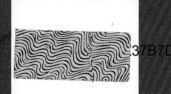

MCMINN'S COLOR ATLAS OF
HEAD AND NECK
ANATOMY

Dedication

To

Arlette Herzig and Robert Logan
Bari Logan

To the memory of Robin Mason, Global Scholar
Patricia Reynolds

Giles Gordon
Scott Rice

Anne, Sam and Isabel
Ralph Hutchings

And

To the Memory of an Esteemed Colleague
Professor R. M. H. (Bob) McMinn

MCMINN'S COLOR ATLAS OF HEAD AND NECK ANATOMY

FIFTH EDITION

Bari M. Logan MA, FMA, Hon MBIE, MAMAA
Formerly University Prosector, Department of Anatomy, University of
Cambridge; Prosector, Department of Anatomy, The Royal College of
Surgeons of England, London and Anatomical Preparator, Department of
Human Morphology, University of Nottingham Medical School, Nottingham, UK

Patricia A. Reynolds BDS, MBBS, MAODE (Open), PhD, FDSRCS (Eng), FDSRCS (Ed), FHEA
Professor Emeritus, Dental Institute, King's College London, London, UK

Scott Rice MBBS, BDS (Hons), MA Clin Ed, AKC, MFDSRCS (Eng), FHEA
Academic Clinical Fellow/Specialist Registrar, Department of Clinical Radiology,
University College London Hospitals NHS Trust/London Deanery, London, UK

Original Photography by Ralph T. Hutchings

Photographer for Visuals Unlimited.com
Formerly Chief Medical Laboratory Scientific Officer, The Royal College of
Surgeons of England, London, UK

For additional online content visit http://expertconsult.inkling.com

ELSEVIER

ELSEVIER

First edition 1981
Second edition 1994
Third edition 2004
Fourth edition 2010
Fifth edition 2017

The right of Bari M. Logan, Patricia A. Reynolds, Scott Rice, Ralph T. Hutchings to be identified as authors of this work has been asserted by them in accordance with the Copyright, Designs and Patents Act 1988.

ISBN: 978-0-7020-7017-4
E-ISBN: 978-0-7020-7043-3

Printed in China
Last digit is the print number: 9   8   7   6   5   4   3   2   1

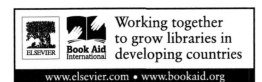

Content Strategist: Jeremy Bowes
Content Development Specialist: Joanne Scott
Content Development Specialist, e-products: Kim Benson
Project Manager: Andrew Riley
Design: Miles Hitchen
Illustration Manager: Karen Giacomucci
Illustrator: MPS North America LLC
Marketing Manager: Melissa Darling

Preface

This fifth edition of *McMinn's Color Atlas of Head and Neck Anatomy* heralds 35 years of publication in eight language editions, of English, French, German, Italian, Japanese, Korean, Portuguese and Spanish; with considerable sales worldwide, it has become an accepted standard text on the subject.

Originally intended as an illustrated reference book for dental students, over the ensuing years it has also proved popular with Radiologists, Neuro, Skull-base, Cranio-facial, Maxillo-facial, Plastic-reconstructive, Ophthalmic, Dental and ENT Surgeons. The book therefore continues to fill an important niche on the medical library bookshelf.

For this fifth edition, a fourth co-author, Scott Rice, joins the team bringing particular specialist knowledge and expertise in the field of head and neck imaging, adding a revised chapter on the subject using state-of-the-art technology.

The chapter on 'Dental Anaesthesia' (Appendix 1) has been revised; whilst the anatomical element remains the same, techniques in the administration of local anaesthesia have been altered in recent years, hence the need to up-date instructive text.

There has been a major boost to the electronic version of the book with the inclusion by Patricia Reynolds and Scott Rice of over 280 new illustrations expanding the imaging of normal and developmental structures, together with some common variations, anomalies, defects and diseases of clinically relevant topics. A newly titled section on teeth is further enhanced by images relating to common dental conditions and diseases. Many of the clinico-pathological images have been sourced from *Cawson, R.A., Binnie, W.H. and Eveson, J.W. Slide Atlas of Oral Disease. 2nd Edition. 1994, Wolfe; and Cawson, R. A., Eveson, J. W. Oral Pathology and Diagnosis. 1987, Gower Medical Publishing Ltd* that are no longer in print. The website also includes an interactive question bank with over 150 multiple choice questions to aid exam preparation and check your understanding.

We hope that all of the above amendments and new additions will be appreciated and that the book will continue in its popularity and important contribution to medical education at both the pre-clinical and postgraduate level.

Bari Logan, Siegershausen, Switzerland
Patricia Reynolds, London
Scott Rice, London
2016

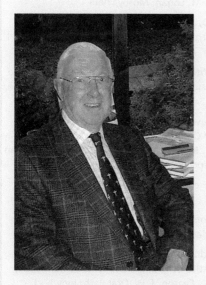

Professor R. M. H. McMinn, MD (Glas), PhD (Sheff), FRCS (Eng)
[b. Sept 23, 1923 – d. July 11, 2012, aged 88]

Robert 'Bob' McMinn was a medical graduate of the University of Glasgow. After leaving hospital posts and service with the Royal Air Force in Iraq and Africa, he began his anatomical career as a Demonstrator in Anatomy in Glasgow in 1950. He became a lecturer in the University of Sheffield and was later Reader and then Titular Professor at King's College, London. In 1970 he was appointed to the Chair of Anatomy at the Royal College of Surgeons of England. Among his publications 'A Colour Atlas of Human Anatomy', with photographer R. T. Hutchings, was first published in 1977 and became a worldwide best-seller, with translations into over 25 languages more than 4 million copies were sold.

For this and other later atlases his co-authors added the name 'McMinn' to the titles in recognition of his contribution to anatomical teaching. He was editor of the eighth and ninth editions of 'Last's Anatomy Regional and Applied' which remains a standard work for surgical trainees. He was programme secretary and later treasurer of the Anatomical Society of Great Britain and Ireland, and was a founder member and first secretary of the British Association of Clinical Anatomists. At the International Anatomical Congress held in Cambridge in 2000 he received a Special Presentation Award from the Anatomical Society for his teaching and research activities. His research interests were in wound healing and tissue repair, and on the association between skin disease and the alimentary tract.

He retired in 1983 and moved with his wife back to their Scottish homeland settling on the west coast in Ardfern, Lochgilphead.

Acknowledgements

The authors are indebted to the following:

- Dr Trevor Coward, Reader in Maxillofacial and Craniofacial Rehabilitation, King's College London Dental Institute, for conservation and mounting of deciduous teeth.
- Mr Robert Bentley, Clinical Director for Major Trauma at King's College Hospital, for the section on Craniosynostosis, images and advice.
- Mr Patrick O'Driscoll, Senior Oral and Maxillofacial Surgeon (retired), Guy's Hospital, King's College London, for clinical and radiographic images.
- Mr Robert Logan for loan of his deciduous teeth.
- Professor Graham Roberts, Professor of Paediatric Dentistry (retired), King's College London, for clinical paedodontic images and advice.
- Dr Ian Parkin, Clinical Anatomist, University of Cambridge, for expert anatomical knowledge.
- Mr Clive Brewis, ENT Registrar, Addenbrooke's Hospital, Cambridge, for advice on the ear.
- Mel Lazenby, Lucie Whitehead and the late Martin Watson, Department of Anatomy, University of Cambridge, for preservation of anatomical material.
- Mr Adrian Newman, Mr Ian Bolton and Mr John Bashford, Anatomy Visual Media Group (AVMG), Department of Anatomy, University of Cambridge, for new edition photographs, digital expertise and advice.

Terminology

Terminology adopted is to the International Anatomical Terminology—Terminologia Anatomica—created in 1988 by the Federative Committee on Anatomical Terminology (FCAT) and approved by the 56 member associations of the International Federation of Associations of Anatomists (IFAA). Stuttgart: Thieme ISBN 3-13-115251-6

Dissection/anatomical preparation credits

The following individuals are credited for their skilled work in preparing the anatomical material illustrated in this book:

- Dr N. Borely—126A, 127B
- Dr T. Coward—22BCD
- Bari M. Logan—5B, 11B, 13C, 15C, 22B, 37EF, 61F, 81EFGH, 89G, 104A, 105B, 106A, 107B, 110, 112, 116A, 117B, 118A, 119C, 120AB, 121C, 122A, 123BCD, 124AB, 128, 134AB, 136ABC, 138A, 140ABCD, 143IJ, 144BCD, 146A, 147BC, 148ABC, 150AB, 151CD, 152ABCD, 154ABC, 155DEF, 158ABCD, 159E, 160ABC, 161D, 166AB, 167C, 168A, 170ABC, 174ABC, 175D, 176ABC, 178AB, 180AB, 182ABC, 184ABCD, 186BC, 187D, 188ABCDEFGH, 190ABCD, 192ABCDE, 196, 198A, 199B, 200, 202A, 203BC, 204ABC, 206A, 207B, 210AC, 211BD, 212A, 213B, 214AB, 215DE, 216AB, 217C, 218, 220A, 221B, 222, 224AB, 226A, 228A, 230AB, 232, 234A, 235B, 236AB, 238A, 239B, 244AB, 246ABCDEF, 248ABC, 276B, 277C, 280B, 282G, 284D, 286I
- Steven F. Logan—(re-painting) 162ABCDEF, 164ABCDEFGH, 165J
- Professor R. M. H. McMinn—240AB, 242A
- Messrs. Adam and Rouilly, for the loan of osteological material.

Clinical photos

Figures 88F, 142E, 192F, 29B, 276A, 277B, 279B are reproduced, with kind permission, from *Imaging Atlas of Human Anatomy*, 3rd Edition, J. Weir and Peter H. Abrahams. Mosby, 2003.

Figures 135C, 169C are reproduced with kind permission from the Gordon Museum, King's College, London, UK.

Table 213 is reproduced, with permission, from *McMinn's Functional and Clinical Anatomy*, R. M. H. McMinn, P. Gaddum-Rosse, R. T. Hutchings, B. M. Logan. Mosby, 1995.

Figures 278A, 281C, 281D, 283H, 285E, 287J are redrawn, with kind permission, from *Introduction to Dental Local Anaesthesia*, H. Evers and G. Haegerstam. Astra/Mediaglobe, 1990.

Figures 269CD from *Griffiths PD. Chapter 19, Vascular supply and drainage of the brain. Susan Standring (ed). Gray's Anatomy*, 41e, page 290. 2016, Elsevier.

Figures 30AB, 31CD redrawn from *Ash M. Wheeler's Dental Anatomy Physiology and Occlusion*, 7th Edition. WB Saunders, originally from Schour L., Massler M.: The development of human dentition. *J Am Dent Assoc* 28:1153, 1941.

Figures 33D, E, F and 35F courtesy of eHuman, Inc; www.ehuman.com.

Figures 27ABC from *Histology and Cell Biology*, 2nd Edition, A.L. Kierszenbaum. Elsevier, 2007.

Online images are reproduced from Cawson, R. A., Binnie, W. H. and Eveson, J. W. Slide Atlas of Oral Disease. 2nd Edition. 1994, Wolfe; and Cawson, R. A., Eveson, J. W. Oral Pathology and Diagnosis. 1987, Gower Medical Publishing Ltd, with kind permission from Prof. John Eveson, Professor Emeritus, School of Dental and Oral Sciences, University of Bristol.

Preservation of Cadavers

Long-term preservation of the cadavers utilised for anatomical dissections (prosections) illustrated in this book, was by standard embalming technique, using an electric motor pump set at a constant pressure rate of 15 p.s.i. Perfusion was achieved through the arterial system via femoral artery cannulation of one leg and return drainage of the accompanying vein.

On the acceptance of 20 litres of preservative fluid by pump, local injection of those areas not visibly affected, was carried out by automatic syringe.

On average 30 litres of preservative fluid was used to preserve each cadaver.

Immediately following perfusion, cadavers were encapsulated in thick gauge clear polythene bags and cold stored at a temperature of 10.6° C at 40% humidity for a minimum period of 16 weeks before dissection. This period of storage allowed the preservative fluid to thoroughly saturate the body tissues, resulting in a highly satisfactory state of preservation.

The chemical formula for the preservative fluid (Logan *et al.,* 1989) is:

Methylated spirit 64 over proof	12.5 litres
Phenol liquefied 80%	2.5 litres
Formaldehyde solution 38%	1.5 litres
Glycerine BP	3.5 litres
	Total = 20 litres

The resultant working strength of each constituent is:

Methylated spirit	55%
Glycerine	12%
Phenol	10%
Formaldehyde solution	3%

The advantages of using this particular preservative fluid are:

(i) A state of soft preservation is achieved, benefiting dissection techniques.
(ii) The low formaldehyde solution content obviates excessive noxious fumes during dissection.
(iii) A degree of natural tissue colour is maintained, benefiting photography.
(iv) Mould growth does not occur on either whole cadavers thus preserved or their subsequent dissected (prosected) and stored parts.

SAFETY FOOTNOTE

Since the preparation of the anatomical material used in this book, there have been substantial changes to health and safety regulations concerning the use of certain chemical constituents in preservative fluids. It is essential therefore, to seek official local health and safety advice and guidance if intending to adopt the above preservative fluid.

Orientation Image

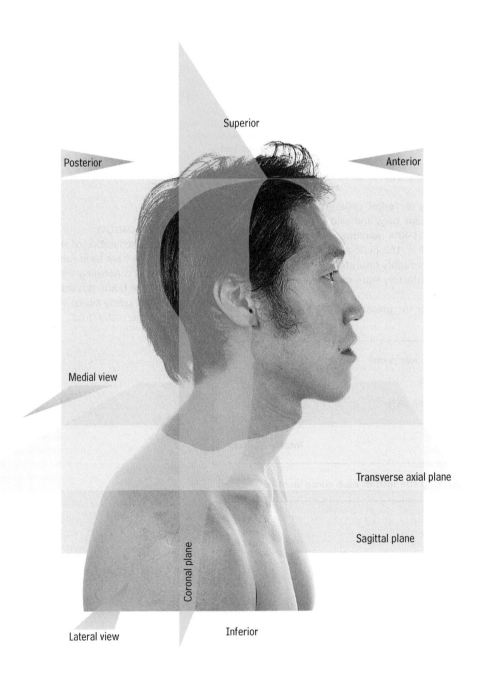

Superior

Posterior

Anterior

Medial view

Transverse axial plane

Sagittal plane

Coronal plane

Lateral view

Inferior

McMinn's Legacy of Illustrated Anatomy Books

Bari Logan entered the academic post of Prosector to the Department of Anatomy, The Royal College of Surgeons of England, London, in January 1977. At that time, 'Bob' McMinn held the Chair as Sir William Collins Professor of Human and Comparative Anatomy and Ralph Hutchings was the Chief Medical Scientific Officer and departmental photographer.

In April of the same year, an evening reception was held at the College for a group of distinguished medical fraternity by Wolfe Medical Publications to launch a new book entitled **A Colour Atlas of Human Anatomy** by the authors McMinn and Hutchings who had spent the previous two years working on the project.

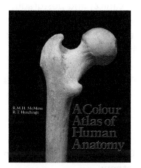

1977—ISBN 0-7234-0709-6
First Ed.   *– 1977*
Second Ed. *– 1988*
Third Ed.   *– 1993*
Fourth Ed. *– 1998*
Fifth Ed.   *– 2003*
Sixth Ed.   *– 2008*
Seventh Ed. – 2013

First Edition dust cover wrap

Instantly considered by many to be a visually stunning production, it was without doubt a pioneering book in the field of human anatomy having many novel concepts in both composition and design that would later be adopted by other authors and become standard format in many new illustrated texts on the subject.

The book, 352 pages, was unusually large in size and contained over 700 high quality colour photographs of almost natural size, of bones, detailed dissections (prosections), and exquisite anatomical preparations depicting the entire human body taken of specimens hitherto unseen beyond the closely guarded confines of the dissecting room and anatomical museum.

Essentially designed as a general reference work for the medical profession, the book rapidly became a best-seller, quickly producing 25 foreign language editions and attaining over four million copies in sales worldwide, it won numerous awards and gained much international academic acclaim.

The book remains in print today, 39 years on and in its seventh edition (2013), but since the fourth edition, under entirely new

authorship, direction and content, although the name 'McMinn' remains in the title for posterity.

Following on from the enormous success of **A Colour Atlas**, the publisher Peter Wolfe approached 'Bob' McMinn and Ralph Hutchings in early 1979 with the idea of producing a new illustrated text to suit the specific educational needs of dental students, for whom the Royal College of Surgeons ran popular postgraduate courses.

Wolfe's proposal was timely because within the College, the renovation and re-organisation of the Wellcome Museum of Anatomy and Physiology, founded by the famous Australian Anatomist R. (Ray) J. Last in 1947, was well underway; and a particular pressing need, identified by Bari Logan, was to prepare for display a range of detailed head and neck prosections and preparations, for which the collection was lacking.

Thus, the co-authorship trio of McMinn, Hutchings and Logan was formed and within a two year period produced their first book together in 1981.

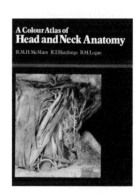

1981—ISBN 0-7234-0755-X
A Colour Atlas of Head and Neck Anatomy
Wolfe Medical Publications: McMinn/ Hutchings/Logan
Designed for dental students
English, French, German, Italian, Japanese, Korean, Portuguese, Spanish
Second Ed.– 1994
Third Ed. – 2004
Fourth Ed. – 2009
Fifth Ed.   – 2016

Over the next seventeen years, there followed a fairly rapid succession of books, despite the retirement of Ralph Hutchings in 1981 and of 'Bob' McMinn in 1983, academic career move of Bari Logan to Cambridge in 1987, further complications along the way of various changes to publishers through company takeovers; and each having additional authorship commitments on other new books.

Key to this speedy turnover, was the ability to combine individual talent in a very harmonious way, work to a logical regime and keep within a strict timeframe.

1982—ISBN 0-7234-0782-7
A Colour Atlas of Foot and
  Ankle Anatomy
Wolfe Medical Publications:
McMinn/Hutchings/Logan
Designed for Podiatrists and
  Chiropodists
English, Chinese, Dutch, French,
  Japanese, Russian, Spanish
Second Ed. – 1995
Third Ed.   – 2004
Fourth Ed. – 2012

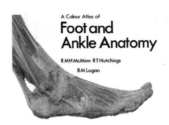

1995—ISBN 0-7234-0967-6
McMinn's Functional and Clinical
  Anatomy
Mosby: McMinn/Gaddum-Rosse/
  Hutchings/Logan
Designed for medical students
English, Italian, Greek
Out of Print

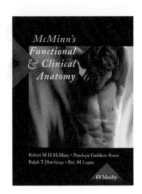

1984—ISBN 0-7234-0831-9
A Colour Atlas of Applied Anatomy
Wolfe Medical Publications: McMinn/
  Hutchings/Logan
Designed for clinicians (The anatomy
  of approaches for
surgical and clinical procedures)
English, Japanese
Out of Print

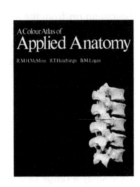

Functional and Clinical included a fourth co-author, Penelope Gaddum-Rosse, a distinguished physiologist, and work began on the project in 1987 as a text originally intended for the nursing profession and appropriately entitled, *Anatomy and Physiology for Nurses,* with the publishers Wolfe.

However, following a takeover of Wolfe Medical Publications by Mosby Year Book Europe, who already had an extensive nursing book list which included both physiology and anatomy titles, the manuscript was shelved for a number of years until a decision on its fate was finally reached in 1993 with the proposal for 'Bob' McMinn to re-edit the entire text and tailor it more to the needs of pre-clinical and postgraduate medical students.

'Bob' completed the task in just under one year and interestingly, it is considered to be the best written of all the McMinn books.

Their final book together was published in 1998.

1986—ISBN 0-7234-0911-0
Picture Tests in Human Anatomy
Wolfe Medical Publications: McMinn/
  Hutchings/Logan
Designed for medical students taking
  practical exams
English, French, German, Japanese,
  Portuguese, Serbo-Croation, Spanish
Out of Print

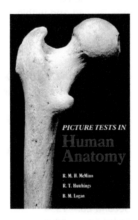

1998—ISBN 1-874545-52-9
The Concise Handbook of Human
  Anatomy
Manson Publishing: McMinn/
  Hutchings/Logan
Designed for sixth form students
  entering a medical career
English, German, Portuguese

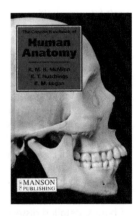

1986—ISBN 0-7234-0958-7
The Human Skeleton: a Photographic
  Manual in Colour
Wolfe Medical Publications: McMinn/
  Hutchings/Logan
Designed for medical students (fold
  out, full size skeleton
pictures and individual bones)
English, Danish, French, German,
  Greek, Japanese, Portuguese
  Spanish
Second Edition: 2007

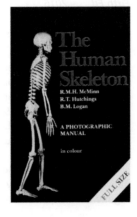

'Bob' was the inspirational driving force behind each book and from the start of the project would clearly outline overall content and specific illustrative requirements for each chapter producing rough sketches or photocopies with accompanying detailed lists of all the most important anatomical structures needed to be clearly seen in the resulting pictures.

Bari would interpret this information, produce his own notes and drawings and carry out the various detailed prosections or anatomical preparations working to the specific camera lens angle and overall framed view required.

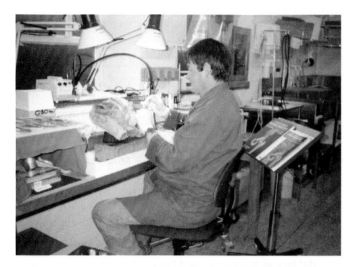

Bari M. Logan Prosector

Sporadic photographic sessions were held, often late evenings and weekends, under the 'Eagle Eye' of 'Bob' who would advise on the camera angle and ensure that all the structures essential to identify were displayed in their correct anatomical positions.

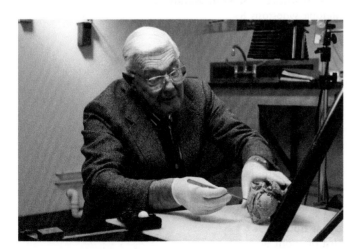

Professor R. ('Bob') H. McMinn Anatomist

Ralph spent infinite time setting-up lighting, establishing correct camera exposure settings and by using full format colour film, produced images of exceptional quality and depth in detail.

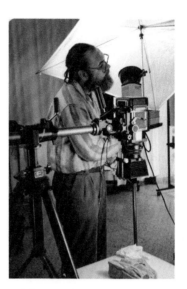

Ralph T. Hutchings Photographer

Since first publication, over the ensuing years to date (2016), the seven books produced by the 'trio', have thus far, created 14 foreign language editions: English, Chinese, Danish, Dutch, French, German, Greek, Italian, Japanese, Korean, Portuguese, Russian, Serbo-Croation and Spanish, with total sales exceeding well over 1 million copies worldwide.

Four of the books remain popular and still in print, **Head and Neck**, fifth edition, **Foot and Ankle**, fourth edition, **Human Skeleton,** second edition, and the **Concise Handbook**, which is currently under revision by new authorship and publisher.

Overall, a remarkable literary achievement in such a specialised field and only made possible by the unique visionary authorship and guidance of 'Bob' McMinn whose legacy of illustrated books on the subject of human anatomy has not only made a significant contribution to medical education in general, but also led to the grateful appreciation and applause of thousands of aspiring students throughout the World.

Bari M. Logan and *Ralph T. Hutchings*
April 2016

Contents

6 Clinical Imaging 251

Appendices 275

Skull, skull bone articulations and teeth

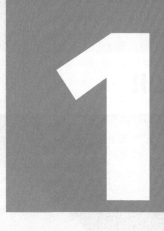

Skull

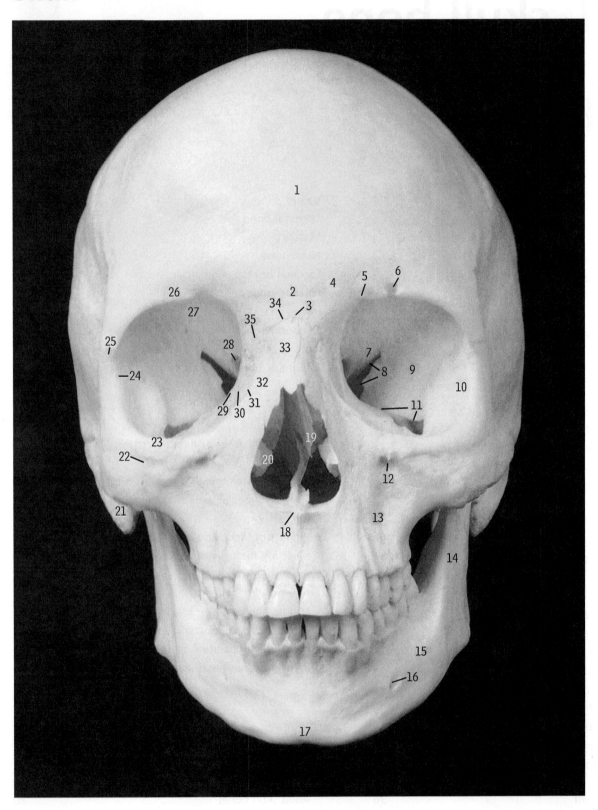

Skull *From the front*

This is the standard view from the front. The most obvious features are the two orbits and the central opening of the nasal cavity.

1 Frontal bone
2 Glabella
3 Nasion
4 Superciliary arch
5 Frontal notch
6 Supra-orbital foramen
7 Lesser wing of sphenoid bone
8 Superior orbital fissure
9 Greater wing of sphenoid bone
10 Zygomatic bone
11 Inferior orbital fissure
12 Infra-orbital foramen
13 Maxilla
14 Ramus
15 Body ⎫
16 Mental foramen ⎬ of mandible
17 Mental protuberance ⎭
18 Anterior nasal spine
19 Nasal septum
20 Inferior nasal concha
21 Mastoid process
22 Zygomaticomaxillary suture
23 Infra-orbital margin
24 Marginal tubercle
25 Frontozygomatic suture
26 Supra-orbital margin
27 Orbital part of frontal bone
28 Optic canal
29 Posterior lacrimal crest
30 Fossa for lacrimal sac
31 Anterior lacrimal crest
32 Frontal process of maxilla
33 Nasal bone
34 Frontonasal suture
35 Frontomaxillary suture

The term *skull* includes the *mandible*, while the cranium is the skull without the mandible; these definitions, however, are not always strictly observed.

The calvaria (a term not often used) is the upper part of the skull that encloses the brain (i.e. the cranial cavity); it has a roof or skull cap (cranial vault) and a floor—the base of the skull.

The anterior part of the skull forms the facial skeleton.

The cavities of the skull
- Cranial cavity, which contains the brain and its membranes.
- Nasal cavity, which is divided into right and left halves by the nasal septum (19, seen here through the pear-shaped opening, the anterior nasal or piriform aperture).
- Orbital cavities or orbits, right and left, which contain the eyes.

The bones of the skull

Unpaired	*Paired*
Frontal bone	Maxilla
Ethmoid bone	Nasal bone
Sphenoid bone	Lacrimal bone
Vomer	Inferior nasal concha
Occipital bone	Palatine bone
Mandible	Temporal bone
	Zygomatic bone
	Parietal bone

For details of individual bones, see pages 36-57.

The supra-orbital, infra-orbital and mental foramina (6, 12 and 16) lie in approximately the same vertical plane.

The supra-orbital foramen (or notch, 6) in the frontal bone lies just above (or at) the supra-orbital margin (26) about 2.5 cm from the midline.

The infra-orbital foramen (12) in the maxilla is 0.5 cm below the infra-orbital margin (23), directly in line below the pupil (with the eye looking straight ahead) and in the long axis of the upper second premolar tooth.

The mental foramen (16) in the mandible lies either below the apex of the lower second premolar tooth or in the interval between the apices of the first and second premolars (as on page 36, B10).

Ossification of the skull

Bones developed by endochondral ossification:
- Ethmoid bone
- Inferior nasal concha
- Sphenoid bone (except for lateral part of greater wing)
- Petromastoid and styloid parts of temporal bone
- Occipital bone (below superior nuchal line)

The rest of the skull bones develop by intramembranous ossification.

Skull *Muscle attachments, from the front*

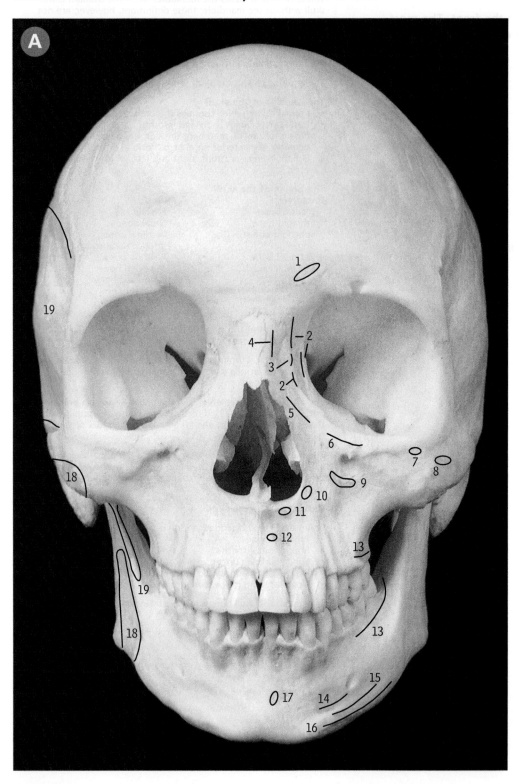

A

1   Corrugator supercilii
2   Orbicularis oculi
3   Medial palpebral ligament
4   Procerus
5   Levator labii superioris
    alaeque nasi
6   Levator labii superioris
7   Zygomaticus minor
8   Zygomaticus major
9   Levator anguli oris
10 Nasalis (transverse part)
11 Nasalis (alar part)
12 Depressor septi
13 Buccinator
14 Depressor labii inferioris
15 Depressor anguli oris
16 Platysma
17 Mentalis
18 Masseter
19 Temporalis

Orbicularis oculi (A2) is
attached partly in front of
and partly behind the fossa
for the lacrimal sac (page 8,
39).

The attachment of levator
labii superioris (A6) is above
the infra-orbital foramen
(page 2, 12), and that of
levator anguli oris (A9)
below the foramen.

The attachment of depressor
labii inferioris (A14) is in
front of the mental foramen
(page 2, 16), and that of
depressor anguli oris (A15)
below the foramen.

The attachments of the muscles belonging to the group commonly called the
muscles of the face or muscles of facial expression are shown on the left side of the
skull. On the right side are shown parts of the attachments of temporalis and
masseter, which belong to the muscles of mastication and are seen more extensively
in the lateral view (page 10).

Skull *Left half from the front*

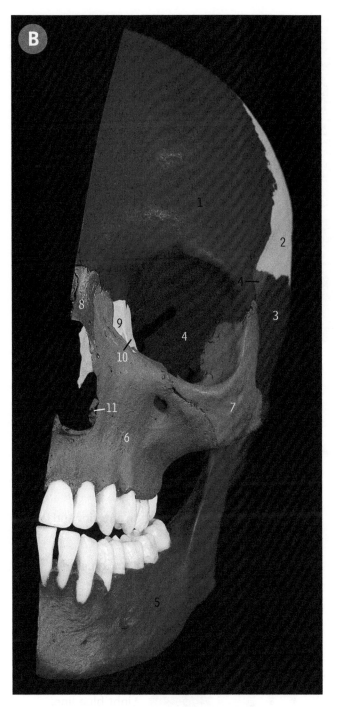

B with individual
bones coloured

1 Frontal bone
2 Parietal bone
3 Temporal bone
4 Sphenoid bone
5 Mandible
6 Maxilla
7 Zygomatic bone
8 Nasal bone
9 Lacrimal bone
10 Ethmoid bone
11 Inferior nasal concha

Skull *Le Fort facial fractures*

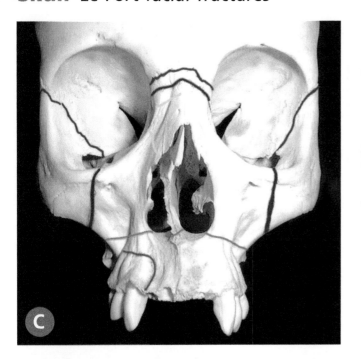

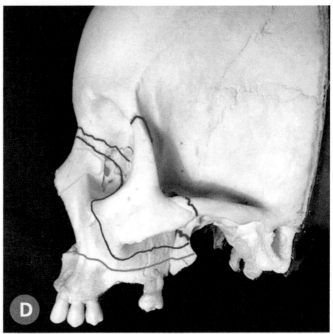

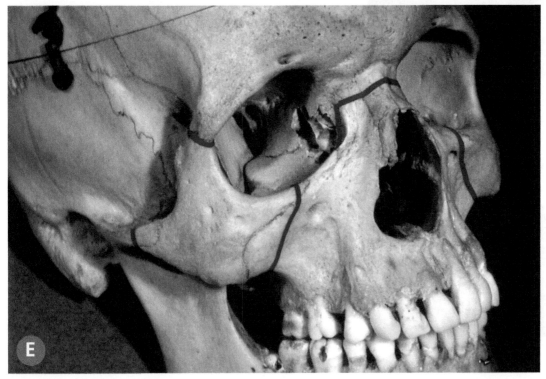

 Anterior and lateral views showing Le Fort fracture lines

E **Le Fort II and III fracture lines**

In anterior and lateral views C D

Dark blue line: Dentoalveolar fracture

Green line: Le Fort I fracture

Purple line: Le Fort II fracture

Light blue line: Pyramidal Le Fort II fracture

Red line: Le Fort III fracture

René Le Fort described the three levels of middle third facial fractures in 1901. Le Fort fractures are lines of weakness of the facial skeleton unable to resist forces from lateral and anterior directions.

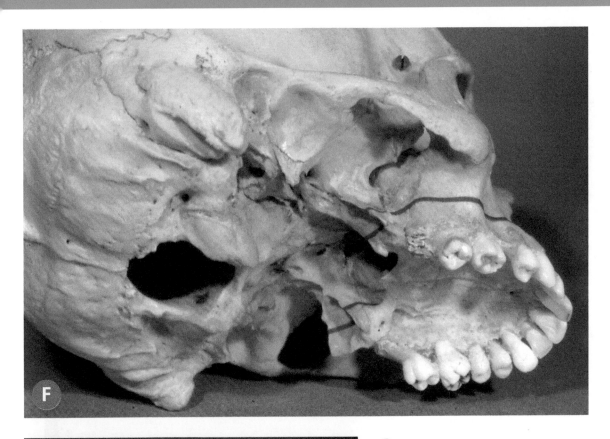

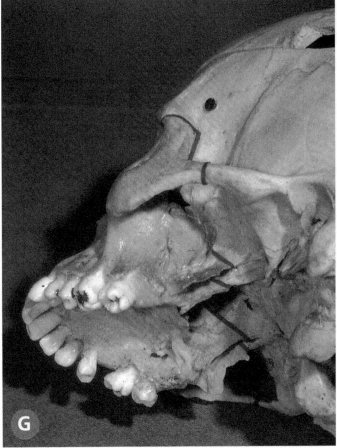

F Le Fort I fracture line

G Le Fort III fracture line

Skull *From the left*

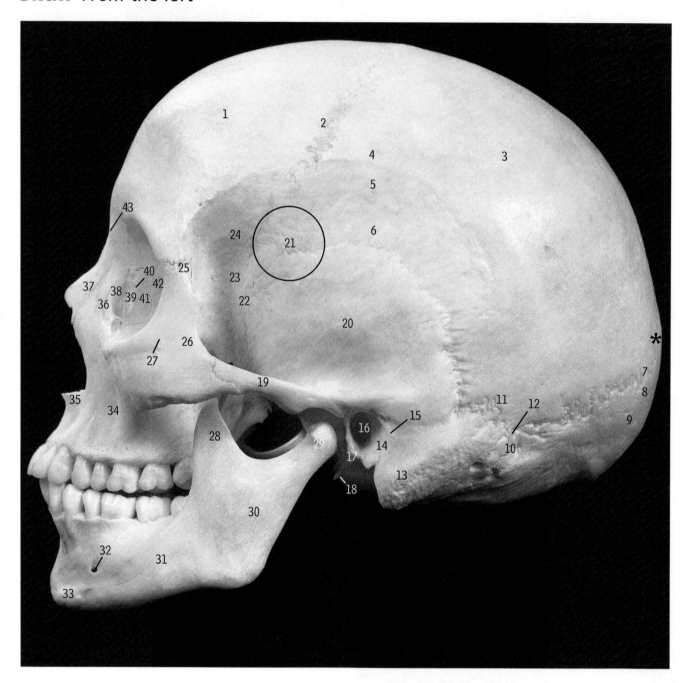

This is the standard view from the side. Prominent features include the zygomatic bone (cheek bone, 26) and zygomatic arch (19), the ramus of the mandible (30) with the coronoid and condylar processes (28 and 29), the external acoustic meatus (16) and the mastoid process (13). An asterisk (*) marks the most posterior part of the skull (the occiput), which is above and behind the external occipital protuberance (9).

1 Frontal bone
2 Coronal suture
3 Parietal bone
4 Superior ⎫
5 Inferior ⎬ temporal line
6 Squamosal suture
7 Lambdoid suture
8 Occipital bone
9 External occipital protuberance
10 Occipitomastoid suture
11 Parietomastoid suture
12 Asterion
13 Mastoid process
14 Tympanic part of temporal bone
15 Suprameatal triangle
16 External acoustic meatus
17 Sheath of styloid process
18 Styloid process
19 Zygomatic arch
20 Squamous part of temporal bone
21 Pterion
22 Sphenosquamosal suture
23 Greater wing of sphenoid bone
24 Sphenofrontal suture
25 Frontozygomatic suture
26 Zygomatic bone
27 Zygomaticofacial foramen
28 Coronoid process ⎫
29 Condylar process ⎪
30 Ramus ⎬ of mandible
31 Body ⎪
32 Mental foramen ⎪
33 Mental protuberance ⎭
34 Maxilla
35 Anterior nasal spine
36 Frontal process of maxilla
37 Nasal bone
38 Anterior lacrimal crest
39 Fossa for lacrimal sac
40 Posterior lacrimal crest
41 Lacrimal bone
42 Orbital part of ethmoid bone
43 Nasion

Some anatomical points of the skull

Nasion (43): the point of articulation between the two nasal bones and the frontal bone.

Inion (9): the central point of the external occipital protuberance.

Bregma (page 14, 10): the junction of the sagittal and coronal sutures (i.e. between the frontal and the two parietal bones). In the newborn skull the anterior fontanelle is in this region (page 78, A1 and D1).

Lambda (page 14, 2): the junction of the sagittal and lambdoid sutures (i.e. between the occipital and the two parietal bones). In the newborn skull the posterior fontanelle is in this region (page 72, C30 and D30).

Pterion (21): an H-shaped area (not a single point) where the frontal, parietal, squamous part of the temporal and greater wing of the sphenoid bones articulate. It is an important landmark since it overlies the anterior branch of the middle meningeal artery (page 32, 2), which may be ruptured by blows on the side of the head, giving rise to extradural haemorrhage (page 199). In the newborn skull the sphenoidal fontanelle is in this region (page 72, B27).

Asterion (12): the junction of the lambdoid, parietomastoid and occipitomastoid sutures (i.e. between the occipital, parietal and temporal bones). In the newborn skull the mastoid fontanelle is in this region (page 78, B20).

Skull *Muscle attachments, from the left*

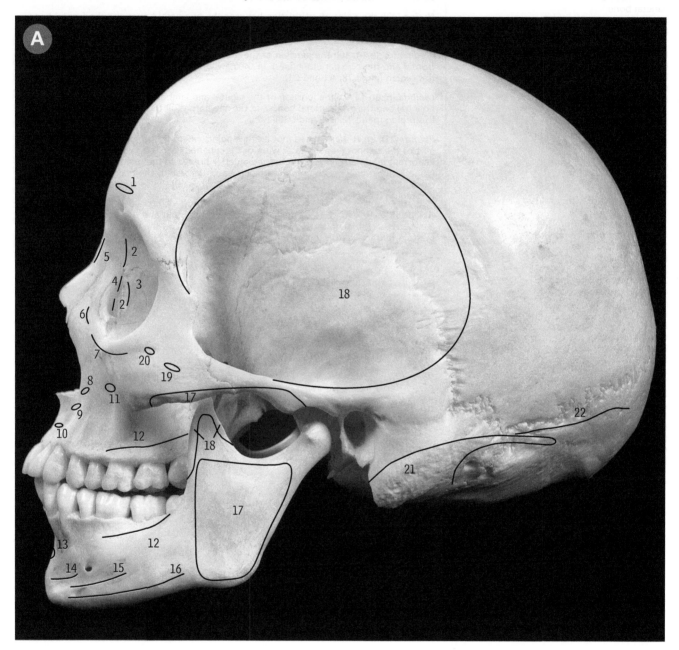

1 Corrugator supercilii
2 Orbicularis oculi (orbital and palpebral parts)
3 Orbicularis oculi (lacrimal part)
4 Medial palpebral ligament
5 Procerus
6 Levator labii superioris alaeque nasi
7 Levator labii superioris
8 Nasalis (transverse part)

9 Nasalis (alar part)
10 Depressor septi
11 Levator anguli oris
12 Buccinator
13 Mentalis
14 Depressor labii inferioris
15 Depressor anguli oris
16 Platysma

17 Masseter
18 Temporalis
19 Zygomaticus major
20 Zygomaticus minor
21 Sternocleidomastoid
22 Occipital belly of occipitofrontalis

Skull *With individual bones coloured, from the left*

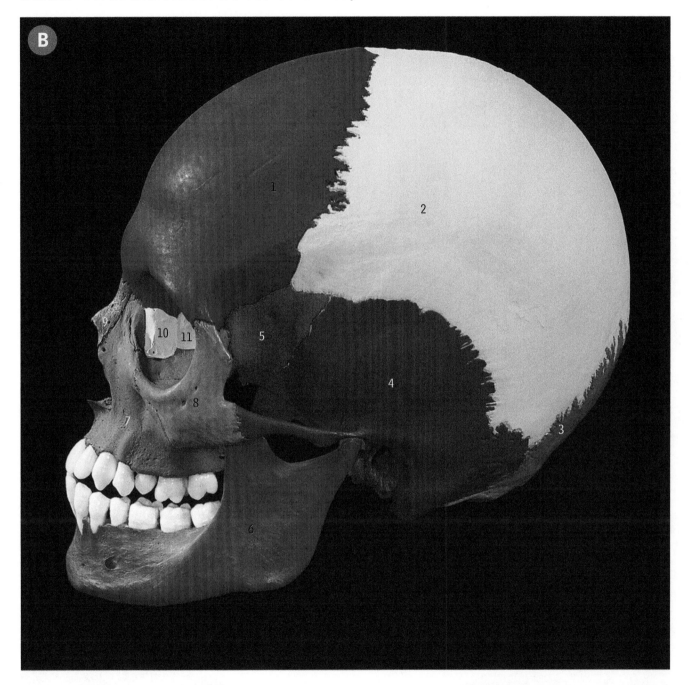

1 Frontal bone
2 Parietal bone
3 Occipital bone
4 Temporal bone
5 Sphenoid bone
6 Mandible
7 Maxilla
8 Zygomatic bone
9 Nasal bone
10 Lacrimal bone
11 Ethmoid bone

The buccinator (A12) has bony attachments to the upper and lower jaws opposite the three molar teeth.

The medial palpebral ligament (A4) and the orbital and palpebral parts of orbicularis oculi (A2) are attached to the anterior lacrimal crest; the lacrimal part of orbicularis oculi (A3) is attached to the posterior lacrimal crest.

The area occupied by the upper attachment of temporalis (A18) is the temporal fossa. The lowest fibres of the muscle run horizontally (page 136, A2) and turn down over the front of the root of the zygomatic process of the temporal bone to reach the mandibular attachment.

The attachment of sternocleidomastoid (A21) to the mastoid process extends well back on to the occipital bone, a feature not expected from the name of the muscle—which suggests it is limited above to the mastoid process alone.

Skull *From behind*

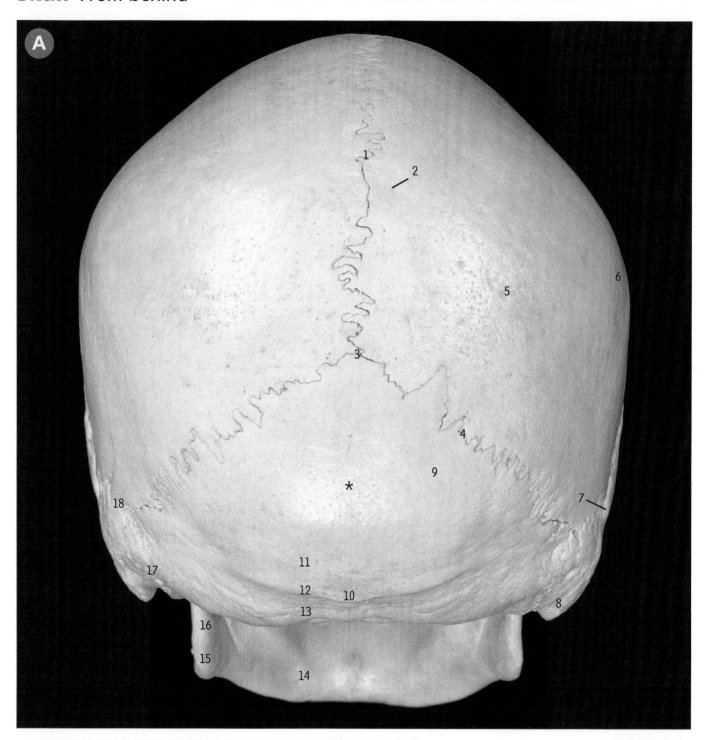

A with the mandible in place

This is the standard view from behind, showing the sagittal and lambdoid sutures (1 and 4) and the external occipital protuberance (10). An asterisk (*) marks the occiput (as on page 8). In the skull in B there are some sutural bones (19) and there has been bony fusion in some sutural areas.

1 Sagittal suture	**6** Parietal tuberosity	**11** Supreme ⎱	**17** Occipitomastoid suture
2 Parietal foramen	**7** Temporal bone	**12** Superior ⎬ nuchal line	**18** Parietomastoid suture
3 Lambda	**8** Mastoid process	**13** Inferior ⎰	**19** Sutural bones
4 Lambdoid suture	**9** Squamous part of occipital bone	**14** Body ⎱	
5 Parietal bone	**10** External occipital protuberance (inion)	**15** Angle ⎬ of mandible	
		16 Ramus ⎰	

Skull *From behind*

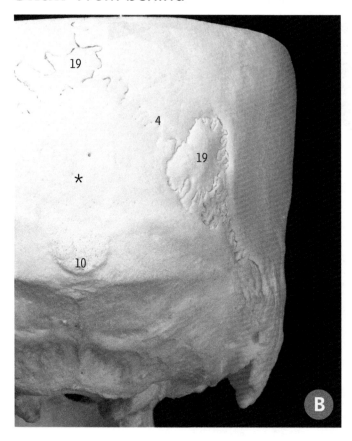

B a different specimen without the mandible

Sutural bones (B19) arise from separate centres of ossification that may occur within cranial sutures. They are commonest in the lambdoid suture (4). See also pages 80-81.

The occiput (*) is the most posterior part of the skull; it is situated in the midline of the occipital bone a few centimetres above the external occipital protuberance (10 and page 8, 8), and is the part struck when falling on the back of the head.

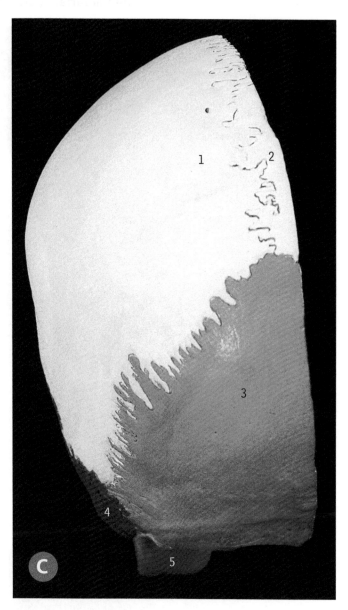

C left half of skull from behind, with individual bones coloured

1 Left parietal bone
2 Right parietal bone*
3 Occipital bone
4 Temporal bone
5 Mandible

* Note that although the skull has been cut through the median sagittal plane, the meandering nature of the suture lines displays both the left and a portion of the right parietal bones.

Vault of skull

A external surface (left half)   **B** internal surface (left half)

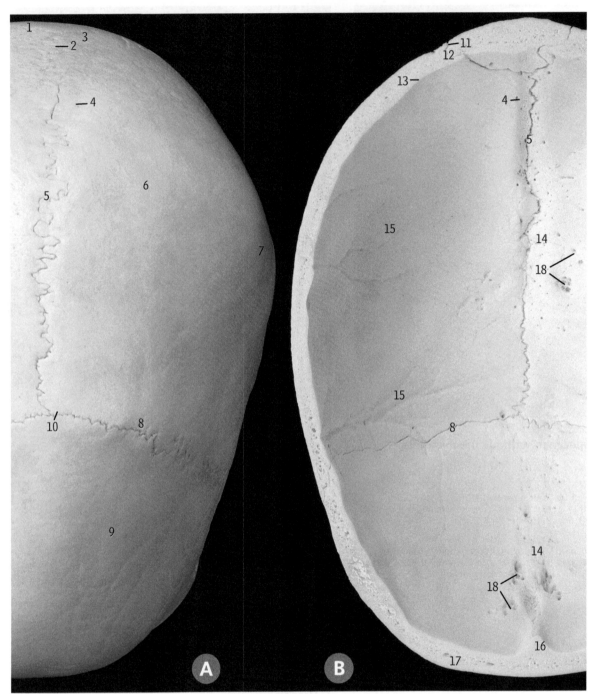

1 Occipital bone
2 Lambda
3 Lambdoid suture
4 Parietal foramen
5 Sagittal suture
6 Parietal bone
7 Parietal tuberosity

8 Coronal suture
9 Frontal bone
10 Bregma
11 Outer table ⎫
12 Diploë   ⎬ of parietal bone
13 Inner table ⎭

14 Groove for superior sagittal sinus
15 Grooves for middle meningeal vessels
16 Frontal crest
17 Frontal sinus
18 Depressions for arachnoid granulations

Vault of skull 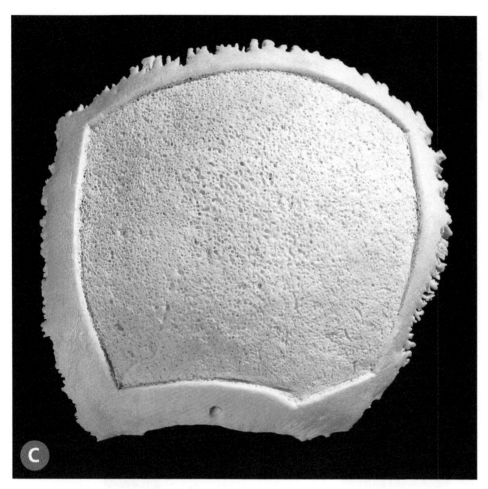 diploë of the right parietal bone

The standard view from above is shown in A, with the sagittal suture (5) in the midline and the coronal suture at the front (8). Internally in B there are grooves and impressions for the superior sagittal sinus (14; page 196, 2), the middle meningeal vessels (15; page 199, B16 and 17) and arachnoid granulations (page 200, 5).

In C the outer layer (outer table) of compact bone has been dissected away to show the 'honeycomb' of cancellous (spongy) bone, known in the skull as the diploë.

The vertex of the skull is the central uppermost part, approximately where the sagittal suture is labelled (5).

The parietal tuberosity (7) is the most lateral part of the cranial vault; it is particularly prominent in this specimen.

Suture lines on the inside of the skull (as in B5 and 8) are less convoluted than on the outside (as in A5 and 8).

Base of skull *External surface* Ⓐ from below

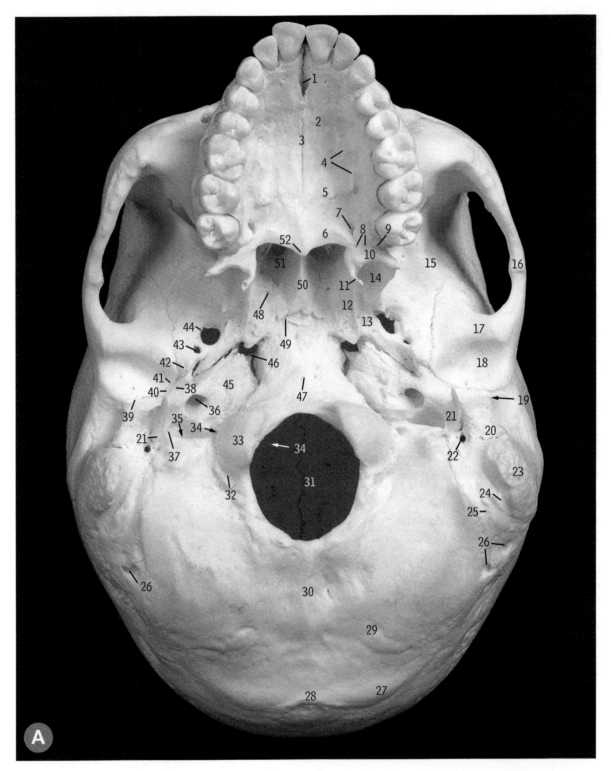

Ⓐ

In A, the standard view of the external surface of the base, the most important foramina (apart from the very large foramen magnum, 31) are the foramen lacerum (46), foramen ovale (44, unusually round where labelled but of more typical oval shape on the unlabelled opposite side), the foramen spinosum (43), the stylomastoid foramen (22), the jugular foramen (35) and the carotid canal (36).

The angled view in B shows parts of the nasal conchae (58-60), visible through the posterior nasal apertures (choanae, A51).

B **from below and behind**

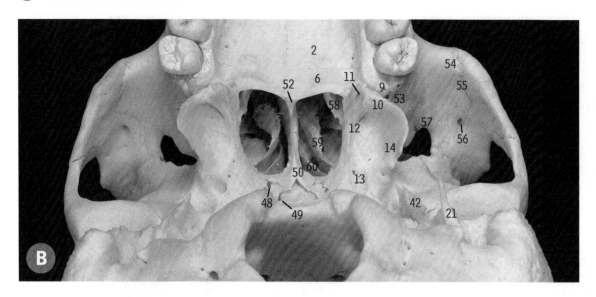

1 Incisive fossa	**31** Foramen magnum
2 Palatine process of maxilla	**32** Condylar canal
3 Median palatine suture	**33** Occipital condyle
4 Palatine grooves and spines	**34** Hypoglossal canal
5 Transverse palatine suture	**35** Jugular foramen
6 Horizontal plate of palatine bone	**36** Carotid canal
7 Greater palatine foramen	**37** Sheath of styloid process
8 Lesser palatine foramina	**38** Petrotympanic fissure
9 Tuberosity of maxilla	**39** Squamotympanic fissure
10 Pyramidal process of palatine bone	**40** Tegmen tympani
11 Pterygoid hamulus	**41** Petrosquamous fissure
12 Medial pterygoid plate	**42** Spine of sphenoid bone
13 Scaphoid fossa	**43** Foramen spinosum
14 Lateral pterygoid plate	**44** Foramen ovale
15 Infratemporal crest	**45** Apex of petrous part of temporal bone
16 Zygomatic arch	**46** Foramen lacerum
17 Articular tubercle	**47** Pharyngeal tubercle
18 Mandibular fossa	**48** Palatovaginal canal
19 External acoustic meatus	**49** Vomerovaginal canal
20 Tympanic part of temporal bone	**50** Vomer
21 Styloid process	**51** Posterior nasal aperture (choana)
22 Stylomastoid foramen	**52** Posterior nasal spine
23 Mastoid process	**53** Infratemporal surface ⎱
24 Mastoid notch	**54** Zygomatic process ⎰ of maxilla
25 Occipital groove	**55** Zygomaticomaxillary suture
26 Mastoid foramen (double on left)	**56** Zygomaticotemporal foramen
27 Superior nuchal line	**57** Inferior orbital fissure
28 External occipital protuberance	**58** Inferior ⎱
29 Inferior nuchal line	**59** Middle ⎰ nasal concha
30 External occipital crest	**60** Superior ⎰

The palatine processes of the maxillae (2) and
the horizontal plates of the palatine bones (6)
form the hard palate.

Base of skull *External surface, muscle attachments*

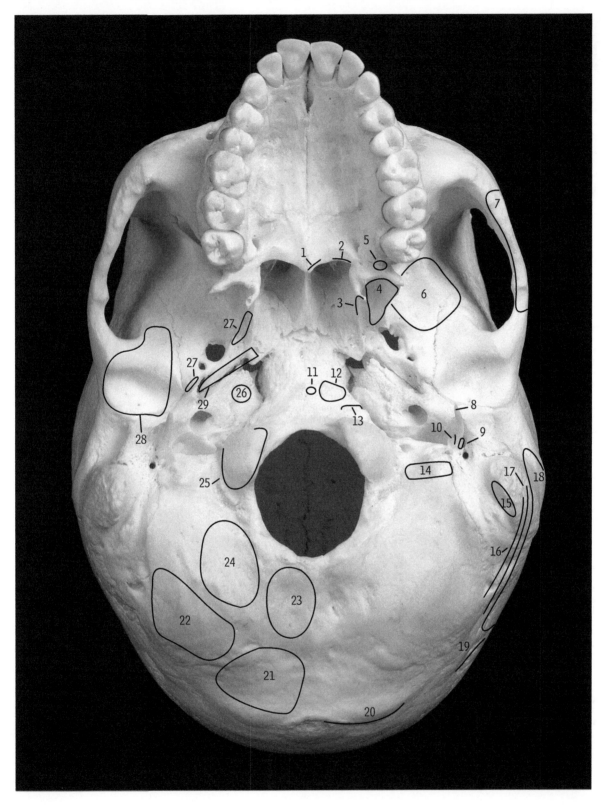

The main origins of the medial and lateral pterygoid muscles (4 and 6) are from the respective sides of the lateral pterygoid plate, with the lateral pterygoid also arising from the infratemporal surface of the greater wing of the sphenoid (6). The uppermost part of the superior constrictor of the pharynx (3) is attached to the lower part of the posterior border of the medial pterygoid plate. Sternocleidomastoid (18) is on the outer side of the mastoid process, with the posterior belly of digastric (15) on the inner side. Trapezius (20) reaches the back of the skull behind semispinalis (21) and the suboccipital muscles (22-24).

1 Musculus uvulae
2 Palatopharyngeus
3 Superior constrictor of pharynx
4 Medial pterygoid (deep head)
5 Medial pterygoid (superficial head)
6 Lateral pterygoid (upper head)
7 Masseter
8 Styloglossus
9 Stylohyoid
10 Stylopharyngeus
11 Pharyngeal raphe
12 Longus capitis
13 Rectus capitis anterior
14 Rectus capitis lateralis
15 Posterior belly of digastric
16 Longissimus capitis
17 Splenius capitis
18 Sternocleidomastoid
19 Occipital belly of occipitofrontalis
20 Trapezius
21 Semispinalis capitis
22 Superior oblique
23 Rectus capitis posterior minor
24 Rectus capitis posterior major
25 Capsule of atlanto-occipital joint
26 Levator veli palatini
27 Tensor veli palatini
28 Capsule of temporomandibular joint
29 Cartilaginous part of auditory tube

Principal skull foramina and their contents
(for more precise details see pages 286-287)

Supra-orbital foramen
Supra-orbital nerve and vessels

Infra-orbital foramen
Infra-orbital nerve and vessels

Mental foramen
Mental nerve and vessels

Mandibular foramen
Inferior alveolar nerve and vessels

Optic canal
Optic nerve
Ophthalmic artery

Superior orbital fissure
Ophthalmic nerve and veins
Oculomotor, trochlear and abducent nerves

Inferior orbital fissure
Maxillary nerve

Sphenopalatine foramen
Sphenopalatine artery
Nasal branches of pterygopalatine ganglion

Foramen rotundum
Maxillary nerve

Foramen ovale
Mandibular and lesser petrosal nerves

Foramen spinosum
Middle meningeal vessels

Foramen lacerum
Internal carotid artery (entering from behind and emerging above)
Greater petrosal nerve (entering from behind and leaving anteriorly as the nerve of the pterygoid canal)

Carotid canal
Internal carotid artery and nerve

Jugular foramen
Inferior petrosal sinus
Glossopharyngeal, vagus and accessory nerves
Internal jugular vein (emerging below)

Internal acoustic meatus
Facial and vestibulocochlear nerves
Labyrinthine artery

Hypoglossal canal
Hypoglossal nerve

Stylomastoid foramen
Facial nerve

Foramen magnum
Medulla oblongata and meninges
Vertebral and anterior and posterior spinal arteries
Accessory nerves (spinal parts)

Base of skull *Internal surface, from above*

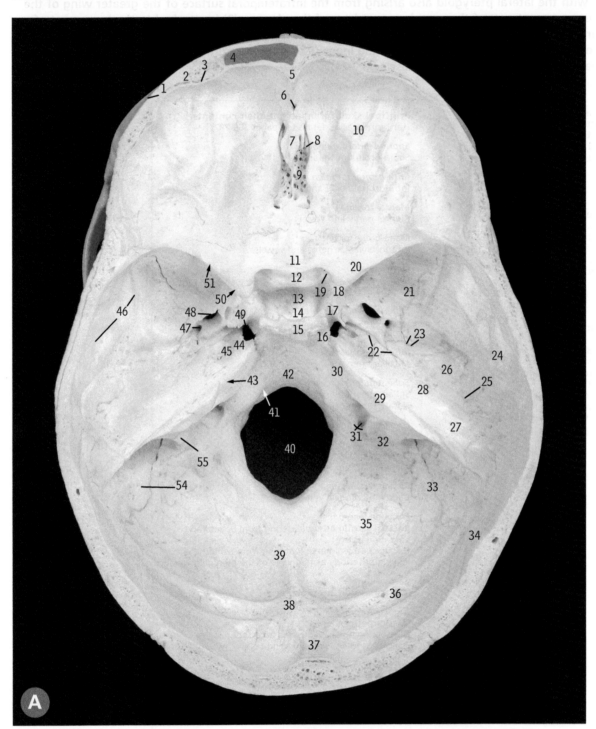

A anterior, middle and posterior cranial fossae, from above

The standard view directly from above is shown in A. In B the skull has been tilted downwards and forwards to bring into view the right superior orbital fissure (51) and foramen rotundum (50) which are not seen when looking straight down from above. The specimen in C shows the left venous and petrosal foramina (52 and 53) which are not often present.

1 Outer table	**21** Greater wing of sphenoid bone	**38** Internal occipital protuberance
2 Diploë	**22** Hiatus and groove for greater petrosal nerve	**39** Internal occipital crest
3 Inner table		**40** Foramen magnum
4 Frontal sinus (upper extremity)	**23** Hiatus and groove for lesser petrosal nerve	**41** Hypoglossal canal
5 Frontal crest		**42** Clivus
6 Foramen caecum	**24** Squamous part of temporal bone	**43** Internal acoustic meatus
7 Crista galli	**25** Petrosquamous fissure	**44** Apex of petrous part of temporal bone
8 Groove for anterior ethmoidal nerve and vessels	**26** Tegmen tympani	
	27 Arcuate eminence	**45** Trigeminal impression
9 Cribriform plate of ethmoid bone	**28** Petrous part of temporal bone	**46** Grooves for middle meningeal vessels
10 Orbital part of frontal bone	**29** Groove for superior petrosal sinus	
11 Jugum of sphenoid bone	**30** Groove for inferior petrosal sinus and petro-occipital suture	**47** Foramen spinosum
12 Prechiasmatic groove		**48** Foramen ovale
13 Tuberculum sellae	**31** Jugular foramen	**49** Foramen lacerum
14 Pituitary fossa (sella turcica)	**32** Groove for sigmoid sinus	**50** Foramen rotundum
15 Dorsum sellae	**33** Occipitomastoid suture	**51** Superior orbital fissure
16 Posterior clinoid process	**34** Mastoid (postero-inferior) angle of parietal bone	**52** Venous (emissary sphenoidal) foramen (of Vesalius)
17 Carotid groove		
18 Anterior clinoid process	**35** Occipital bone	**53** Petrosal (innominate) foramen
19 Optic canal	**36** Groove for transverse sinus	**54** Mastoid emissary foramen
20 Lesser wing of sphenoid bone	**37** Groove for superior sagittal sinus	**55** Aqueduct of vestibule

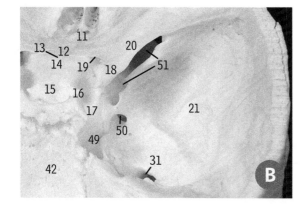

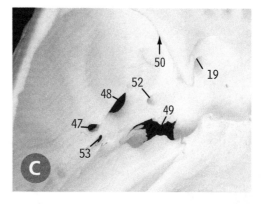

B the right half of the middle cranial fossa, from above, right and behind

C the left half of the middle cranial fossa, from above

For details of the bones of the cranial fossae see pages 68–71.

The foramina rotundum, ovale and spinosum (50, 48 and 47) are always present within the greater wing of the sphenoid bone; the venous (emissary sphenoidal) foramen (of Vesalius, C52) and the petrosal (innominate) foramen (C53) are occasional additions.

The openings in the *anterior cranial fossa* are:
* the foramen caecum (6)
* the foramina of the cribriform plate of the ethmoid bone (9)

The openings in the *middle cranial fossa* are:
* the optic canal (19)
* the superior orbital fissure (51)
* the foramen rotundum (50)
* the foramen ovale (48)
* the foramen spinosum (47)
* the venous (emissary sphenoidal) foramen (of Vesalius) (52) (occasional)
* the petrosal (innominate) foramen (53) (occasional)
* the foramen lacerum (49)
* the hiatus for the greater and lesser petrosal nerves (22 and 23)

The openings in the *posterior cranial fossa* are:
* the foramen magnum (40)
* the internal acoustic meatus (43)
* the aqueduct of the vestibule (55)
* the jugular foramen (31)
* the hypoglossal canal (41)
* the mastoid foramen (54)

For the contents of skull foramina see pages 19 and 286–287.

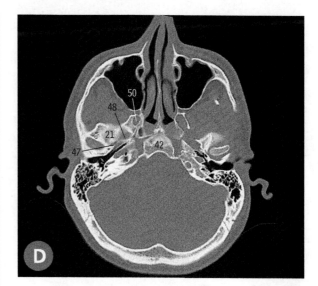

D axial CT image through the middle cranial fossa, similar to the level shown in Figure B

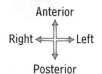

Interior of skull *Left half*

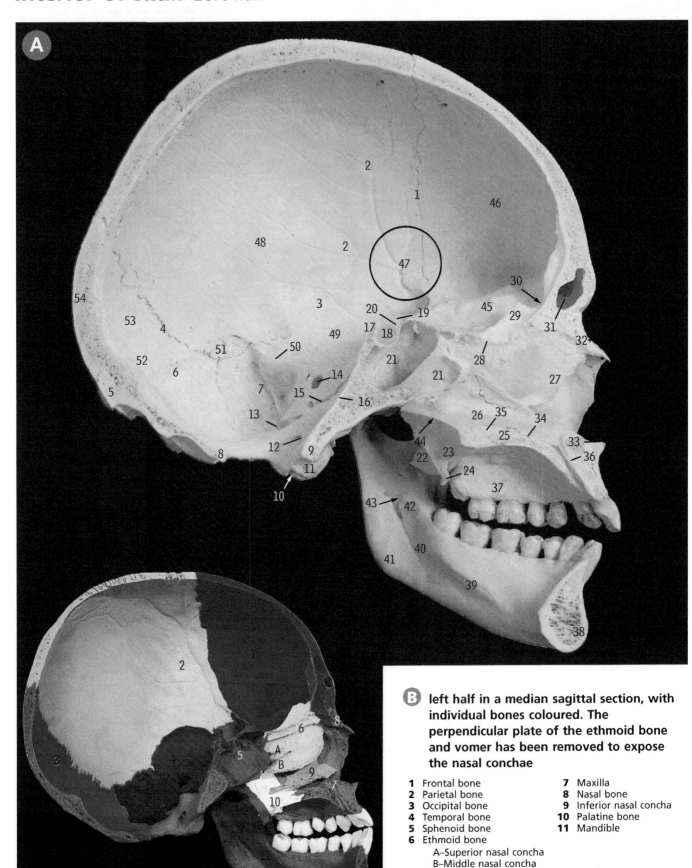

B left half in a median sagittal section, with individual bones coloured. The perpendicular plate of the ethmoid bone and vomer has been removed to expose the nasal conchae

1 Frontal bone
2 Parietal bone
3 Occipital bone
4 Temporal bone
5 Sphenoid bone
6 Ethmoid bone
    A–Superior nasal concha
    B–Middle nasal concha

7 Maxilla
8 Nasal bone
9 Inferior nasal concha
10 Palatine bone
11 Mandible

The inside of the left half of the skull is seen from the right, with the bony part of the nasal septum intact (the vomer, 26, and the perpendicular plate of the ethmoid bone, 27). The encircled area (47) indicates the position of pterion (see the notes on pages 9 and 199).

A in a median sagittal section

1 Coronal suture
2 Grooves for middle meningeal vessels
3 Squamosal suture
4 Lambdoid suture
5 External occipital protuberance
6 Groove for transverse sinus
7 Groove for sigmoid sinus
8 Posterior ⎫
9 Anterior ⎬ margin of foramen magnum
10 Mastoid process
11 Occipital condyle
12 Hypoglossal canal
13 Jugular foramen
14 Internal acoustic meatus
15 Groove for inferior petrosal sinus
16 Clivus
17 Dorsum sellae
18 Pituitary fossa
19 Anterior clinoid process
20 Optic canal
21 Sphenoidal sinus
22 Lateral plate ⎫
23 Medial ⎬ of pterygoid bone
24 Pterygoid hamulus
25 Hard palate
26 Vomer
27 Perpendicular plate ⎫
28 Cribriform plate ⎬ of ethmoid bone

29 Crista galli
30 Foramen caecum
31 Frontal sinus
32 Nasal bone
33 Anterior nasal spine
34 Nasal crest of maxilla
35 Nasal crest of palatine bone
36 Incisive canal
37 Alveolar process of maxilla
38 Mental protuberance
39 Mylohyoid line of mandible
40 Groove for mylohyoid nerve
41 Angle of mandible
42 Lingula
43 Mandibular foramen
44 Posterior nasal aperture (choana)
45 Orbital part ⎫
46 Squamous part ⎬ of frontal bone
47 Pterion (encircled)
48 Parietal bone
49 Squamous part of temporal bone
50 Groove for superior petrosal sinus
51 Mastoid (posterior inferior) angle of parietal bone
52 Internal occipital protuberance
53 Occipital bone
54 Occiput

The grooves for the middle meningeal vessels (2) on the inside of the cranial vault pass upwards and backwards.

The groove for the transverse sinus (6) runs forwards on the occipital bone, crosses the mastoid angle of the parietal bone (51) and then turns downwards on the temporal bone to become the groove for the sigmoid sinus (7) which leads into the jugular foramen (13; compare with the views in page 30, A36, 34, 32 and 31).

The pituitary fossa (18) lies above the sphenoidal sinus (21).

The hypoglossal canal (12) in the occipital bone is above the occipital condyle (11), with the internal acoustic meatus (14) at a higher level in the temporal bone. In this view the occipital condyle obscures the mastoid process (10).

Cavities of skull *Orbit and nasal cavity*

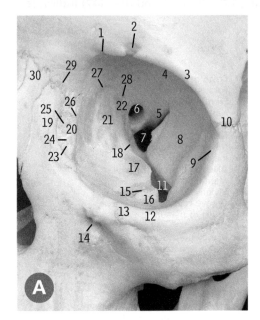

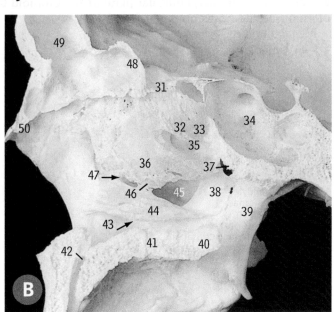

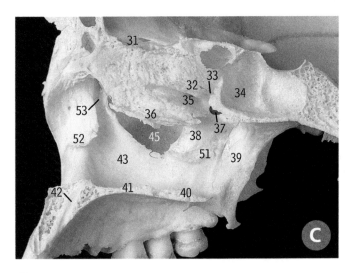

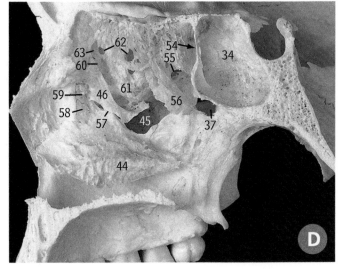

A left orbit

B right half of the nasal cavity, with the lateral wall intact

C lateral wall, with the inferior nasal concha removed

D lateral wall, with the middle nasal concha removed

In A, looking into the left orbit slightly from the left and above, the roof, lateral wall, floor and medial wall can all be seen. The bones taking part in these boundaries are bracketed together in the key and are described further on pages 58-63.

B-E all show the lateral wall of the right half of the nasal cavity. In B the wall is complete. Removal of the inferior nasal concha (B44) in C enables more of the medial wall of the maxilla to be seen (43). Removal of the middle nasal concha (B36) in D displays the ethmoidal bulla (61) and semilunar hiatus (60). The oblique view in E shows the opening in the anterior wall of the sphenoidal sinus (54).

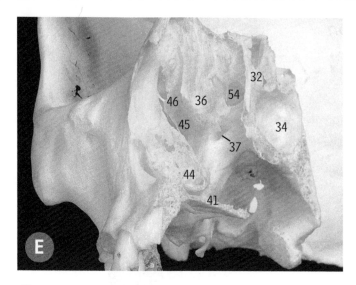

E oblique view, from the front and the left, with the nasal septum removed

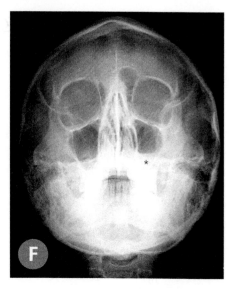

F fractures of the zygomatic complex or maxilla can cause blood to collect in the maxillary sinus giving rise to a dependent fluid level (*), as shown in the occipitomental radiograph above

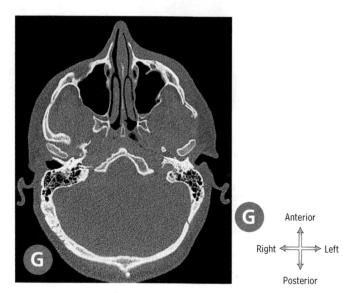

G axial CT imaging through the maxillary sinus demonstrating a left zygomatic complex fracture

1 Frontal notch
2 Supra-orbital foramen
3 Supra-orbital margin
4 Orbital part of frontal bone ⎫ forming roof
5 Lesser wing of sphenoid bone ⎭
6 Optic canal
7 Superior orbital fissure
8 Greater wing of sphenoid bone ⎫ forming lateral
9 Zygomatic bone (with leader to tubercle) ⎭ wall marginal
10 Frontozygomatic suture
11 Inferior orbital fissure
12 Infra-orbital margin
13 Zygomaticomaxillary suture
14 Infra-orbital foramen
15 Infra-orbital groove
16 Zygomatic bone ⎫
17 Maxilla ⎬ forming floor
18 Orbital process of palatine bone ⎭
19 Frontal process of maxilla ⎫
20 Lacrimal bone ⎪
21 Orbital plate of ethmoid bone ⎬ forming medial wall
22 Body of sphenoid bone ⎭
23 Anterior lacrimal crest
24 Lacrimal groove
25 Fossa for lacrimal sac
26 Posterior lacrimal crest
27 Anterior ⎫ ethmoidal foramen
28 Posterior ⎭
29 Frontomaxillary suture
30 Nasal bone
31 Cribriform plate of ethmoid bone
32 Superior nasal concha
33 Spheno-ethmoidal recess
34 Sphenoidal sinus
35 Superior meatus
36 Middle nasal concha
37 Sphenopalatine foramen
38 Perpendicular plate of palatine bone
39 Medial pterygoid plate
40 Horizontal plate of palatine bone
41 Palatine process of maxilla
42 Incisive canal
43 Inferior meatus and medial wall of maxilla
44 Inferior nasal concha

45 Maxillary hiatus
46 Uncinate process of ethmoid bone
47 Middle meatus
48 Crista galli
49 Frontal sinus
50 Nasal bone
51 Conchal crest of perpendicular plate of palatine bone
52 Conchal crest of maxilla
53 Nasolacrimal canal
54 Aperture of sphenoidal sinus into spheno-ethmoidal recess
55 Aperture of posterior ethmoidal air cell into superior meatus
56 Base of middle nasal concha
57 Ethmoidal process ⎫ of inferior nasal concha
58 Lacrimal process ⎭
59 Descending process of lacrimal bone
60 Semilunar hiatus
61 Ethmoidal bulla
62 Apertures of middle ethmoidal air cells
63 Frontonasal duct

For further details of the bones of the orbit see pages 58-63, and of the nose pages 58 and 64-66.

In B the crista galli (48) is large and the frontal sinus (49) has extended into it.

Cavities of skull *Infratemporal region*

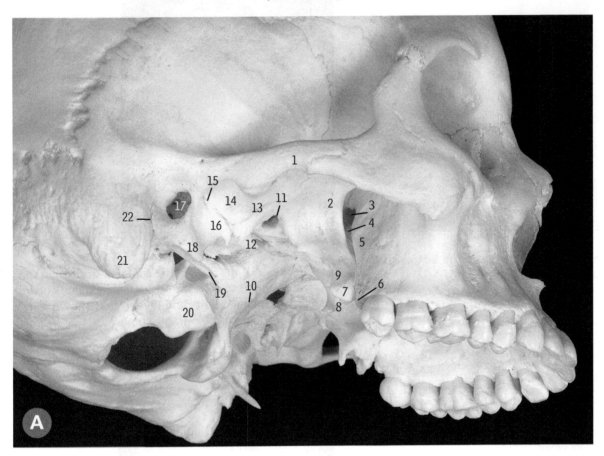

A

A the right infratemporal region, obliquely from below

1 Zygomatic arch
2 Lateral pterygoid plate
3 Sphenopalatine foramen
4 Pterygomaxillary fissure
5 Infratemporal surface of maxilla
6 Tuberosity of maxilla
7 Pyramidal process of palatine bone
8 Pterygoid hamulus
9 Medial pterygoid plate
10 Pharyngeal tubercle
11 Foramen ovale
12 Spine of sphenoid bone
13 Articular tubercle
14 Mandibular fossa
15 Squamotympanic fissure
16 Tympanic part of temporal bone
17 External acoustic meatus
18 Sheath of styloid process
19 Styloid process
20 Occipital condyle
21 Mastoid process
22 Tympanomastoid fissure

The main reason for examining the tilted view in A is to note the pterygomaxillary fissure (4), behind the maxilla (5) and in front of the pterygoid process whose lateral pterygoid plate (2) is shown throughout its length. In the depth of the fissure, i.e. in the medial wall of the pterygopalatine fossa (pages 74 and 75), the sphenopalatine foramen (3) is seen. (In the normal lateral view, as on page 8, the fissure and plate are largely obscured by the zygomatic arch and the coronoid process of the mandible—see pages 8, 16 and 34.)

Teeth *Histology of dental tissues*

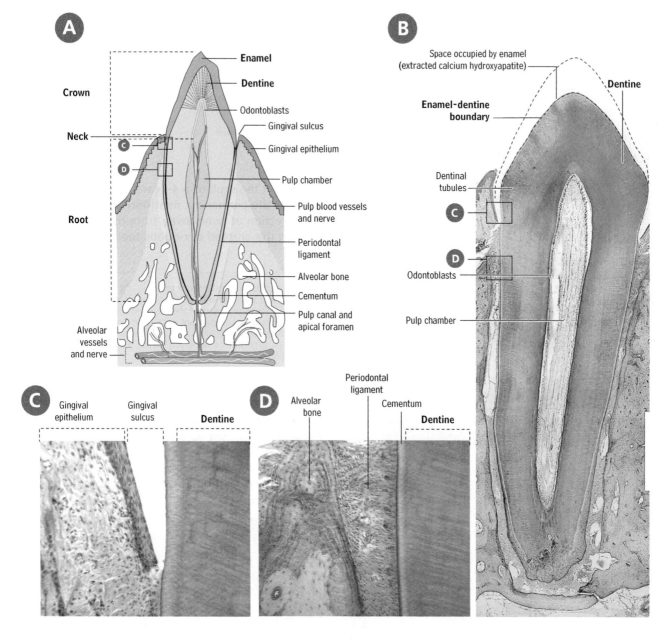

A Enamel
Dentine
Odontoblasts
Gingival sulcus
Gingival epithelium
Pulp chamber
Pulp blood vessels and nerve
Periodontal ligament
Alveolar bone
Cementum
Pulp canal and apical foramen

Crown
Neck
Root
Alveolar vessels and nerve

B Space occupied by enamel (extracted calcium hydroxyapatite)
Enamel–dentine boundary
Dentine
Dentinal tubules
Odontoblasts
Pulp chamber

C Gingival epithelium
Gingival sulcus
Dentine

D Alveolar bone
Periodontal ligament
Cementum
Dentine

A Diagram of longitudinal section of incisor tooth showing supportive tissue and neurovascular supply

B Histological section of partially decalcified incisor tooth

C Histological section of epithelial attachment (high-power section of region in B)

D Histological section of periodontal ligament (high-power section of region in B)

Deciduous dentition

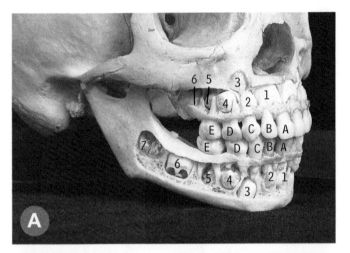
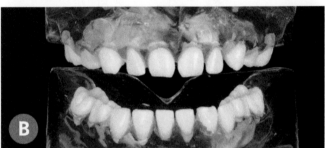

A

erupted and unerupted teeth, right side, in the skull of a child aged 4. Deciduous teeth lettered A-E, permanent teeth numbered 1-6

A	Central	} incisor
B	Lateral	
C	Canine	
D	First	} molar
E	Second	

permanent dentition, right side

1	Central	} incisor
2	Lateral	
3	Canine	
4	First	} premolar
5	Second	
6	First	} molar

In A, from the skull of a 4-year-old child, the unerupted teeth of the permanent dentition have been displayed by dissection of bone away from the jaws, which still contain the erupted deciduous teeth (lettered).

In the deciduous dentition of the child ('milk teeth'), there are central and lateral incisors and canines in corresponding positions to the permanent teeth of the same name, but the first and second deciduous molars are in the positions of the first and second permanent premolars. To distinguish them from the permanent teeth, the deciduous teeth are given letters instead of numbers (as in A).

B C D

B is an anterior view of upper and lower exfoliated deciduous teeth set up on a clear plastic model. C and D are the occlusal views of the upper and lower arches, respectively. The roots are resorbed in the normal processes of exfoliation as the permanent dentition erupts

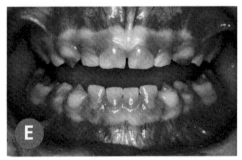

This clinical image of the deciduous dentition demonstrates chronological hypoplasia following a systemic insult that would have occurred post-natally. See also anomalies and abnormalities page 28 D and E.

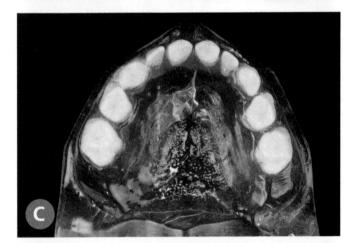

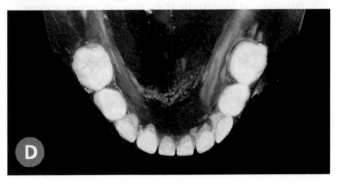

Eruption dates of deciduous and permanent dentitions

Eruption dates of deciduous dentition

Tooth		Calcification begins (months in utero [miu])	Crown completed (months)	Date of eruption (months)	Root completed (years)
UPPER	A	4	4	7	1½,-2
	B	4½	5	8	1½-2
	C	5	9	16-20	2½-3
	D	5	6	12-16	2-2½
	E	6-7	10-12	20-30	3
LOWER	A	4½	4	6½	1½-2
	B	4½	4½	7	1½-2
	C	5	9	16-20	2½-3
	D	5	6	12-16	2-2½
	E	6	10-12	20-30	3

Eruption dates of permanent dentition

		(months)	(years)	(years)	(years)
UPPER	1	3-4	4-5	7-8	10
	2	10-12	4-5	8-9	11
	3	4-5	6-7	11-12	13-15
	4	18-21	5-6	10-11	12-13
	5	24-30	6-7	10-12	12-14
	6	Birth	2-3	6-7	9-10
	7	2-3 yrs	7-8	12-13	14-16
	8	7-9 yrs	12-16	17-21	18-25
LOWER	1	3-4	4-5	6-7	9
	2	3-4	4-5	7-8	10
	3	4-5	6-7	9-10	12-14
	4	20-24	5-6	10-12	12-13
	5	27-30	6-7	11-12	13-14
	6	Birth	2-3	6-7	9-10
	7	2-3 yrs	7-8	12-13	14-15
	8	8-10 yrs	12-16	17-21	18-25

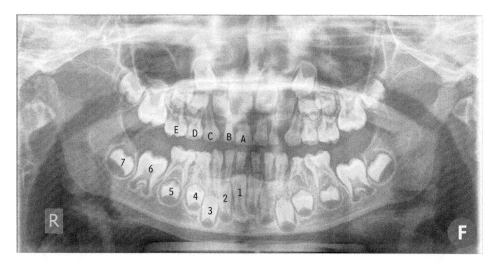

 dental panoramic tomograph of a child in the mixed dentition demonstrating the deciduous dentition, similar in appearance to Figure A

 Bonus E-Book Content Online

Stages of tooth eruption *Development, form, eruption and timelines*

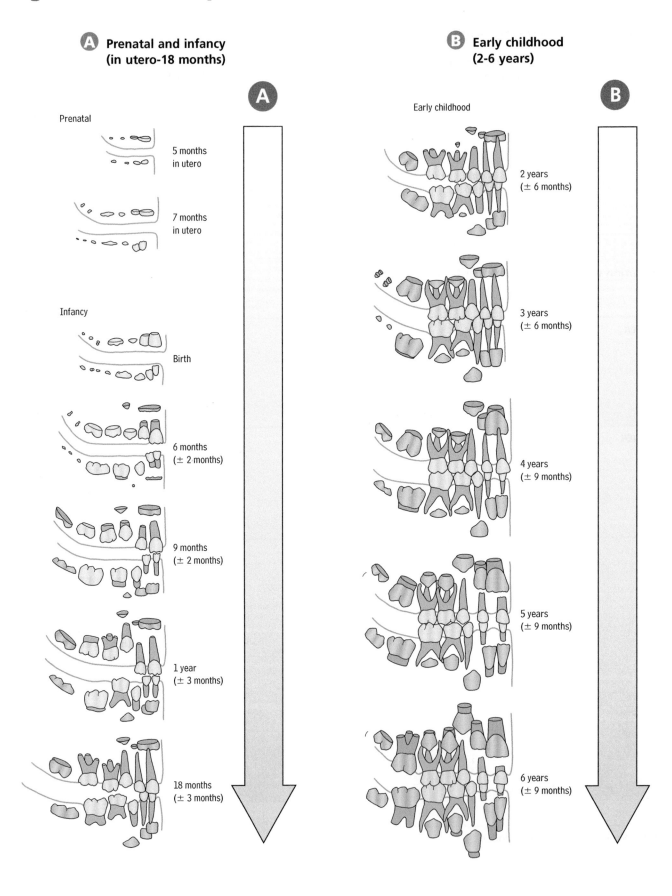

A Prenatal and infancy (in utero-18 months)

Prenatal

5 months in utero

7 months in utero

Infancy

Birth

6 months (± 2 months)

9 months (± 2 months)

1 year (± 3 months)

18 months (± 3 months)

B Early childhood (2-6 years)

Early childhood

2 years (± 6 months)

3 years (± 6 months)

4 years (± 9 months)

5 years (± 9 months)

6 years (± 9 months)

C **Mixed dentition**
Late childhood
(7-10 years)

D **Permanent dentition**
Adolescence and adulthood
(11-35 years)

Late childhood

Adolescence and adulthood

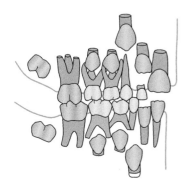

7 years
(± 9 months)

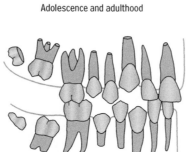

11 years
(± 9 months)

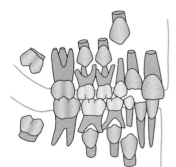

8 years
(± 9 months)

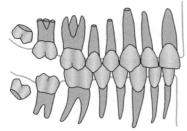

12 years
(± 6 months)

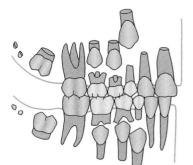

9 years
(± 9 months)

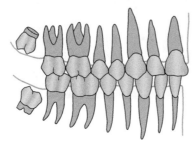

15 years
(± 6 months)

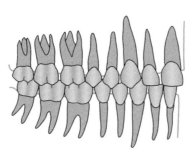

21 years

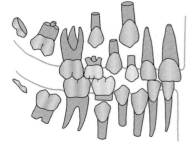

10 years
(± 9 months)

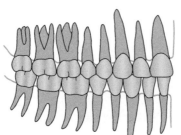

35 years

Permanent dentition

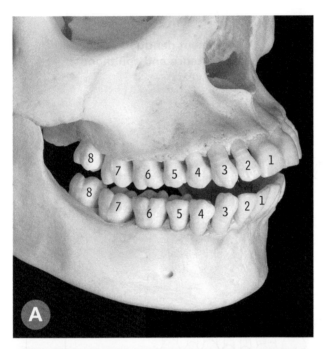

The corresponding teeth of the upper and lower jaws have corresponding names. In dentistry the teeth are often referred to by the numbers 1-8 as listed, rather than by name. Thus, 'right upper six' refers to the right upper first molar.

A permanent dentition, right side

1 Central	} incisor	6 First	} molar
2 Lateral		7 Second	
3 Canine		8 Third	
4 First	} premolar		
5 Second			

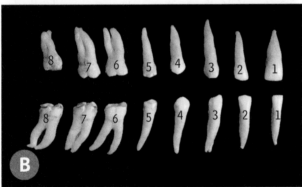

B adult right upper and lower teeth, from the right, shown from their outer (labial or buccal) sides, to illustrate their roots

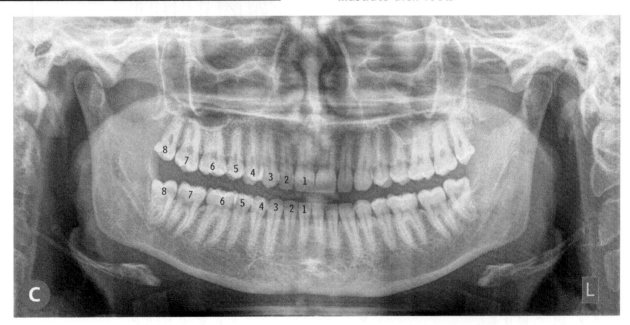

C dental panoramic tomograph of the permanent dentition corresponding to Figure A

Three-dimensional surface models from CT images

These images are two-dimensional images of three-dimensional polygon surface models created from micro-CT scans. The voxel radiodensity data generated by the scanner are processed to determine the junction between the tooth, pulp space and bone. This junction is mapped to create the polygon models. They are highly interactive when viewed on a computer allowing for viewer-controlled angle and opacity.

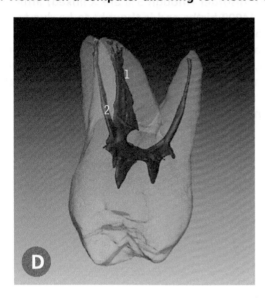

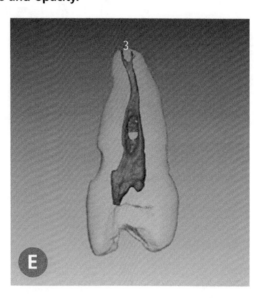

D Transparent computer model of an upper first molar created from a micro-CT scan of a real tooth. The mesial buccal root contains a single but very broad canal space (1). Some of these roots have two canals (2). Image courtesy of eHuman, Inc; www.ehuman.com

E Transparent computer model of an upper right first premolar. Note the presence of two apical foramina (3). Image courtesy of eHuman, Inc; www.ehuman.com

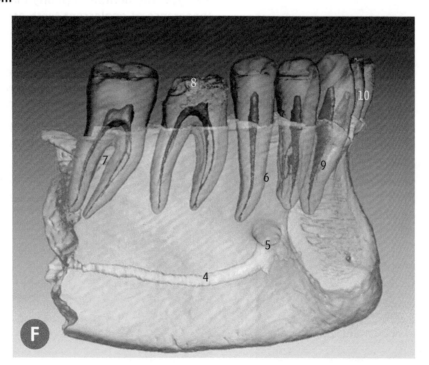

F Transparent computer model of the right side of a mandible showing the relationship of the inferior alveolar canal (4) and the mental foramen (5) to the roots of the premolar teeth (6). The figure shows fully formed lower right seven (7), loss of crown on lower right six (8) and the presence of the lower right canine (9) and incisors (10) (hidden in this view). Image courtesy of eHuman, Inc; www.ehuman.com

Anomalies and abnormalities

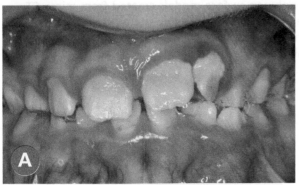

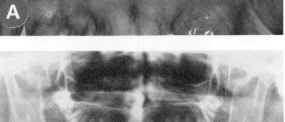

Amelogenesis imperfecta is an inherited autosomal dominant disorder (though 5% are X linked) affecting 1:400–1:14000 births and is thought to be due to abnormal production of enamel proteins such as ameloblastin and enamelin. The teeth have a higher risk of caries, are hypersensitive and any number of teeth can be involved. A is a clinical photo of affected teeth and B is an orthopantomographic view of such a dentition

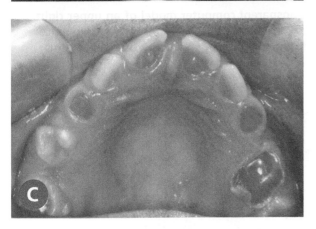

C Dentinogenesis imperfecta is an autosomal dominant disorder affecting 1:5000–1:8000 births. It has three main types, the first of which is associated with osteogenesis imperfecta with characteristic blue-coloured sclerae of the eyes. The dentine is poorly mineralised and gives the appearance of opalescent teeth as the enamel is translucent. The enamel is poorly supported with resultant severe attrition of the teeth

D Chronological hypoplasia of the teeth is the result of abnormal tooth development following a time-limited serious disease or environmental insult

E Tetracycline staining results from the use of this antibiotic when the teeth are developing

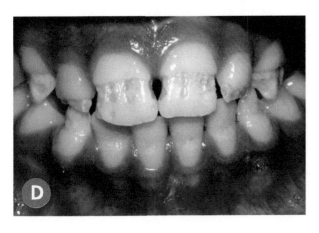

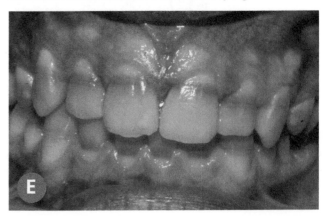

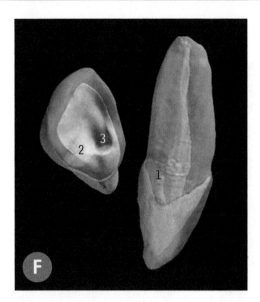

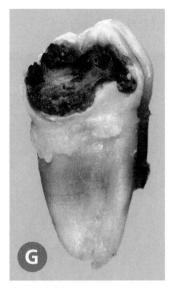

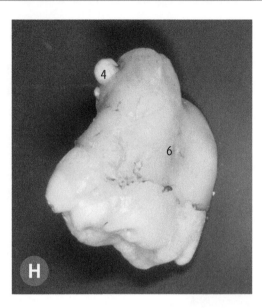

F Occasionally the enamel organ invaginates into the dental papilla during odontogenesis resulting in an enamel-lined cavity (1). This is usually seen on the cingulae (2) of the central and lateral incisors and may present as a small pit (3) or extend to the apex producing the so-called dens in dente. Image courtesy of eHuman, Inc; www.ehuman.com

G This deep carious cavity led to irreversible pulpitis and extraction of the molar

H There are several anomalies of tooth development including enamel pearls (4), bigeminated teeth (6), and supernumerary, supplemental and missing teeth. Enamel pearls (4) are small focal overgrowths of enamel seen on the root surface often close to the ameloentinal junction most commonly in maxillary molars. Occasionally a core of dentine and a small pulp horn are found within them. H is both bigeminated (6) and has an associated enamel pearl (4)

I The eruptive patterns of teeth can become disrupted leading to impacted teeth which are notably seen in the lower third molars. Such impactions are classically described as vertical (7), horizontal (8), mesioangular (9) and distoangular (10) depending on their position relative to the normal dental arch. The apices of lower third molars are closely related to the inferior dental nerve

1 Dens in dente
2 Cingulum
3 Pit on cingulum
4 Enamel pearl
5 Ameloentinal junction
6 Bigeminated upper molars
7 Vertical impaction, lower right third molar
8 Horizontal impaction, lower right third molar
9 Mesioangular impaction, lower left third molar
10 Distoangular impaction, lower right third molar

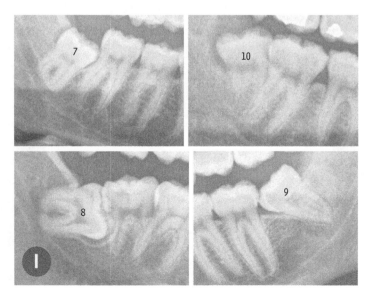

Bones of the skull Mandible

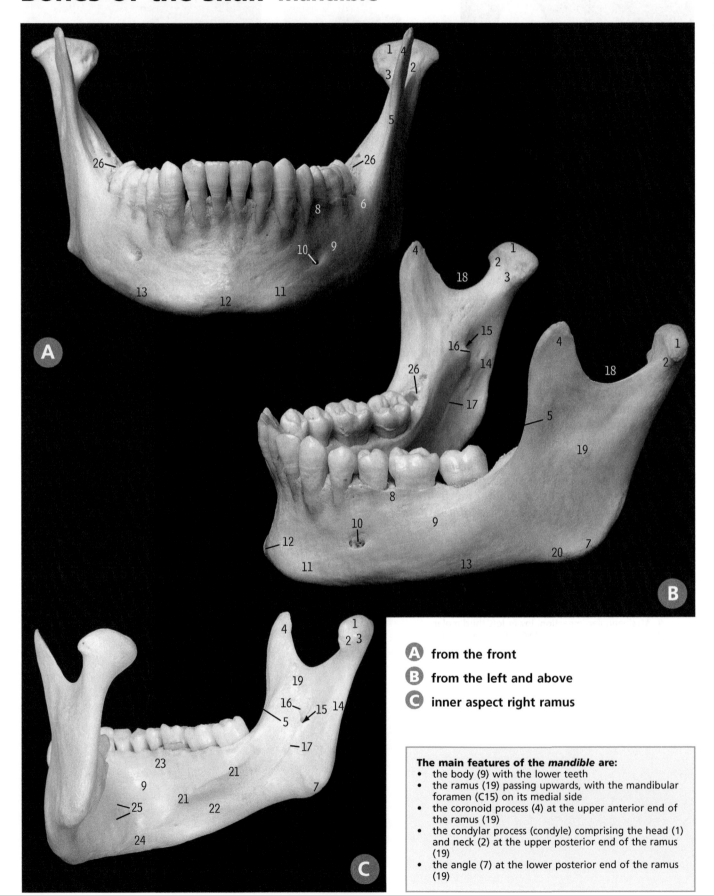

A from the front

B from the left and above

C inner aspect right ramus

The main features of the *mandible* are:
- the body (9) with the lower teeth
- the ramus (19) passing upwards, with the mandibular foramen (C15) on its medial side
- the coronoid process (4) at the upper anterior end of the ramus (19)
- the condylar process (condyle) comprising the head (1) and neck (2) at the upper posterior end of the ramus (19)
- the angle (7) at the lower posterior end of the ramus (19)

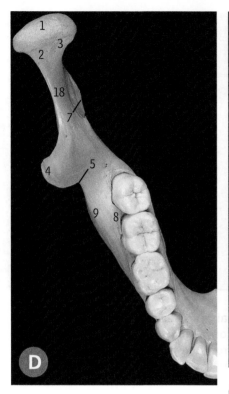

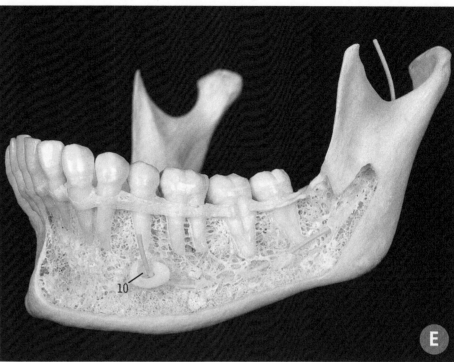

D from above

E from the left

The *mandible* is the bone of the lower jaw, bearing the lower teeth and forming the temporomandibular joints with the temporal bones.

In mandible A and B, (26) the third molar teeth are unerupted. In mandible C, D, E and F the third molar teeth are present.

In E and F compact bone has been removed to expose the underlying cancellous bone and canal in which a yellow marker has been placed to indicate the course of the inferior alveolar nerve which enters the mandibular foramen (15) and exits the mental foramen (10) as the mental nerve.

1 Head ⎫
2 Neck ⎬ forming
3 Pterygoid fovea ⎭ condylar process
4 Coronoid process
5 Anterior border of ramus and coronoid notch
6 Oblique line
7 Angle
8 Alveolar part
9 Body
10 Mental foramen
11 Mental tubercle
12 Mental protuberance
13 Base
14 Posterior border of ramus
15 Mandibular foramen
16 Lingula
17 Mylohyoid groove
18 Mandibular notch
19 Ramus
20 Inferior border of ramus
21 Mylohyoid line
22 Submandibular fossa
23 Sublingual fossa
24 Digastric fossa
25 Superior and inferior mental spines
26 Unerupted third molar tooth

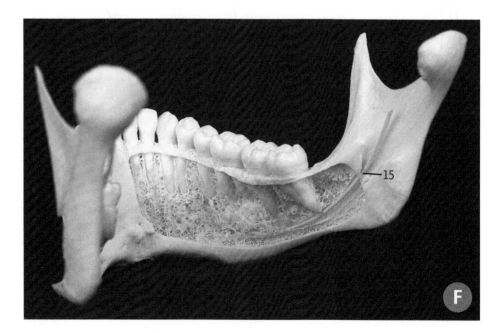

F from the left, behind and below

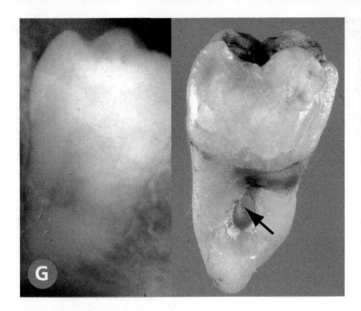

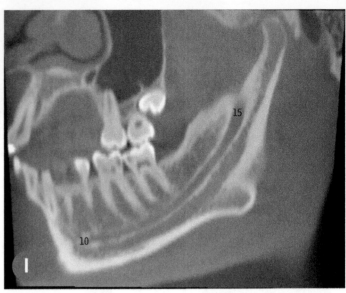

G The inferior dental nerve (IDN) passes adjacent to the roots of the lower molar in variable patterns. In extreme cases it may pass through the roots of the tooth itself as shown here in the radiograph and extracted tooth specimen (arrow)

I Oblique sagittal cone beam CT image of the mandible demonstrating the course of the inferior dental nerve from the mandibular foramen to the mental foramen

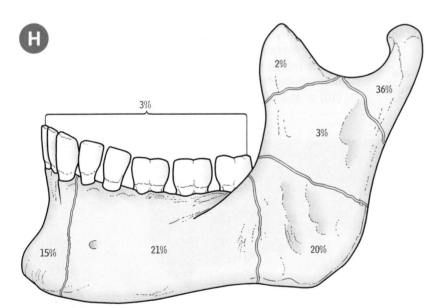

H The most commonly presenting fracture of the mandible is that of the condyle, followed by those of the body. However, there are often combinations of fractures such as the guardsman fracture of the symphysis and bilateral condyles. Percentages may vary depending on reported series

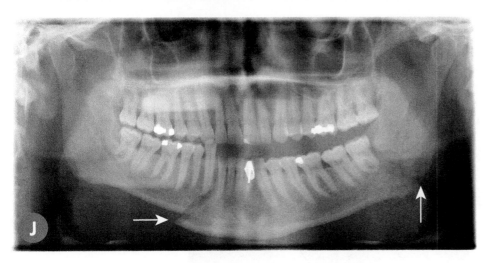

J Dental panoramic tomograph demonstrating a displaced fracture of the mandible at the left angle and right parasymphysis

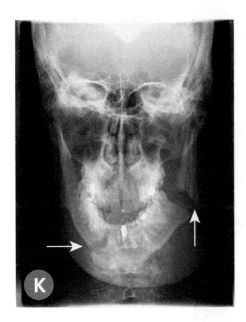

K Posteroanterior radiograph of the mandible in the same patient. Note the distraction of the proximal segment of the mandible due to the pull of masseter, temporalis, and medial pterygoid muscles

Mandible *Muscle attachments and age changes*

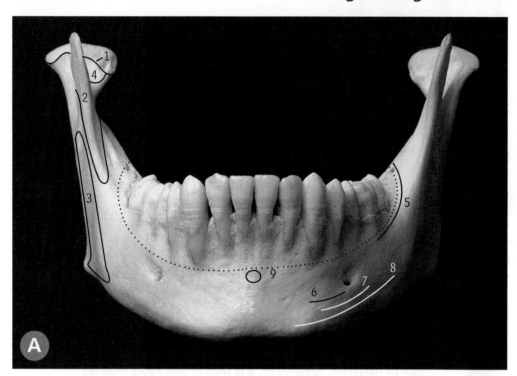

A from the front

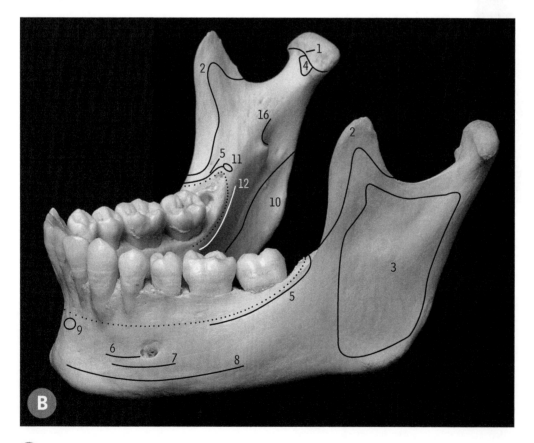

B from the left and above

In C the yellow marker indicates where the lingual nerve lies in contact with the periosteum—below and behind the third molar tooth (here unerupted). The side view of the edentulous (toothless) mandible in old age (D) should be compared with B and C. Note that the angle between the ramus and the body has become more obtuse, and that alveolar bone has become resorbed so that the mental foramen comes to lie nearer the upper surface of the edentulous body.

The attachment of the buccinator muscle (5, to the alveolar bone opposite the molar teeth—the third molar is here unerupted) extends back to the pterygomandibular raphe (11).

The attachment of the temporalis tendon (2) extends from the lowest part of the mandibular notch, over the coronoid process, and down the front of the ramus almost as far as the third molar tooth (here unerupted).

1 Capsule of temporomandibular joint
2 Temporalis
3 Masseter
4 Lateral pterygoid
5 Buccinator
6 Depressor labii inferioris
7 Depressor anguli oris
8 Platysma
9 Mentalis
10 Medial pterygoid
11 Pterygomandibular raphe and superior constrictor of pharynx
12 Mylohyoid
13 Anterior belly of digastric
14 Geniohyoid
15 Genioglossus
16 Sphenomandibular ligament
17 Stylomandibular ligament

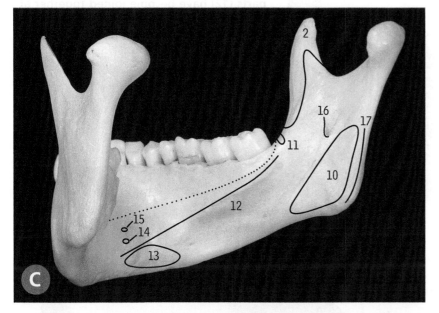

C medial aspect of right body and ramus

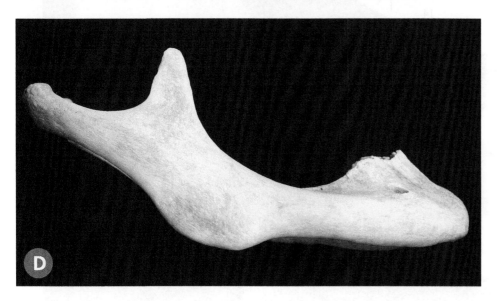

D mandible in old age, from the right

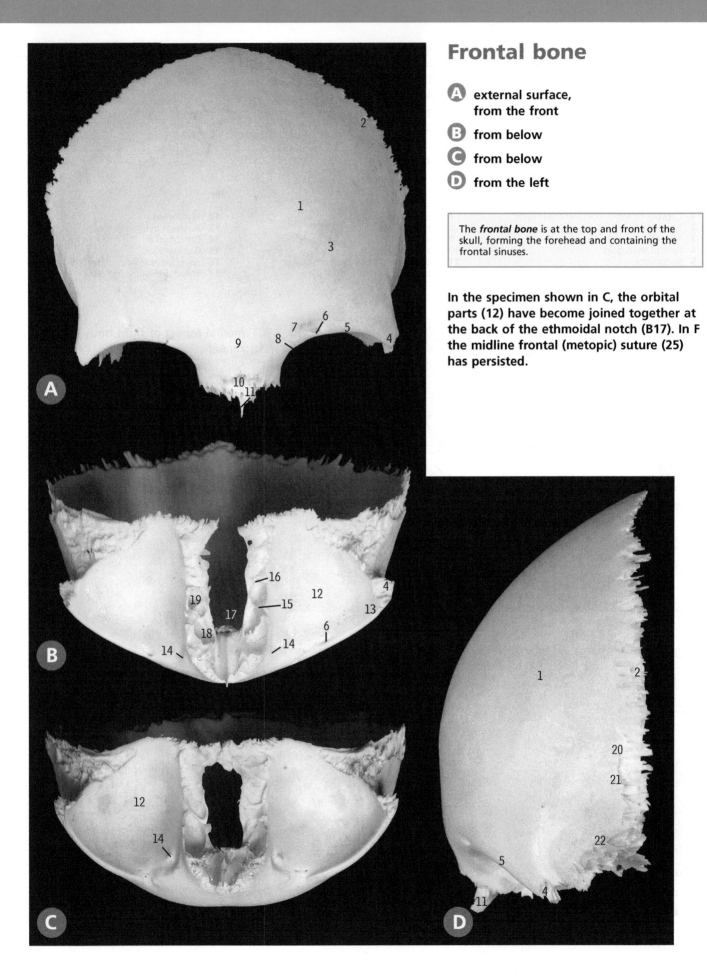

Frontal bone

A external surface, from the front

B from below

C from below

D from the left

> The *frontal bone* is at the top and front of the skull, forming the forehead and containing the frontal sinuses.

In the specimen shown in C, the orbital parts (12) have become joined together at the back of the ethmoidal notch (B17). In F the midline frontal (metopic) suture (25) has persisted.

1 Squamous part
2 Parietal margin
3 Frontal tuberosity
4 Zygomatic process
5 Supra-orbital margin
6 Supra-orbital foramen
7 Superciliary arch
8 Position of frontal notch or foramen
9 Glabella
10 Nasal part
11 Nasal spine
12 Orbital part
13 Fossa for lacrimal gland
14 Trochlear fovea (tubercle in C)
15 Anterior ethmoidal foramen
16 Posterior ethmoidal foramen
17 Ethmoidal notch
18 Frontal sinus
19 Roof of ethmoidal air cells
20 Superior temporal line
21 Inferior temporal line
22 Temporal surface
23 Frontal crest
24 Foramen caecum
25 Frontal (metopic) suture

The main features of the *frontal bone* are:
- the squamous part (1) curving upwards and backwards above
- the nose and orbits
- the orbital parts (12) passing backwards as the roofs of the orbits
- the nasal part (10) with the nasal spine (11) passing downwards.

In the intact skull, the ethmoidal notch (B17) is filled by the cribriform plate of the ethmoid bone and crista galli (page 30, A7 and 9; page 44, A2 and 3).

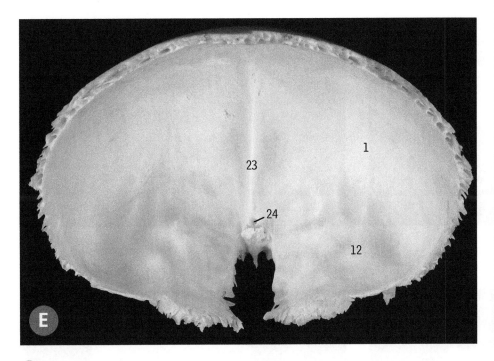
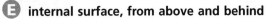

E internal surface, from above and behind

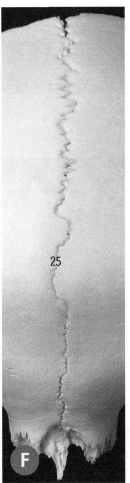

F external surface, from the front

Ethmoid bone

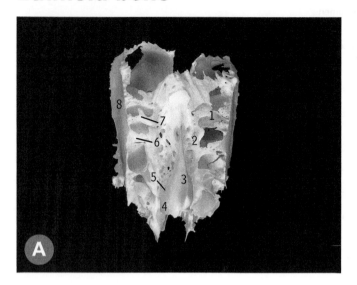

A from above

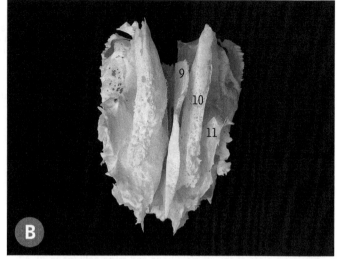

B from below

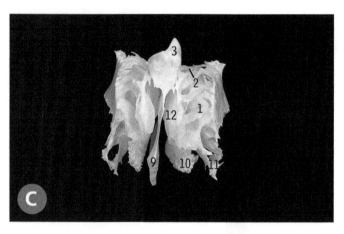

C from the front

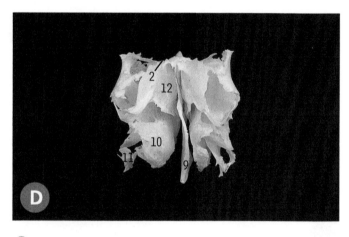

D from behind

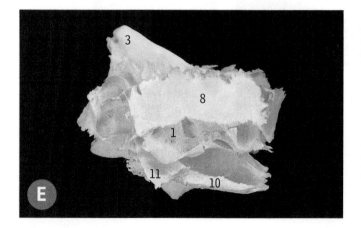

E from the left

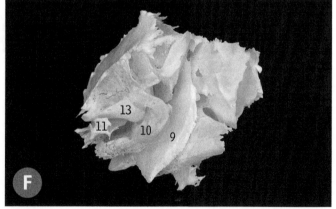

F from the left, below and behind

The specimen in F has been tilted obliquely upwards to show how the (left) ethmoidal bulla (F13) is overlapped by the middle nasal concha (F10).

The *ethmoid bone* is in the centre of the skull between the orbits, containing the ethmoidal sinuses and forming parts of the nasal and orbital cavities.

The main features of the *ethmoid bone* are:
- the perpendicular plate (B, C, D and F, 9) with the crista galli (A and C, 3) at the upper end
- the cribriform plate (A, C and D, 2) on each side at right angles to the perpendicular plate
- the ethmoidal labyrinth (sinus, A and C, 1) on each side hanging down from the outer edge of the cribriform plate
- superior and middle nasal conchae (C and D, 12 and 10) on the medial side of each labyrinth

The crista galli and cribriform plates (A3 and 2) form the central part of the floor of the anterior cranial fossa (page 30, A7 and 9).

The perpendicular plate forms part of the bony nasal septum (page 32, 27).

The superior and middle nasal conchae (C and D, 12 and 10) project from the medial wall of the ethmoidal labyrinth as part of the lateral wall of the nasal cavity (page 34, B32 and 36). (The inferior nasal concha is a separate bone, not part of the ethmoid: page 34, B44 and page 53, G and H.)

The lateral wall of the ethmoidal labyrinth is the orbital plate (A and E, 8), forming part of the medial wall of the orbit (page 34, A21 and page 63, D and E, 20). This orbital plate is paper-thin and hence often called the lamina papyracea; the outlines of ethmoidal air cells are usually visible through it (as in E8).

The ethmoidal bulla (F13, a bulging air cell) is under cover of the middle nasal concha (F10). When this concha is removed (as in page 34, D) a groove is seen between the bulla and the uncinate process of the ethmoid (F10 and 11). This groove, lined by mucous membrane in the intact nasal cavity, is the semilunar hiatus (page 34, D60, between 61 and 46, and page 160, B12, between 11 and 14).

---

1 Ethmoidal labyrinth and air cells
2 Cribriform plate
3 Crista galli
4 Ala of crista galli
5 Slit for anterior ethmoidal nerve and vessels
6 Groove for anterior ethmoidal nerve and vessels
7 Groove for posterior ethmoidal nerve and vessels
8 Orbital plate
9 Perpendicular plate
10 Middle nasal concha
11 Uncinate process
12 Superior nasal concha
13 Ethmoidal bulla

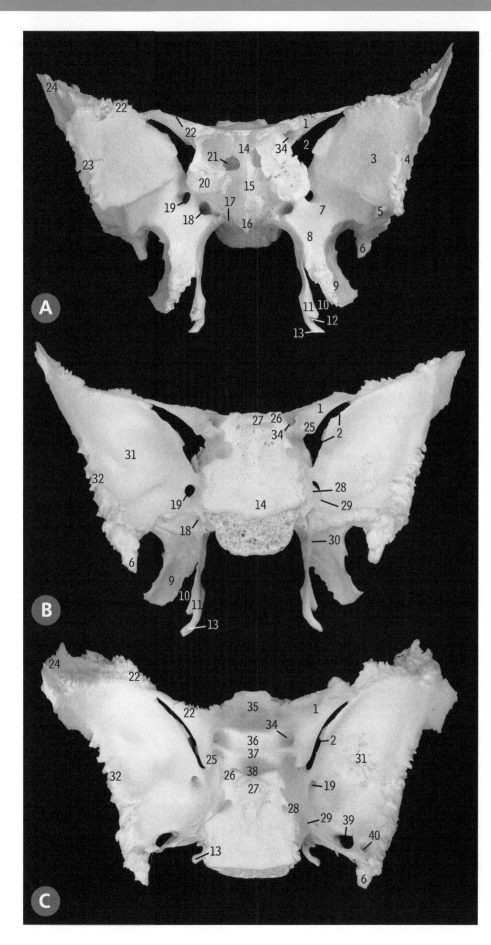

Sphenoid bone

A from the front
B from behind
C from above and behind

The **sphenoid bone** is in the middle of the base of the skull, extending to each side and containing the pituitary fossa and the sphenoidal sinuses.

1 Lesser wing
2 Superior orbital fissure
3 Orbital surface ⎤
4 Temporal surface ⎥ of greater
5 Infratemporal   ⎥ wing crest
6 Spine   ⎥
7 Maxillary surface ⎦
8 Pterygoid process
9 Lateral pterygoid plate
10 Pterygoid notch
11 Medial pterygoid plate
12 Groove of pterygoid hamulus
13 Pterygoid hamulus
14 Body
15 Crest
16 Rostrum
17 Vaginal process
18 Pterygoid canal
19 Foramen rotundum
20 Concha
21 Aperture of sphenoidal sinus
22 Frontal margin
23 Zygomatic margin
24 Parietal margin
25 Anterior clinoid process
26 Posterior clinoid process
27 Dorsum sellae
28 Carotid groove
29 Lingula
30 Scaphoid fossa
31 Cerebral surface of greater wing
32 Squamous margin
33 Groove for auditory tube
34 Optic canal
35 Jugum
36 Prechiasmatic groove
37 Tuberculum sellae
38 Pituitary fossa (sella turcica)
39 Foramen ovale
40 Foramen spinosum
41 Ala
42 Posterior border
43 Groove for nasopalatine nerve and vessels

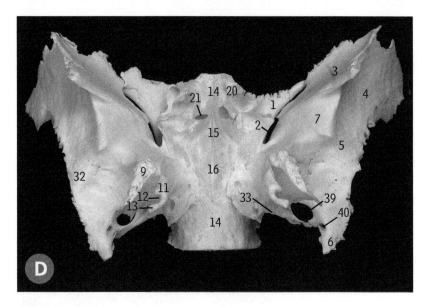

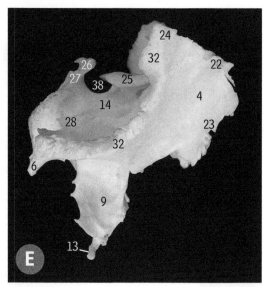

D from below

E from the right

Vomer

The *vomer* is in the midline of the base of the skull, forming the posterior part of the nasal septum.

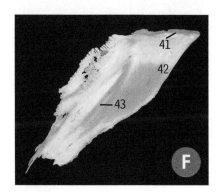

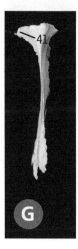

F from the left
G from behind

The main features of the *sphenoid bone* are:
- the body (A14) containing the two sphenoidal air sinuses with their apertures anteriorly (A21)
- the pituitary fossa (C and E, 38) indenting the upper surface of the body
- the lesser wing (1) on each side passing laterally with the optic canal between its roots (C34)
- the greater wing (A3; B31) on each side passing laterally below the lesser wing, with the superior orbital fissure (A and B, 2) between the lesser and greater wings, and the foramina rotundum, ovale and spinosum within the greater wing
- the pterygoid process (A8) on each side passing downwards to divide into the medial and lateral pterygoid plates (A and B, 9 and 11)

The posterior part of the body which joins the occipital bone at the spheno-occipital synchondrosis (page 71) is commonly known as the basisphenoid (B14 and the lower 14 in D).

The main features of the *vomer* are the alae (41) which project laterally at the upper margin.

Occipital bone

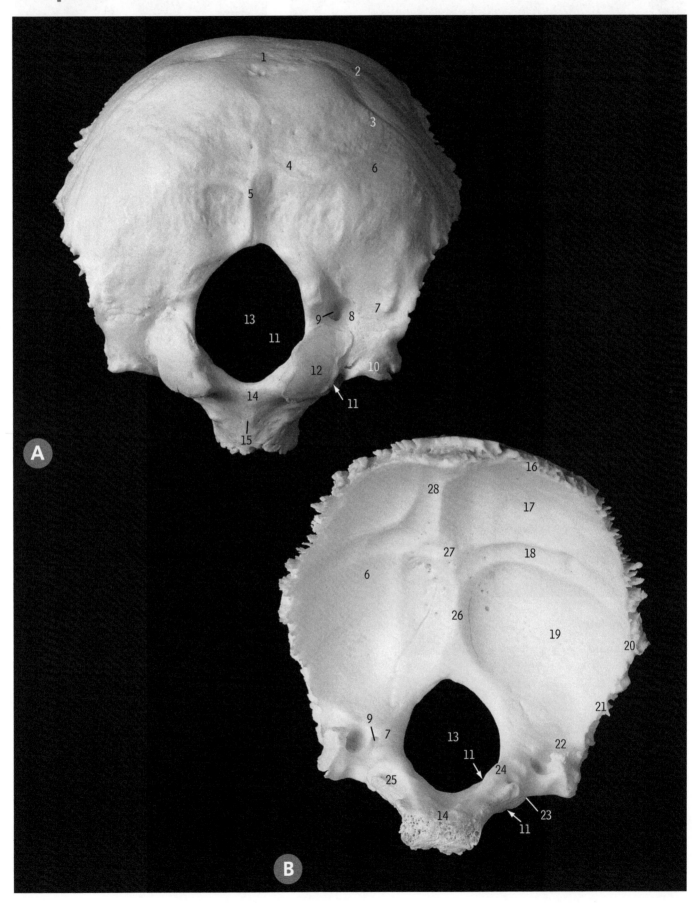

A external surface, from below

B internal surface

C external surface, from the right and below

1 External occipital protuberance	**15** Pharyngeal tubercle
2 Supreme nuchal line	**16** Lambdoid margin
3 Superior nuchal line	**17** Cerebral fossa
4 Inferior nuchal line	**18** Groove for transverse sinus
5 External occipital crest	**19** Cerebellar fossa
6 Squamous part	**20** Lateral angle
7 Lateral part	**21** Mastoid margin
8 Condylar fossa	**22** Groove for sigmoid sinus
9 Condylar canal	**23** Jugular notch
10 Jugular process	**24** Jugular tubercle
11 Hypoglossal canal	**25** Groove for inferior petrosal sinus
12 Condyle	**26** Internal occipital crest
13 Foramen magnum	**27** Internal occipital protuberance
14 Basilar part	**28** Groove for superior sagittal sinus

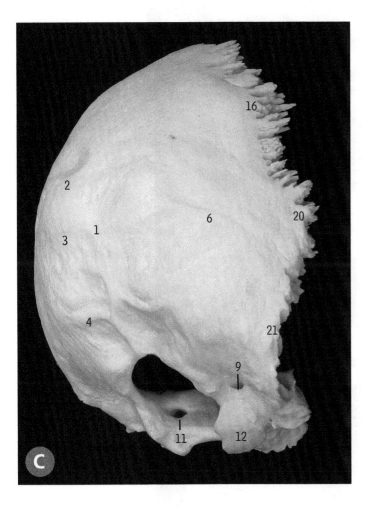

The *occipital bone* is at the back of the base of the skull, containing the foramen magnum and bearing the condyles for the atlanto-occipital joints by which the skull is attached to the vertebral column.

The main features of the *occipital bone* are:
- the foramen magnum (13) in the lower part
- the squamous part (6) curving upwards and backwards behind the foramen magnum
- the lateral parts (7), with condyles on the lower surfaces (A and C, 12)
- the basilar part (A and B, 14) in front of the foramen magnum

The anterior end of the basilar part (B14) which joins the sphenoid bone at the spheno-occipital synchondrosis (page 71) is commonly known as the basi-occiput (compare with the basisphenoid—see the note on page 47).

The hypoglossal canal (A and C, 11) passes approximately above the middle of the occipital condyle (A12), but is only seen when viewed from the side (as in C, 11). The hypoglossal nerve runs through it.

The condylar canal (A9), which is not always present, opens behind the occipital condyle. An emissary vein passes through it connecting the sigmoid sinus (inside the skull) to veins in the suboccipital region (outside the skull).

Maxilla *Left*

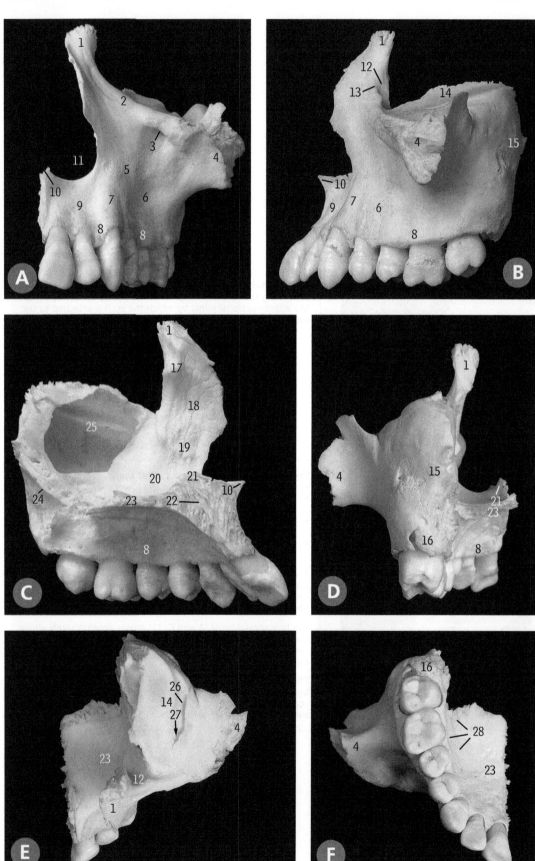

Ⓐ from the front

Ⓑ from the lateral side

Ⓒ from the medial side

Ⓓ from behind

Ⓔ from above

Ⓕ from below

In D and F, 16 the third molar tooth is unerupted

> The *maxilla* forms half of the upper jaw, bearing the upper teeth of one side and containing the maxillary sinus.

Nasal bone *Left*

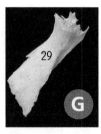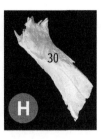

> The *nasal bone* forms with its fellow the bridge of the nose.

Ⓖ from the lateral side

Ⓗ from the medial side

Lacrimal bone *Left*

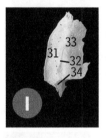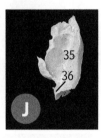

> The *lacrimal bone* is at the front of the medial wall of the orbit.

Ⓘ from the lateral side

Ⓙ from the medial side

1 Frontal process	**20** Inferior meatus
2 Infra-orbital margin	**21** Nasal crest
3 Infra-orbital foramen	**22** Incisive canal
4 Zygomatic process	**23** Palatine process
5 Anterior surface	**24** Greater palatine groove
6 Canine fossa	**25** Maxillary hiatus and sinus
7 Canine eminence	**26** Infra-orbital groove
8 Alveolar process	**27** Infra-orbital canal
9 Incisive fossa	**28** Palatine grooves and
10 Anterior nasal spine	spines
11 Nasal notch	**29** Lateral surface and vascular
12 Lacrimal groove	foramen
13 Anterior lacrimal crest	**30** Internal surface and
14 Orbital surface	ethmoidal groove
15 Infratemporal surface	**31** Lacrimal groove
16 Tuberosity (over unerupted	**32** Posterior lacrimal crest
third molar tooth)	**33** Orbital surface
17 Ethmoidal crest	**34** Lacrimal hamulus
18 Middle meatus	**35** Nasal surface
19 Conchal crest	**36** Descending process

The main features of the *maxilla* are:
- the maxillary sinus with the hiatus in the medial wall (C25)
- the alveolar process (A-D, 8) at the lower margin with the upper teeth
- the frontal process (A-D, 1) passing upwards
- the palatine process (C-F, 23) passing medially
- the zygomatic process (A, B, D and F, 4) passing laterally to articulate with the zygomatic process of the temporal bone to form the zygomatic arch

In the intact skull, the two maxillae unite with one another below the nasal notch (A11), but the frontal processes (A1) are separated from one another by the two nasal bones (page 2, 33)

The palatine process (F23) articulates at the back with the horizontal plate of the palatine bone (page 52, F15). They both articulate with their fellows of the opposite side to form the hard palate (page 16, A2 and 6).

For articulations forming the lateral wall of the nasal cavity, see pages 64-65.

The main features of the *nasal bone* are:
- the smooth lateral surface (G29)
- the ethmoidal groove (H30) on the internal surface

The main features of the *lacrimal bone* are:
- the orbital (lateral) surface with the lacrimal groove (I31) at the front
- the descending process (J36) pointing downwards

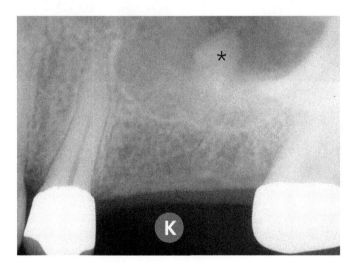

Ⓚ The apices of the maxillary molars are closely related to the maxillary sinus. Fractured roots of these teeth (*) may become dislodged into the antrum during extraction

Palatine bone *Left*

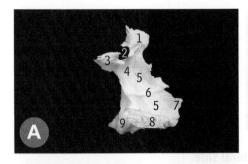

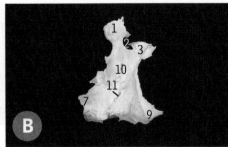

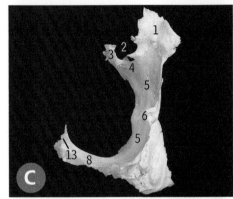

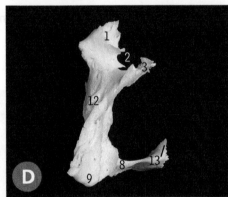

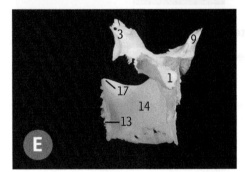

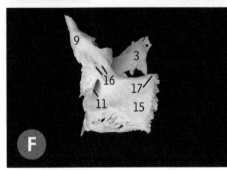

A from the medial side

B from the lateral side

C from the front

D from behind

E from above

F from below

1 Orbital process
2 Sphenopalatine notch
3 Sphenoidal process
4 Ethmoidal crest
5 Perpendicular plate, nasal surface
6 Conchal crest
7 Maxillary process
8 Horizontal plate
9 Pyramidal process
10 Perpendicular plate, maxillary surface
11 Greater palatine groove
12 Perpendicular plate
13 Nasal crest
14 Horizontal plate, nasal surface
15 Horizontal plate, palatal surface
16 Lesser palatine canals
17 Posterior nasal canals
18 Anterior end
19 Lacrimal process
20 Medial surface
21 Ethmoidal process
22 Posterior end
23 Maxillary process
24 Lateral surface

The *palatine bone* is at the back of the lateral wall of the nasal cavity and forms part of the roof of the mouth (hard palate).

Inferior nasal concha *Left*

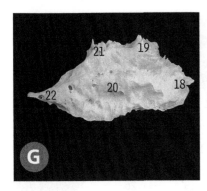

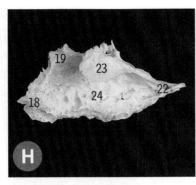

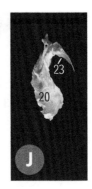

G from the medial side

H from the lateral side

J from the front

The *inferior nasal concha* is in the lower part of the lateral wall of the nasal cavity.

The main features of the *palatine bone* are:
- the perpendicular plate (A and C, 5; B10), the largest part of the bone
- the orbital and sphenoidal processes (A-D, 1 and 3) at the upper end of the perpendicular plate, with the sphenopalatine notch in between (A-D, 2)
- the horizontal plate (C and D, 8) passing medially at the lower end of the perpendicular plate
- the maxillary process (A and B, 7) passing forwards at the lower end of the perpendicular plate
- the pyramidal process (A, B and D-F, 9) passing backwards at the lower end of the perpendicular plate

The upper surface of the orbital process of the palatine bone (E1) forms the most posterior part of the floor of the orbit (page 34, A18).

The sphenopalatine notch (A2), at the upper end of the perpendicular plate (A5) between the orbital and sphenoidal processes (A1 and 3), is converted into the sphenopalatine foramen (in the lateral wall of the nasal cavity) by articulation with the body of the sphenoid bone (page 74, B6).

For articulations forming the lateral wall of the nose see pages 64-65, and the floor of the orbit, pages 62-63.

The main features of the *inferior nasal concha* are:
- the convex medial surface (G20) with a sharp posterior end (G22)
- the lacrimal and ethmoidal processes (G19 and 21), passing upwards
- the maxillary process (H and J, 23) passing downwards on the lateral side

The anterior and posterior ends of the lateral surface (H18 and 22) articulate with the conchal crests of the maxilla and palatine bone, respectively (page 50, C17 and page 52, A6).

Temporal bone *Right*

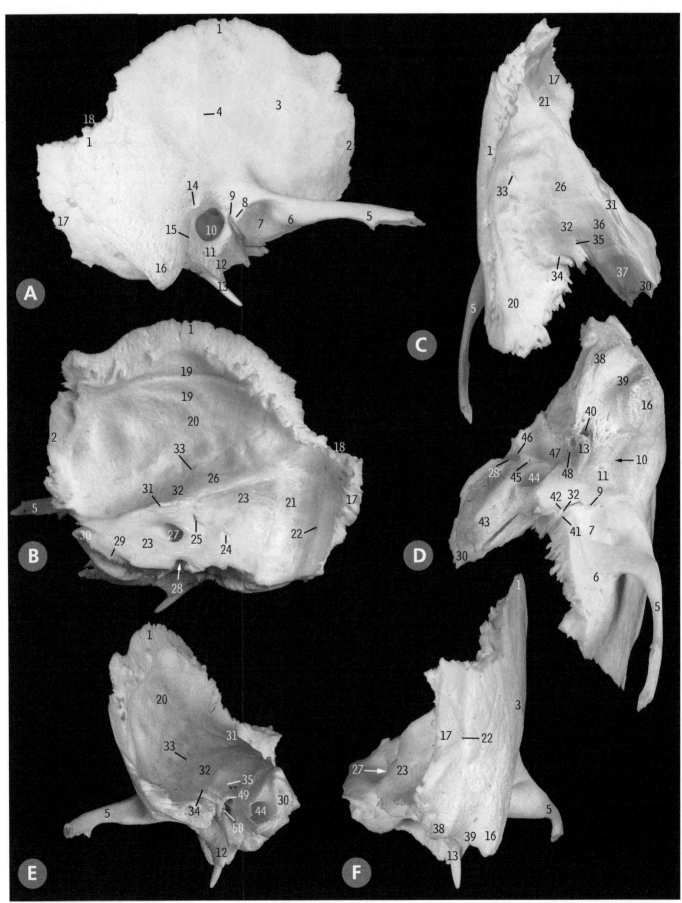

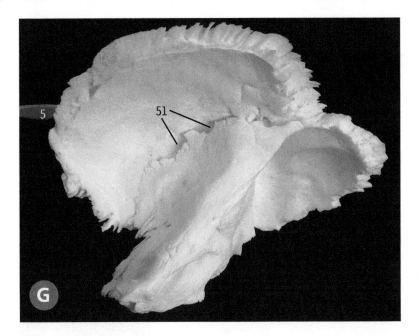

51

5

G

Ⓐ from the lateral side

Ⓑ from the medial side

Ⓒ from above

Ⓓ from below

Ⓔ from the front

Ⓕ from behind

Ⓖ from the medial side and above

The *temporal bone* is at the side and base of the skull, containing the ear and making the temporomandibular joint with the mandible.

The main features of the *temporal bone* are:
- the petrous part (C31; D43) including the mastoid process (A and F, 16)
- the squamous part (A and F, 3) passing upwards but including the mandibular fossa (A and D, 7) facing downwards and the zygomatic process (A and D, 5) passing forwards
- the styloid process (A and F, 13) passing downwards and forwards
- the tympanic part (A11) surrounding the external acoustic meatus (A10) opening laterally
- the internal acoustic meatus (B27) in the petrous part opening medially

The suprameatal triangle (A14) overlies the mastoid antrum (page 182, F50) which lies medially about 1.25 cm from the surface.

The mastoid foramen (F22, above and behind the mastoid process, F16) transmits an emissary vein from the sigmoid sinus to the posterior auricular or occipital vein.

The mastoid canaliculus (D48, in the lateral part of the jugular fossa, D47) transmits the auricular branch of the vagus nerve.

The arcuate eminence (B26) in the petrous part overlies the anterior semicircular canal.

In G the petrosquamous fissure (51) has remained open, so forming a groove for the petrosquamous sinus. The fissure is normally almost closed, as in B33. The sinus is present in fetal life but usually disappears in the adult; if it persists it may receive small veins from the tympanic cavity and form a venous communication between the inside and the outside of the skull.

For further details of the temporal bone and ear see pages 182-185.

1 Parietal margin
2 Sphenoidal margin
3 Temporal surface of squamous part
4 Groove for middle temporal artery
5 Zygomatic process
6 Articular tubercle
7 Mandibular fossa
8 Postglenoid tubercle
9 Squamotympanic fissure
10 External acoustic meatus
11 Tympanic part
12 Sheath of styloid process
13 Styloid process
14 Suprameatal pit and spine (suprameatal triangle)
15 Tympanomastoid fissure
16 Mastoid process
17 Occipital margin
18 Parietal notch
19 Groove for parietal branches of middle meningeal vessels
20 Cerebral surface of squamous part
21 Groove for sigmoid sinus
22 Mastoid foramen
23 Posterior surface of petrous part
24 External opening of aqueduct of vestibule
25 Subarcuate fossa
26 Arcuate eminence
27 Internal acoustic meatus
28 External opening of cochlear canaliculus in jugular notch
29 Groove for inferior petrosal sinus
30 Apex of petrous sinus
31 Superior margin of petrous part and groove for superior petrosal sinus
32 Tegmen tympani
33 Petrosquamous fissure (upper part)
34 Hiatus and groove for lesser petrosal nerve
35 Hiatus and groove for greater petrosal nerve
36 Anterior surface of petrous part
37 Trigeminal impression
38 Occipital groove
39 Mastoid notch
40 Stylomastoid foramen
41 Petrosquamous fissure (lower part)
42 Petrotympanic fissure
43 Inferior surface of petrous part
44 Carotid canal
45 Tympanic canaliculus
46 Intrajugular process
47 Jugular fossa
48 Mastoid canaliculus
49 Semicanal for tensor tympani
50 Semicanal for auditory tube
51 Groove for petrosquamous sinus

Parietal bone *Right*

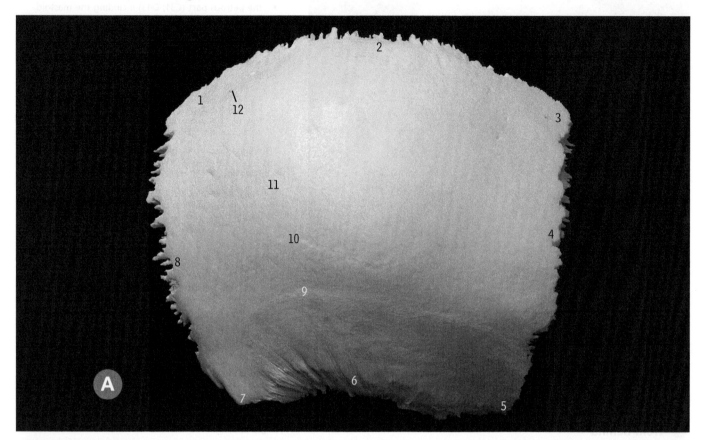

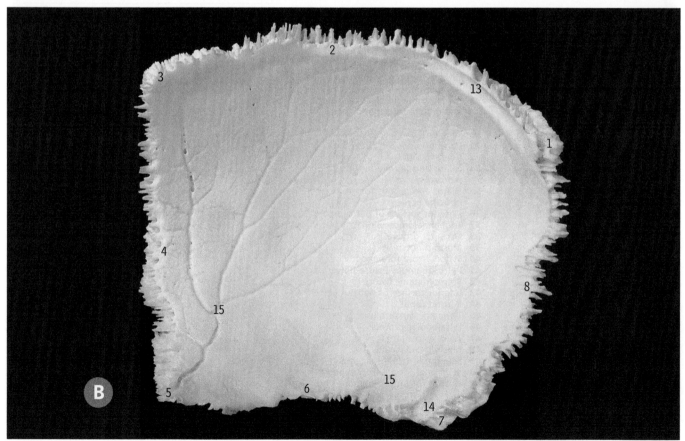

A external surface

B internal surface

The *parietal bone* is at the side and top of the skull.

1 Occipital (posterosuperior) angle
2 Sagittal (superior) margin
3 Frontal (anterosuperior) angle
4 Frontal (anterior) margin
5 Sphenoidal (antero-inferior) angle
6 Squamous (inferior) margin
7 Mastoid (postero-inferior) angle
8 Occipital (posterior) margin
9 Inferior temporal line
10 Superior temporal line
11 Parietal tuberosity
12 Parietal foramen
13 Groove for part of superior sagittal sinus
14 Groove for sigmoid sinus at mastoid angle
15 Grooves for middle meningeal vessels
16 Frontal process
17 Temporal margin
18 Temporal process
19 Lateral surface
20 Maxillary margin
21 Zygomaticofacial foramen
22 Orbital margin
23 Orbital surface
24 Zygomaticofacial foramen
25 Temporal surface
26 Zygomaticotemporal foramen
27 Sphenoidal margin
28 Marginal tubercle

The main features of the *parietal bone* are:
- the convex external surface (A)
- the concave internal surface with grooves for the middle meningeal vessels (B15) passing upwards and backwards, and the groove for the sigmoid sinus (B14) at the mastoid (postero-inferior) angle

To assist in orientation of the parietal bone, note that grooves for the middle meningeal vessels run upwards and backwards (B15), and that the groove for a small part of the sigmoid sinus is at the mastoid (postero-inferior) angle (B14).

The main features of the *zygomatic bone* are:
- the slightly convex lateral surface (C19)
- the smoothly curved orbital margin (C22) and orbital surface (D23)
- the frontal process (C and D, 16) passing upwards
- the temporal process (C and D, 18) passing backwards

Official nomenclature does not recognise the margins of the zygomatic bone (C17 and 22) but they are helpful terms for orientation.

The marginal tubercle (Whitnall's tubercle, D28) lies just inside the orbital margin below the frontozygomatic suture (in the intact skull), and it can often be felt with the fingertip even if not readily visible. It receives the attachment of the lateral palpebral raphe (from orbicularis oculi) and the lateral palpebral ligament.

Zygomatic bone *Left*

C lateral surface

D from the medial side

E from the front

F from behind

The *zygomatic bone* is at the front and side of the skull, forming the prominence of the cheek.

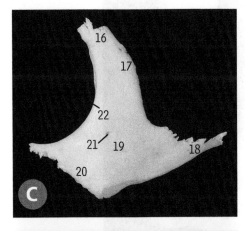

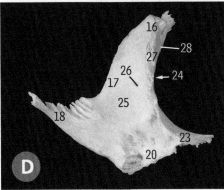

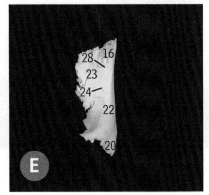

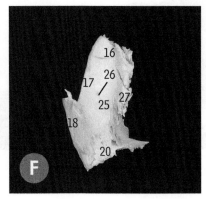

Skull bone articulations Facial skeleton

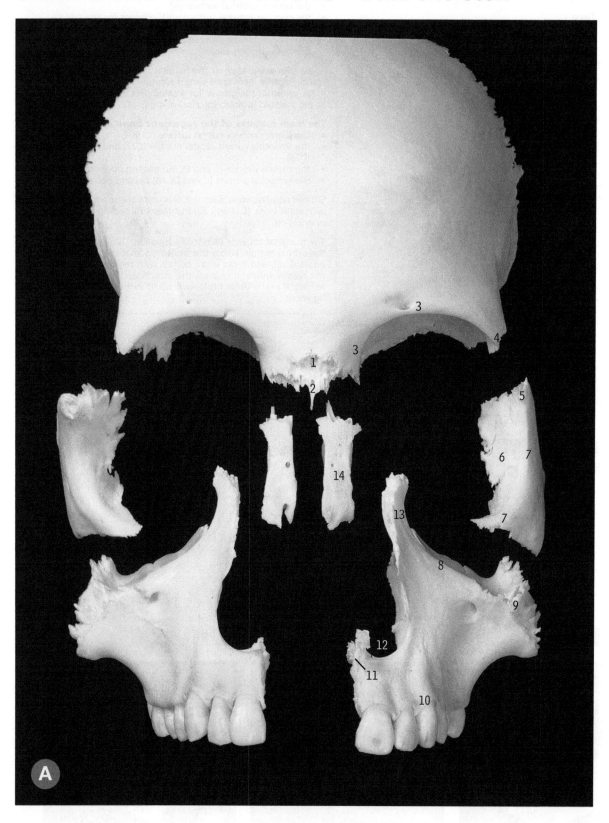

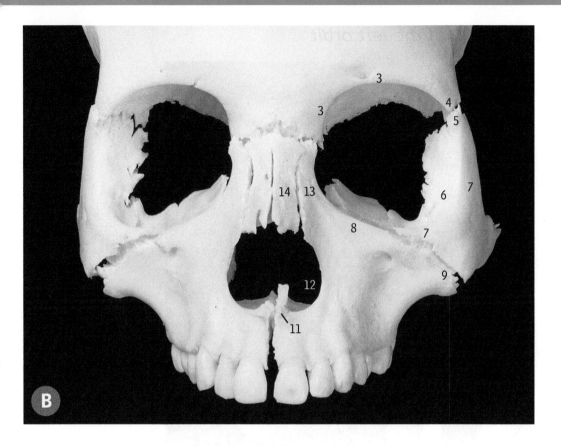

Orbital and anterior nasal apertures

A **B** the frontal, nasal and zygomatic bones and the maxillae, from the front, separated and articulated

Because of the irregular nature of the bone margins that take part in skull sutures, close and precise re-articulation of bones is not usually possible, but the illustrations on pages 58-81 indicate the way that individual skull bones become assembled together to form the complete skull.

1 Nasal part ⎫
2 Nasal spine ⎬ of frontal bone
3 Supra-orbital margin ⎪
4 Zygomatic process ⎭
5 Frontal process ⎫
6 Orbital surface ⎬ of zygomatic bone
7 Orbital margin ⎭
8 Infra-orbital margin ⎫
9 Zygomatic process ⎪
10 Alveolar process ⎪
11 Anterior nasal spine ⎬ of maxilla
12 Nasal notch ⎪
13 Frontal process ⎪
14 Nasal bone ⎭

The **orbital aperture** (aditus of the orbit) is bounded above by the supra-orbital margin of the frontal bone (3), laterally by the zygomatic bone (7) and the zygomatic process of the frontal bone (4), below by the zygomatic bone (7) and the infra-orbital margin of the maxilla (8), and medially by the frontal bone (3) and the anterior lacrimal crest of the orbital process of the maxilla (13).

The **anterior nasal (piriform) aperture** is bounded largely by the nasal notches of the maxillae (12), with the lower margins of the nasal bones above (14).

Orbit *Roof and lateral wall of the left orbit*

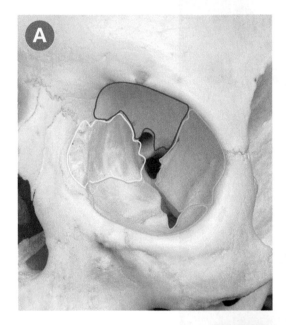

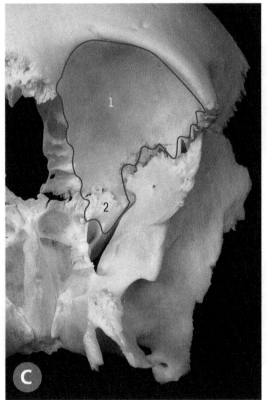

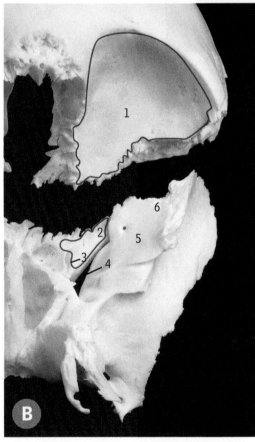

Roof, walls and floor of the orbit: Ⓐ Ⓑ Ⓒ Ⓓ Ⓔ

Green: floor
Yellow: medial wall
Red: roof
Blue: lateral wall

1 Orbital part of frontal bone
2 Lesser wing ⎫
3 Optic canal ⎪
4 Superior orbital fissure ⎪
5 Greater wing ⎪
6 Frontal margin of greater wing ⎪
7 Lesser wing ⎬ of sphenoid bone
8 Lateral wall of body ⎪
9 Pterygoid process ⎪
10 Foramen rotundum ⎪
11 Superior orbital fissure ⎪
12 Orbital surface of greater wing ⎭
13 Zygomatic margin
14 Orbital surface ⎫
15 Frontal process ⎬ of zygomatic bone
16 Marginal tubercle ⎭
17 Orbital margin
18 Infra-orbital margin ⎫ of maxilla
19 Orbital surface ⎬
20 Inferior orbital fissure

Ⓐ the left orbit, from the front, left and above (as in page 34, A)

Ⓑ Ⓒ parts of the frontal and sphenoid bones, from below, separated and articulated, forming the roof of the orbit

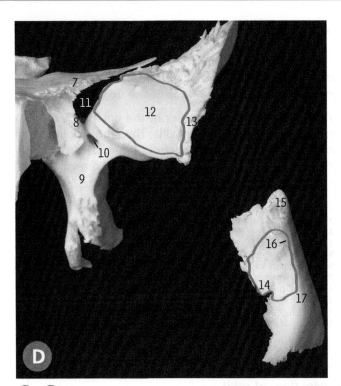

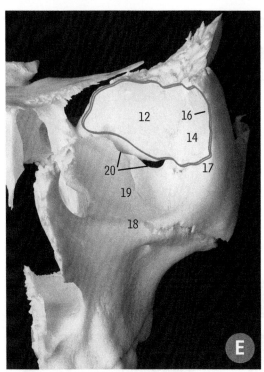

D **E** part of the sphenoid bone and the zygomatic bone, from the front (with the maxilla in E), separated and articulated, forming the lateral wall of the orbit

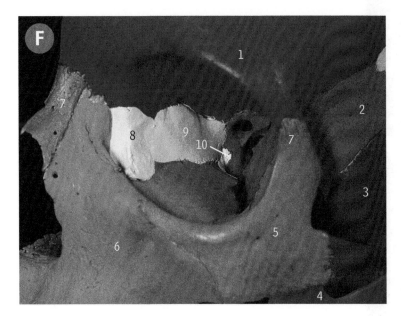

F the left orbit, from the front, left and above, with individual bones coloured

1 Frontal bone
2 Sphenoid bone
3 Temporal bone
4 Mandible
5 Zygomatic bone
6 Maxilla
7 Nasal bone
8 Lacrimal bone
9 Ethmoid bone
10 Palatine bone

The *roof of the orbit* is formed mainly by the orbital part of the frontal bone (B and C, 1), with the lesser wing of the sphenoid bone (2) in the most posterior part. (The greater wing, B5, forms part of the lateral wall of the orbit.)

The *lateral wall of the orbit* is formed by the orbital surfaces of the greater wing of the sphenoid (12) and the zygomatic bone (14). (The zygomatic bone also forms part of the floor of the orbit, with the maxilla—see next page.)

Orbit *Floor and medial wall of the left orbit*

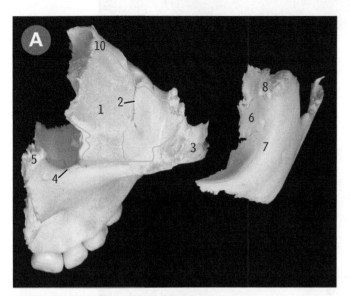

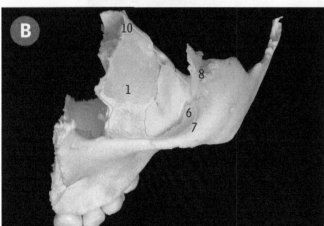

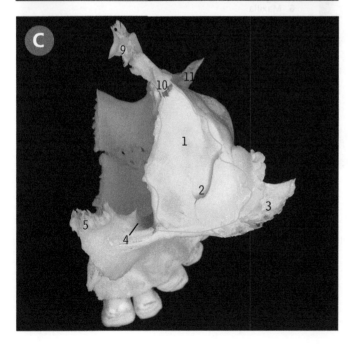

A **B** **C** the left maxilla and the zygomatic and palatine bone from above and in front, separated and articulated, forming the floor of the orbit

In A and B the orbital process of the palatine bone (10) remains adherent to the maxilla; the whole palatine bone is shown in C. The sphenoid bone, part of whose body forms the most posterior part of the medial wall, is not shown here (see page 34, A22).

1	Orbital surface	⎫
2	Infra-orbital groove	⎪
3	Zygomatic process	⎬ of maxilla
4	Lacrimal groove	⎪
5	Frontal process	⎭
6	Orbital surface	⎫
7	Orbital margin	⎬ of zygomatic bone
8	Frontal process	⎭
9	Sphenoidal process	⎫
10	Orbital process	⎬ of palatine bone
11	Pyramidal process	⎭

A **B** **C**

Green: floor of orbit

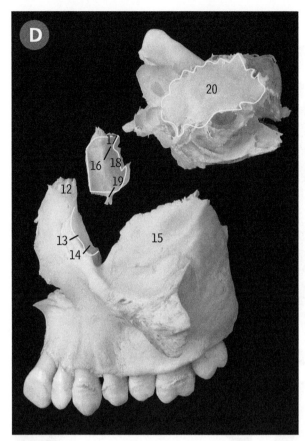

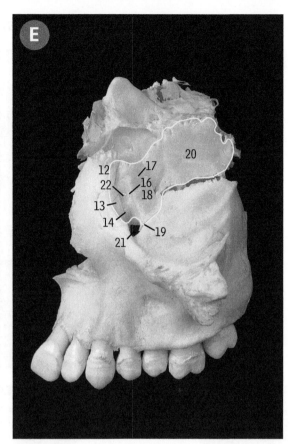

D **E** the left maxilla and the lacrimal bone and the ethmoid bone, from the left, separated and articulated, forming the medial wall of the orbit

12 Frontal process ⎫
13 Anterior lacrimal crest ⎬ of maxilla
14 Lacrimal groove ⎪
15 Orbital surface ⎭
16 Lacrimal groove ⎫
17 Posterior lacrimal crest ⎪
18 Orbital surface ⎬ of lacrimal bone
19 Lacrimal hamulus ⎪
20 Orbital plate of ethmoid bone ⎭
21 Nasolacrimal canal
22 Fossa for lacrimal sac

D **E**

Yellow: medial wall of orbit

The *floor of the orbit* is formed by the orbital surface of the maxilla (1) and zygomatic bone (6), with the orbital process of the palatine bone (10) in the most posterior part.

The upper opening of the nasolacrimal canal (E21), formed by the maxilla and lacrimal bones, is at the front of the junction between the floor and medial wall of the orbit (see also pages 66 and 67).

The **medial wall of the orbit** begins at the anterior lacrimal crest of the frontal process of the maxilla. The lacrimal grooves of this process and of the lacrimal bone form the fossa for the lacrimal sac, and behind the posterior lacrimal crest lies the rest of the orbital surface of the lacrimal bone. The orbital plate of the ethmoid bone then forms much of the medial wall, with a small part of the body of the sphenoid (not shown here but seen in F on page 61) as the most posterior part of this wall.

Nasal cavity *Right roof, floor and lateral wall*

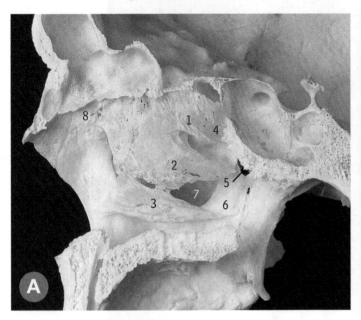

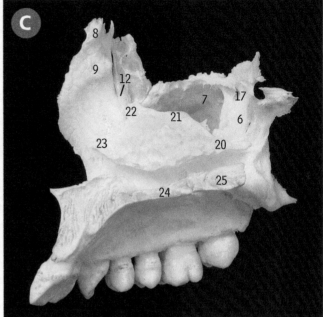

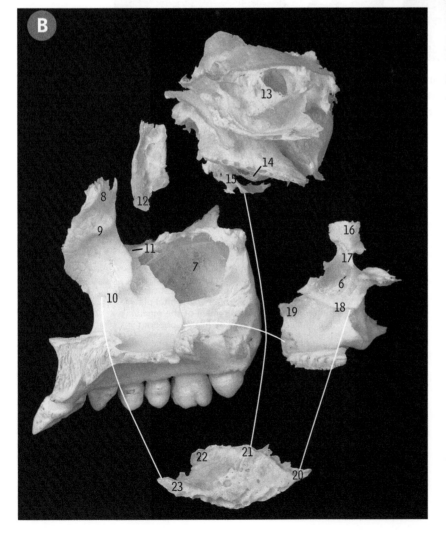

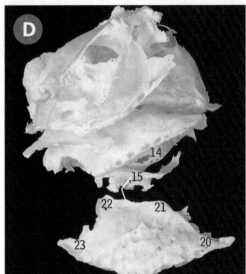

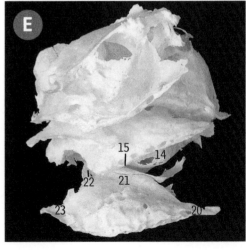

Ⓐ the right half of the nasal cavity, in the intact skull (as in page 34, B)

Ⓑ the right maxilla, the lacrimal, ethmoid and palatine bones and the inferior nasal concha, from the left

Ⓒ the right maxilla with the lacrimal and palatine bones and the inferior nasal concha articulated

Ⓓ **Ⓔ** The ethmoid bone and the right inferior nasal concha, separated and articulated

The white lines in B indicate which parts of the palatine bone and inferior nasal concha overlap and articulate with one another and with the maxilla, as shown in C. In E the uncinate process of the ethmoid bone (15) articulates with the ethmoidal process of the inferior concha (21).

1	Superior ⎫
2	Middle ⎬ nasal concha
3	Inferior ⎭
4	Spheno-ethmoidal recess
5	Sphenopalatine foramen
6	Perpendicular plate of palatine bone
7	Maxillary hiatus
8	Frontal process ⎫
9	Ethmoidal crest ⎬ of maxilla
10	Conchal crest ⎪
11	Lacrimal groove ⎭
12	Descending process of lacrimal bone
13	Left ethmoidal labyrinth ⎫
14	Right ethmoidal bulla ⎬ of ethmoid bone
15	Right uncinate process ⎭
16	Orbital process ⎫
17	Ethmoidal crest ⎬ of palatine bone
18	Conchal crest ⎪
19	Maxillary process ⎭
20	Posterior end ⎫
21	Ethmoidal process ⎬ of inferior concha
22	Lacrimal process ⎪
23	Anterior end ⎭
24	Palatine process of maxilla
25	Horizontal plate of palatine bone

When articulated, the four bones arranged around the maxilla in B (lacrimal, ethmoid and palatine bones and the inferior nasal concha) reduce the size of the maxillary hiatus (B7) to the size shown in A7 or smaller. In life the size is further reduced by mucous membrane (as in page 160, C21).

In B and D the ethmoid bone has been tilted upwards to show the right ethmoidal bulla (14) and uncinate process (15). These bony features are not seen in A because they are under cover of the middle nasal concha (2); they are shown on page 34, D61 and 46, respectively, after removal of the concha.

The roof of each half of the nasal cavity is formed centrally by the cribriform plate of the ethmoid bone (page 32, 28), with anteriorly the nasal bone and the nasal spine of the frontal bone (page 58, A2 and 14), and posteriorly the body of the sphenoid bone overlapped by the ala of the vomer and the sphenoidal process of the palatine bone (page 76, B2 and 11).

The floor is formed by the palatine process of the maxilla and the horizontal plate of the palatine bone (C24 and 25).

The medial wall is the nasal septum, whose bony part consists of the perpendicular plate of the ethmoid bone and the vomer (page 32, 27 and 26), with the nasal crests of the maxilla (page 50, D21) and palatine bone (page 52, C13) at the very base, and (in front) the septal cartilage (page 158, A22).

The lateral wall consists of the medial surface of the maxilla with the large maxillary hiatus (B7) being reduced in size by the overlapping of the lacrimal and ethmoid bones (above), the palatine bone (behind) and the inferior nasal concha (below) (as indicated in B, C and D—see also pages 66 and 67).

In A the left frontal sinus (unlabelled) is large and extends backwards at its lower end into the crista galli.

Nasal cavity *Maxillary hiatus and nasolacrimal canal*

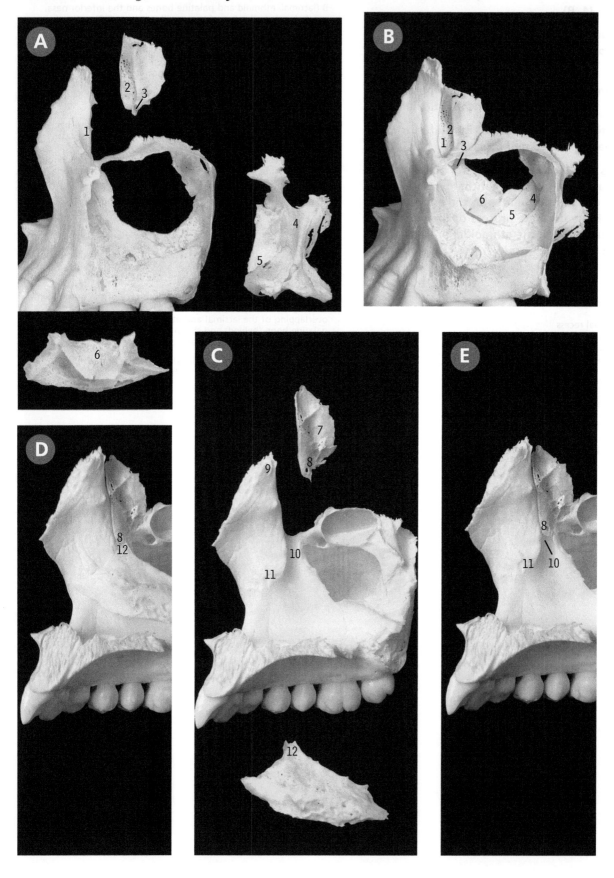

Ⓐ Ⓑ the left maxilla, lacrimal and palatine bones, and the inferior nasal concha, separated and articulated

Ⓒ the right maxilla, lacrimal bone and inferior nasal concha, separated

Ⓓ the right maxilla, lacrimal bone and inferior concha articulated

Ⓔ the right maxilla and lacrimal bone articulated

In A much of the lateral wall and orbital surface of the maxilla have been removed, so that the hiatus can be viewed from the lateral side. In B the hiatus seen in A is shown to be partly filled in by the descending process of the lacrimal bone at the upper anterior corner (3), the maxillary process of the inferior nasal concha below (6), and the maxillary process and perpendicular plate of the palatine bone behind (5 and 4). (The ethmoid bone which covers much of the upper part of the hiatus is not shown.)

In C-E the conversion of the nasolacrimal groove of the maxilla (10) into the nasolacrimal canal is illustrated by its articulation with the lacrimal bone and inferior nasal concha (8 and 12).

 1 Lacrimal groove of maxilla
 2 Lacrimal groove ⎱ of lacrimal bone
 3 Descending process ⎰
 4 Perpendicular plate ⎱ of palatine bone
 5 Maxillary process ⎰
 6 Maxillary process of inferior nasal concha
 7 Nasal surface ⎱ of lacrimal bone
 8 Descending process ⎰
 9 Frontal process ⎱
10 Lacrimal groove ⎬ of maxilla
11 Conchal crest ⎰
12 Lacrimal process of inferior nasal concha

Note that A and B show bones of the left side, with a large hole cut in the lateral wall of the maxilla, so that when articulated in B the lateral sides of the lacrimal and palatine bones and the inferior nasal concha can be seen partly filling the maxillary hiatus (the gap in the medial wall of the maxilla). In C-E the bones are those of the right side, showing their medial surfaces.

Base of the skull *Anterior cranial fossa*

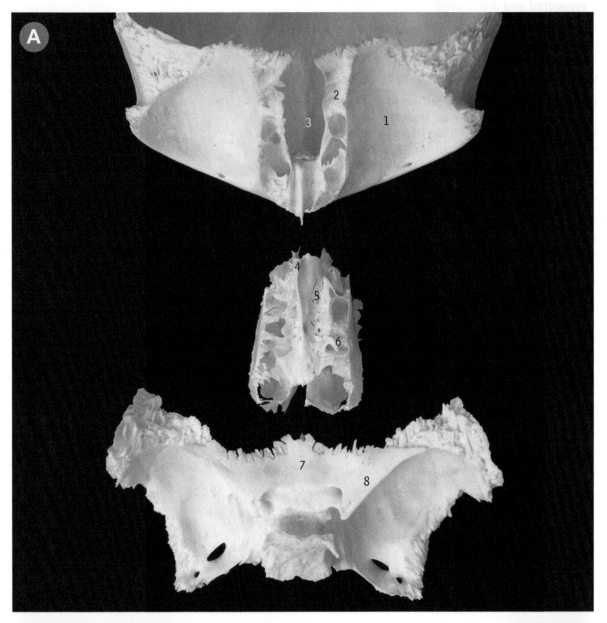

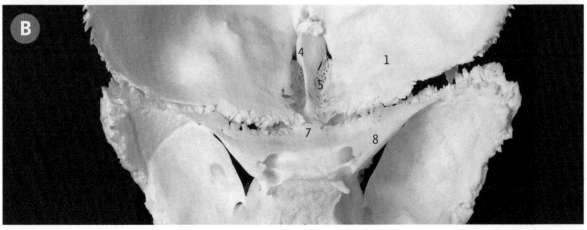

A the frontal, ethmoid and sphenoid bones, from above and behind, with the frontal bone tilted forwards

B the bones articulated

In A the frontal bone has been tilted forwards to show the orbital (lower) surface of the orbital part (1), whose medial edge (2) forms the roof of the ethmoidal labyrinth (6). With the bones articulated in B, the cerebral (upper) surface of the orbital part is seen.

1 Orbital part of frontal bone
2 Roof of ethmoidal air cells
3 Ethmoidal notch
4 Crista galli
5 Cribriform plate of ethmoid bone
6 Ethmoidal labyrinth and air cells
7 Jugum of sphenoid bone
8 Lesser wing of sphenoid bone

The *anterior cranial fossa* is formed by the orbital parts of the frontal bone (1), the crista galli and cribriform plates of the ethmoid bone (4 and 5), and the jugum and lesser wings of the sphenoid bone (7 and 8).

For the contents of the anterior cranial fossa see page 207.

The medial part of the orbital part of the frontal bone (2) forms the roof of the ethmoidal air cells (6), while the anterior wall of the body of the sphenoid completes the posterior wall of the ethmoidal labyrinth.

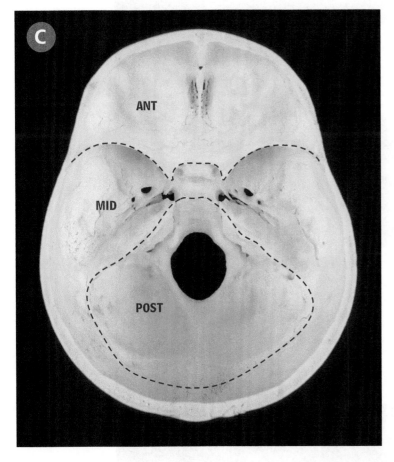

C Base of skull, internal surface, from above

ANT – anterior cranial fossa

MID – middle cranial fossa

POST – posterior cranial fossa

The tentorium cerebelli forms the roof of the posterior cranial fossa; the anterior and middle cranial fossae have no upper boundary (see page 207).

Base of the skull *Middle and posterior cranial fossae*

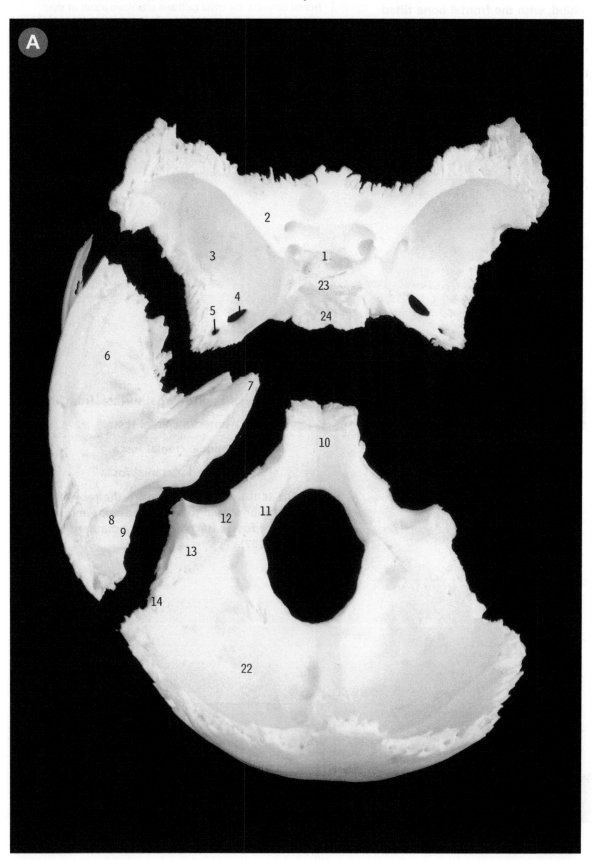

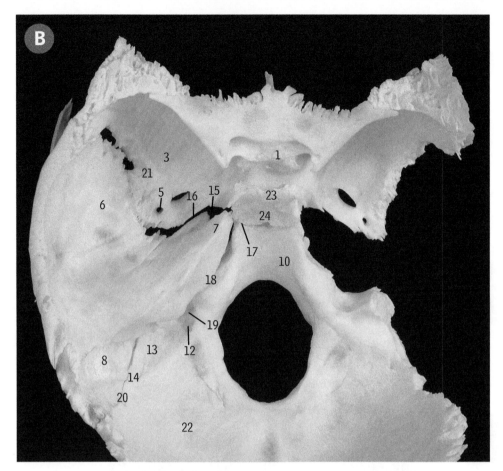

A **B** the sphenoid, left temporal and occipital bones, from above, separated and articulated

The posterior angle of the greater wing of the sphenoid, containing the foramen spinosum (5), fits into the angle between the squamous and petrous parts of the temporal bone (6 and 7).

1	Body
2	Lesser wing
3	Greater wing
4	Foramen ovale
5	Foramen spinosum
6	Squamous part of temporal bone
7	Apex
8	Groove for sigmoid sinus
9	Occipital margin
10	Basilar part
11	Lateral part
12	Jugular notch
13	Groove for sigmoid sinus
14	Mastoid margin
15	Foramen lacerum
16	Sphenopetrosal synchondrosis
17	Spheno-occipital synchondrosis
18	Petro-occipital suture and groove for inferior petrosal sinus
19	Jugular foramen
20	Occipitomastoid suture
21	Sphenosquamosal suture
22	Squamous part of occipital bone
23	Dorsum sellae
24	Basisphenoid

1 Body ⎫
2 Lesser wing ⎪
3 Greater wing ⎬ of sphenoid bone
4 Foramen ovale ⎪
5 Foramen spinosum ⎭

7 Apex ⎫
8 Groove for sigmoid sinus ⎬ of petrous part of temporal bone
9 Occipital margin ⎭

10 Basilar part ⎫
11 Lateral part ⎪
12 Jugular notch ⎬ of occipital bone
13 Groove for sigmoid sinus ⎪
14 Mastoid margin ⎭

The *middle cranial fossa* consists of a central part, formed by the body of the sphenoid bone (1), and right and left lateral parts, each formed by the greater wing of the sphenoid (3) and the squamous and petrous parts of the temporal bone (6 and 7).

The *posterior cranial fossa* is formed by the basilar, lateral and squamous parts of the occipital bone (10, 11 and 22), the petrous parts of the temporal bones (7-9), a small part of the postero-inferior (mastoid) angles of the parietal bones (not shown here but see page 30, A34 and page 56, B14), and the dorsum sellae (23) and posterior part of the body of the sphenoid bone.

The gap between the front of the apex of the petrous part of the temporal bone (7) and the sphenoid bone is the foramen lacerum (B15). A very small portion of the basilar part of the occipital bone (10) is at the medial margin of the foramen.

The gap between the jugular notch of the occipital bone (A12) and the petrous part of the temporal bone forms the jugular foramen (B19).

The junction between the basilar part of the occipital bone (10, often called the basi-occiput) and the posterior part of the body of the sphenoid bone (24, often called the basisphenoid) is a synchondrosis, which becomes a complete bony union by the age of 25 years.

For the contents of the *middle* and *posterior cranial fossae* see page 207.

Base of the skull *External surface, posterior part*

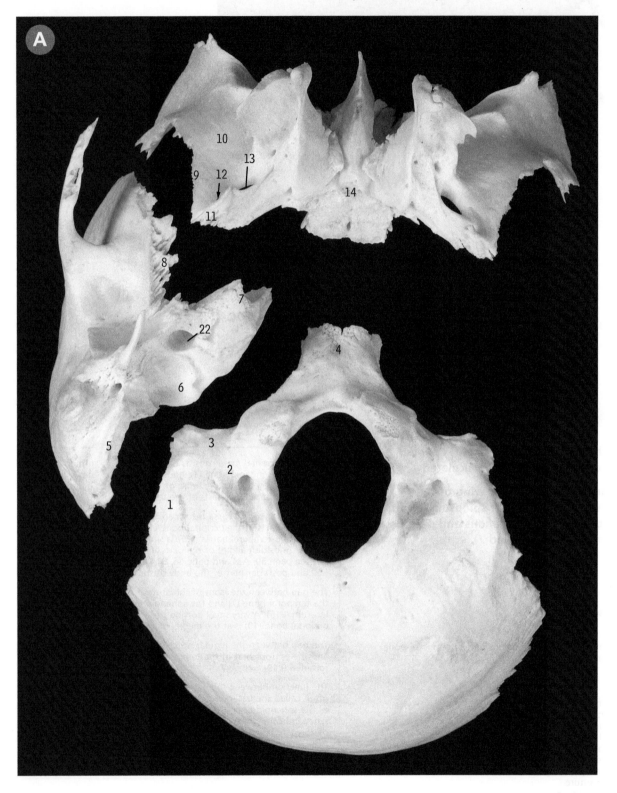

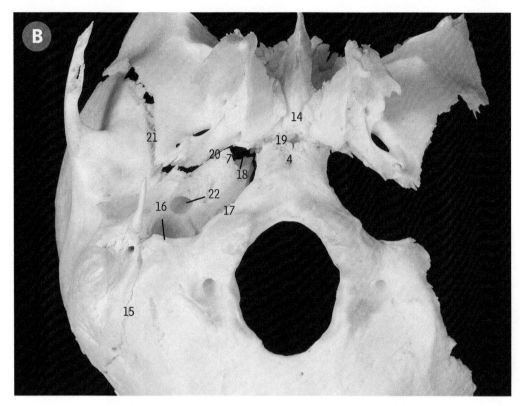

A B the sphenoid, right temporal and occipital bones, from below, separated and articulated

(Compare with the upper surfaces of these bones in pages 70, A and 71, B and the whole base in pages 18 and 30, A.)

1 Mastoid margin ⎫
2 Lateral part   ⎬ of occipital bone
3 Jugular notch   ⎪
4 Basilar part   ⎭
5 Occipital margin ⎫
6 Jugular notch   ⎬ of petrous part of temporal bone
7 Apex   ⎭
8 Sphenoidal margin of squamous part of temporal bone
9 Squamous margin ⎫
10 Greater wing   ⎪
11 Spine   ⎬ of sphenoid bone
12 Foramen spinosum ⎪
13 Foramen ovale   ⎪
14 Body   ⎭
15 Occipitomastoid suture
16 Jugular foramen
17 Petro-occipital suture
18 Foramen lacerum
19 Spheno-occipital synchondrosis
20 Sphenopetrosal synchondrosis and groove for auditory tube
21 Sphenosquamosal suture
22 Carotid canal

The *foramen lacerum* (B18) is the gap between the front of the apex of the petrous part of the temporal bone (A and B, 7) and the sphenoid bone; at its medial margin is a small portion of the basilar part of the occipital bone (A and B, 4).

The *jugular foramen* (B16) is the gap between the jugular notch of the petrous part of the temporal bone (A6) and the jugular notch of the occipital bone (A3).

The *carotid canal* (B22) is within the petrous part of the temporal bone. From its lower opening (as seen here) it turns medially and forwards in the bone to an upper opening in the back part of the foramen lacerum; this upper opening can only be seen when looking very obliquely into the foramen from the front, or when looking 'end-on' at the apex of the petrous temporal (page 54, E44).

Base of the skull *Right pterygopalatine fossa*

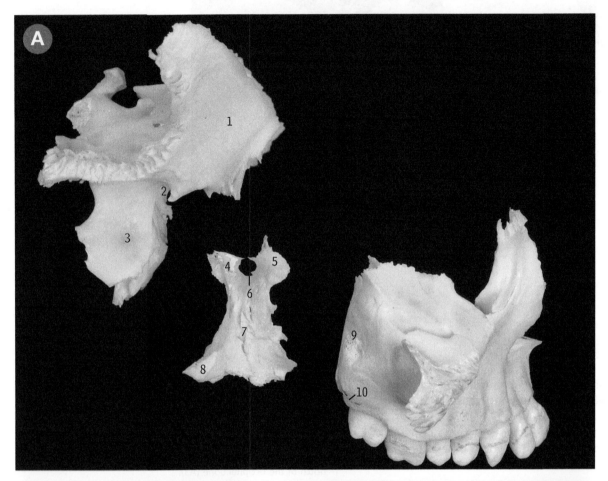

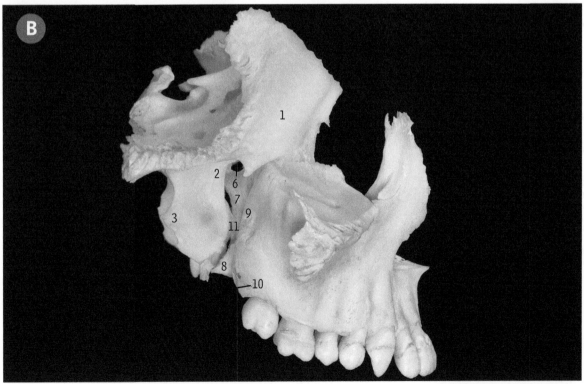

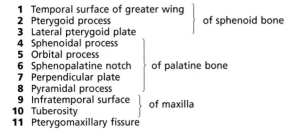

A **B** the right maxilla and palatine bone and the sphenoid bone, from the right, separated and articulated

(Compare with page 20, A)

1 Temporal surface of greater wing
2 Pterygoid process } of sphenoid bone
3 Lateral pterygoid plate
4 Sphenoidal process
5 Orbital process
6 Sphenopalatine notch } of palatine bone
7 Perpendicular plate
8 Pyramidal process
9 Infratemporal surface } of maxilla
10 Tuberosity
11 Pterygomaxillary fissure

The *pterygopalatine fossa* is the space behind the maxilla and in front of the pterygoid process of the sphenoid bone (see the first note on page 21).

The anterior wall of the fossa is formed by the infratemporal (posterior) surface of the maxilla (9).

The posterior wall of the fossa is formed by the pterygoid process of the sphenoid bone (2).

The medial wall of the fossa is formed by the perpendicular plate of the palatine bone (7). The sphenopalatine notch at the upper end of the plate (6) is converted into the sphenopalatine foramen (as in B6) by the overlying body of the sphenoid bone (hidden in this side view by the greater wing, 1).

Laterally, the pterygomaxillary fissure (B11) forms the communication between the pterygopalatine fossa and the infratemporal fossa (see also page 20, A4).

The pyramidal process of the palatine bone (8) articulates with the tuberosity of the maxilla (10) and fills in the triangular gap between the lower ends of the medial and lateral pterygoid plates (page 17, B10).

For the contents of the *pterygopalatine fossa*, see page 141.

Base of the skull *Right posterior nasal aperture*

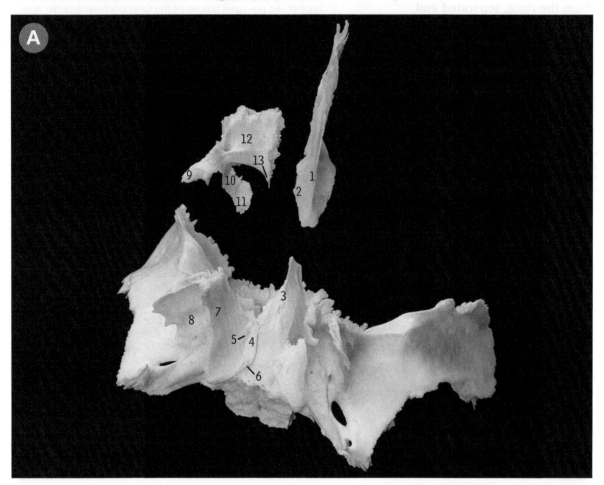

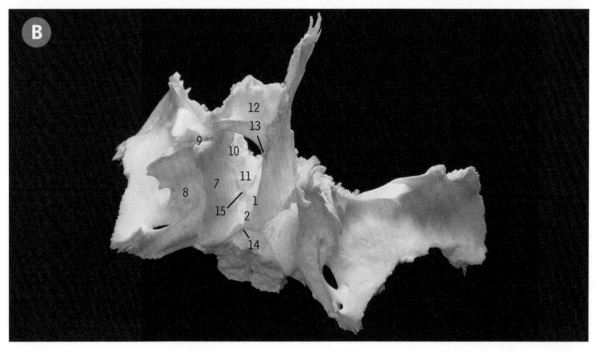

The sphenoid and right palatine bones and the vomer, from the left, below and behind, separated and articulated

The vomer (1) forms the posterior part of the (midline) nasal septum, and parts of the palatine and sphenoid bones form the remaining boundaries of the posterior nasal apertures.

1 Posterior border ⎤
2 Ala   ⎦ of vomer
3 Rostrum
4 Vaginal process
5 Groove that becomes palatovaginal canal (15) when articulated with sphenoidal process of palatine bone (11)
6 Groove that becomes vomerovaginal canal (14) when articulated with ala of vomer (2)   ⎬ of sphenoid bone
7 Medial pterygoid plate
8 Lateral pterygoid plate
9 Pyramidal process ⎤
10 Perpendicular plate
11 Sphenoidal process ⎬ of palatine bone
12 Horizontal plate
13 Posterior nasal spine ⎦
14 Vomerovaginal canal
15 Palatovaginal canal

The *posterior nasal aperture* is commonly called the choana.

The posterior border of the vomer (1) separates the two choanae, forming their medial boundaries.

The other boundaries are:
- laterally—the medial pterygoid plate of the sphenoid bone (7)
- below—the posterior border of the horizontal plate of the palatine bone (12)
- above—the body and vaginal process of the sphenoid bone (4) and the ala of the vomer (2)

A groove on the lower surface of the vaginal process of the sphenoid bone (A5) is converted into the palatovaginal canal (B15) by articulation with the upper surface of the sphenoidal process of the palatine bone (B11).

The vomerovaginal canal (B14) lies between the upper surface of the vaginal process of the sphenoid bone (A6) and the ala of the vomer (2). Anteriorly, the vomerovaginal canal joins the palatovaginal canal (B15).

The pyramidal process of the palatine bone (9) fills in the gap between the lower ends of the medial and lateral pterygoid plates (7 and 8; page 17, B10).

Fetal skull

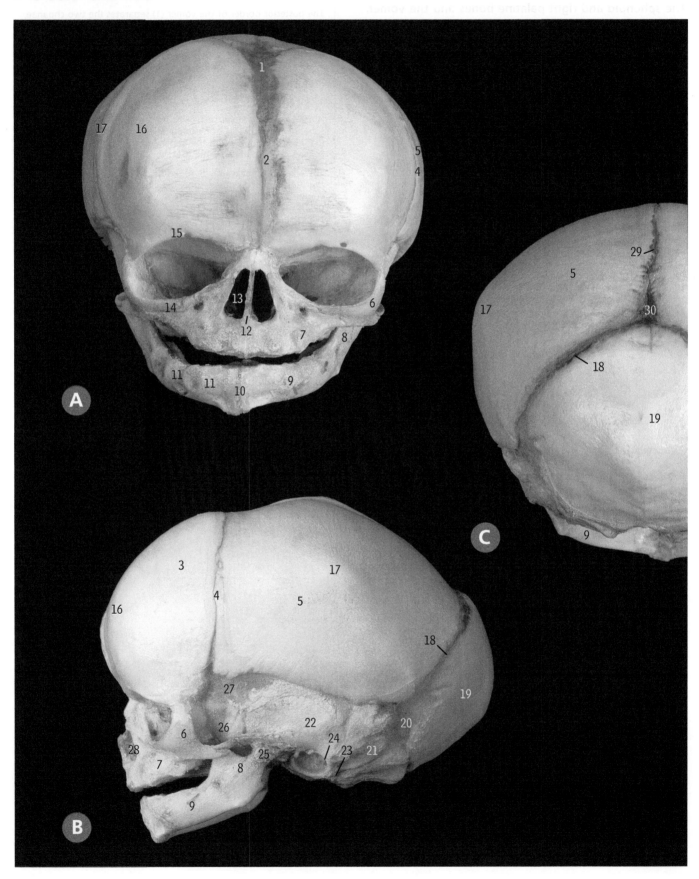

Fetal skull
Skull of a full-term fetus

(A) from the front

(B) from the left

(C) from behind (left side)

(D) from above

Apart from size differences (see notes below) and the lack of erupted teeth, the striking features of the fetal skull compared with the adult are the large sutures (2, 4, 18 and 29) and the fontanelles, the unossified spaces at the four angles of the parietal bone (1, 20, 27 and 30).

 1 Anterior fontanelle
 2 Frontal (metopic) suture
 3 Half (squamous part) of frontal bone
 4 Coronal suture
 5 Parietal bone
 6 Zygomatic bone
 7 Maxilla
 8 Ramus ⎫
 9 Body ⎬ of mandible
10 Symphysis menti
11 Elevations over deciduous teeth
12 Nasal septum
13 Anterior nasal aperture
14 Infra-orbital margin
15 Supra-orbital margin
16 Frontal tuberosity
17 Parietal tuberosity
18 Lambdoid suture
19 Occipital bone
20 Mastoid (posterolateral) fontanelle
21 Petrous part ⎫
22 Squamous part ⎬ of temporal bone
23 Stylomastoid foramen
24 Tympanic ring
25 Condylar process of mandible
26 Greater wing of sphenoid bone
27 Sphenoidal (anterolateral) fontanelle
28 Septal cartilage
29 Sagittal suture
30 Posterior fontanelle

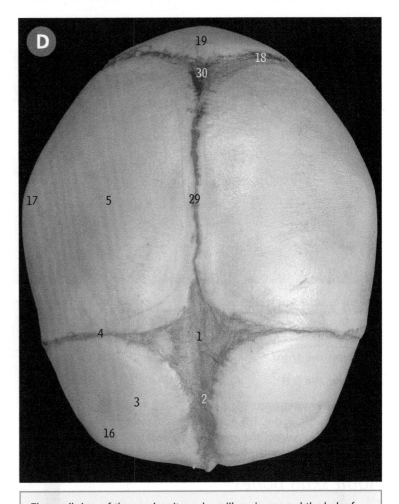

The small sizes of the nasal cavity and maxillary sinuses and the lack of erupted teeth all contribute to the face at birth, forming a relatively smaller proportion of the skull than in the adult. (Compare A with the adult skull on page 2.)

The posterior and sphenoidal fontanelles (30 and 27) close (become bony) within 3 months of birth, the mastoid fontanelle (20) at 1 year and the anterior fontanelle (1) at about 18 months. These provide a helpful window ultrasound in the neonate (see FIGURES.)

The mastoid process does not develop until the second year, so that before then the stylomastoid foramen (23) and the emerging facial nerve are relatively near the surface and unprotected. (Compare with the adult skull on page 16, A22 and 23.)

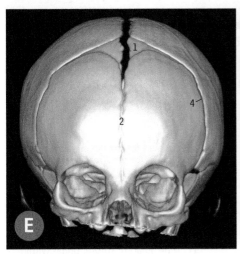

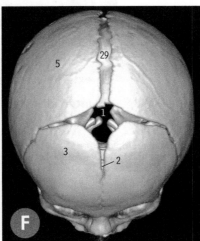

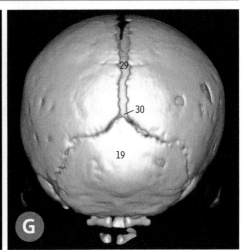

(E)(F)(G) **volume computed tomogram (CT) reconstruction of the neonatal skull demonstrating the fontanelles and the unossified sutures**

Fontanelles, sutures and sutural bones

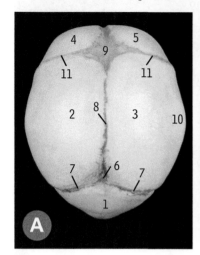

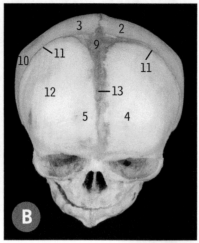

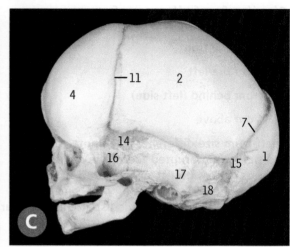

Skull of a full-term fetus

A from above

B from the front

C from the left

Note the large sutures (7, 8, 11, 13) and the fontanelles (6, 9, 14, 15), unossified areas of fibrous membrane between the developing and merging individual skull bones.

Adult skull bones

D Occipital and associated parietal bones from above, arranged in their normal configuration of union but slightly separated to show the fine serrated edges of the bones which when tightly interlocked and fused give the typical (meandering line) appearance of adult skull bone suture lines

Vault of skull, of normal dimensions, containing thirteen sutural bones which have been individually coloured to highlight their position and configuration.

E external surface from above

F internal surface

G external surface from behind

H external surface from the left and above

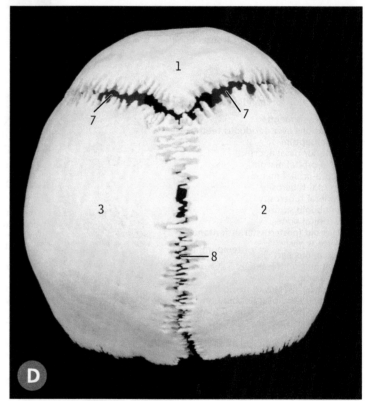

left and right frontal bones with a persistent 'metopic' suture

I external surface from the front

J internal surface from behind

1 Occipital bone	**13** Frontal metopic suture	**25** Grooves for middle meningeal vessels
2 Left parietal bone	**14** Sphenoidal (anterolateral) fontanelle	**26** Groove for superior sagittal sinus
3 Right parietal bone	**15** Mastoid (posterolateral) fontanelle	**27** Frontal crest
4 Left frontal bone	**16** Greater wing of sphenoid bone	**28** Depressions for arachnoid granulations
5 Right frontal bone	**17** Squamous part ⎫ of temporal bone	**29** Single sutural bone within the left side coronal suture
6 Posterior (median) fontanelle	**18** Petrous part ⎭	**30** Three sutural bones within the sagittal suture
7 Lambdoid suture	**19** Lambda	**31** Nine adjacent sutural bones within the lambdoid suture
8 Sagittal suture	**20** Bregma	
9 Anterior (median) fontanelle	**21** Frontal bone	
10 Parietal tuberosity	**22** Outer table ⎫	
11 Coronal suture	**23** Diploë ⎬ of parietal bone	
12 Frontal tuberosity	**24** Inner table ⎭	

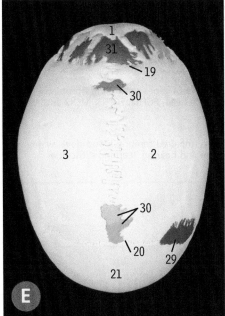

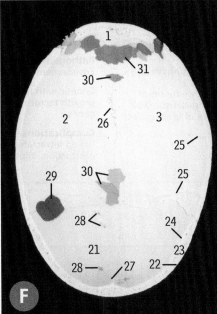

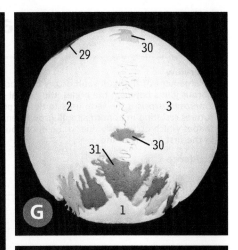

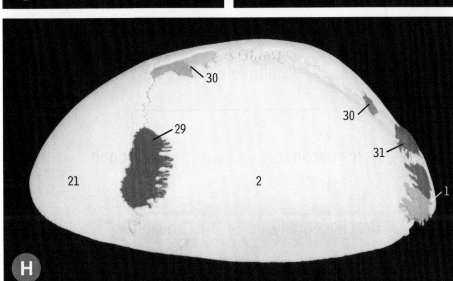

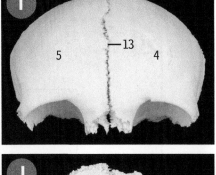

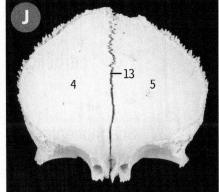

Postnatal closure of the six *fontanelles*

Sphenoidal (anterolateral) fontanelle—left and right	3 months
Posterior (median) fontanelle	3 months
Mastoid (posterolateral) fontanelle—left and right	12 months
Anterior (median) fontanelle	18 months

Postnatal closure of the *cranial sutures*

Sutures narrow by 6 months and begin to interlock within the first year and assume an adult serrated (meandering line) appearance by 2 years of age. They fuse in the second decade and complete ossification in the third decade. The two halves of the fetal frontal bone occasionally fail to fuse, resulting in a persisting anterior mid-line (metopic) suture in the adult. (See [B] 4, 5; [I] 4, 5; [J] 4, 5)

Sutural (Wormian) bones

Sutural bones arise from separate centres of ossification that can occur at fontanelles and within or adjacent to cranial sutures, most frequently found in the (posterior lateral) lambdoid suture. They are usually irregular in shape and size and may be found as a single bone, often referred to as an 'inca' bone, or quite commonly in multiple numbers, the latter associated with hydrocephalic skulls and thought to be a result of rapid cranial expansion. (See [E], [F], [G])

Suture lines on the inside of the skull are less serrated than on the outside. (See [F], [E])

Clinical implications

Sutural bones can be mistaken for skull fractures on radiological images.

Cranial sutures and craniosynostosis

Overview
Enlargement of the skull vault occurs by appositional growth at the fibrous joints between the bones, the cranial sutures.
Craniosynostosis is the term used to define premature fusion of sutures resulting in abnormal skull growth and characteristic skull shapes which occur early due to the enormous rate of brain growth in the first 2 years of life.

Incidence

1 in 2500 live births

Pathogenesis
Environmental (external pressure, lack of underlying brain growth)

Genetic with mutations in several genes controlling fibroblastic growth factor receptors, e.g. FGFR1, FGFR2, FGFR3, MSX2 and twist genes

Complications
Raised intracranial pressure, impaired cerebral blood flow, airway obstruction, impaired vision and hearing, learning difficulties

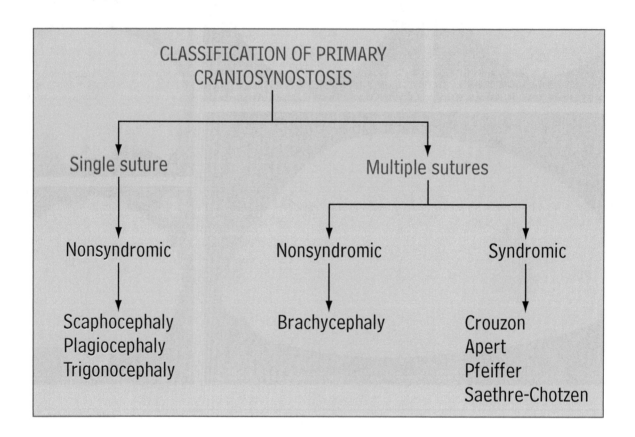

CLASSIFICATION OF PRIMARY CRANIOSYNOSTOSIS

Single suture — Nonsyndromic → Scaphocephaly, Plagiocephaly, Trigonocephaly

Multiple sutures
- Nonsyndromic → Brachycephaly
- Syndromic → Crouzon, Apert, Pfeiffer, Saethre-Chotzen

Examples of suture synostoses include:
Metopic, leading to trigonocephaly
Sagittal, leading to scaphocephaly
Coronal, leading to plagiocephaly
Multiple, often associated with specific syndromes
Syndromes involving other hand and limb abnormalities, e.g. Alpert, Crouzon and Saethre-Chotzen

Metopic synostosis

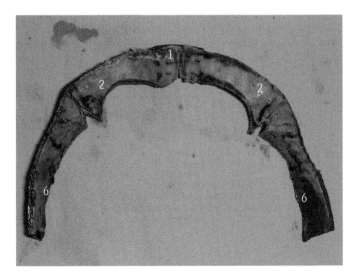

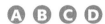

1 Frontonasal suture region
2 Supra-orbital ridge bone
3 Metopic suture line
4 Anterior fontanelle
5 Bi-coronal flap design
6 Posterolateral extension of bandeau

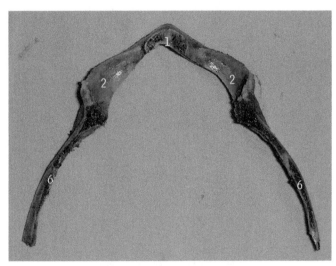

A pre-operative view: triangular-shaped head with narrow bi-temporal width

B peri-operative view: supraorbital bandeau removed at surgery viewed from below

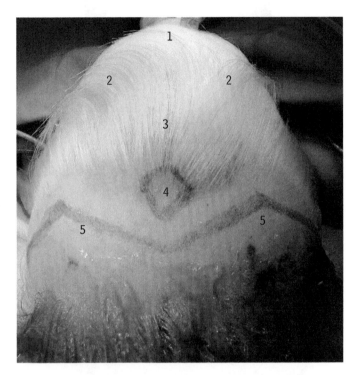

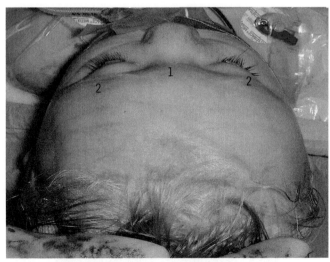

C peri-operative view: osteotomised bandeau to increase bi-temporal width and lateral forehead projection

D post-operative view

Sagittal synostosis

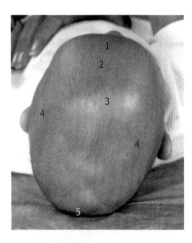

A pre-operative view

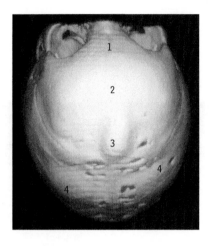

B Computed tomogram (CT) showing fusion and ridging of anterior sagittal suture

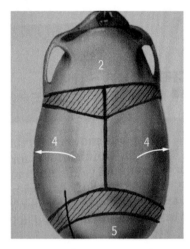

C features of scaphocephaly showing elongated and narrowed skull

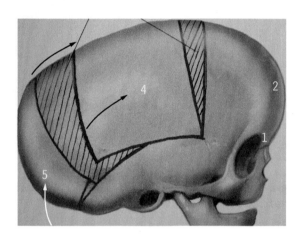

D diagram to show craniectomy cuts to permit increased width and reduction in length of skull

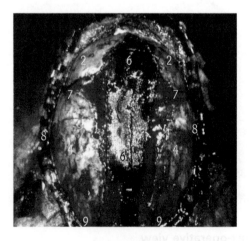

E peri-operative view of sagittal craniectomy and release of lambdoid and coronal sutures

A **B** **C** **D** **E** **G**

1 Frontonasal suture
2 Frontal bone
3 Ridging of bone
4 Parietal bone region
5 Occipital bone region
6 Sagittal craniectomy
7 Coronal suture line
8 Surgical clips on coronal flaps
9 Lambdoid suture region

Coronal synostosis

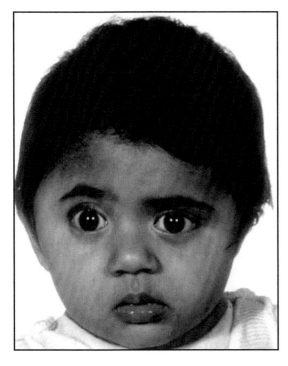

F pre-operative view

Features of plagiocephaly with recession and elevation of the forehead on the affected side with curvature of the face

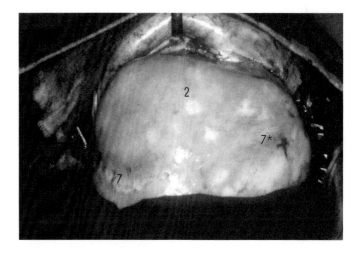

G peri-operative view

Right coronal suture fusion with forehead recession (7*)

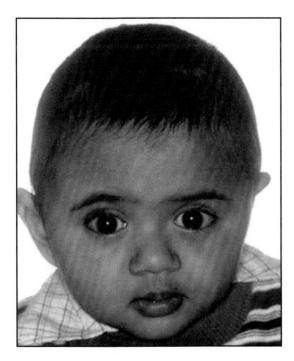

H post-operative view

Cervical vertebrae and neck

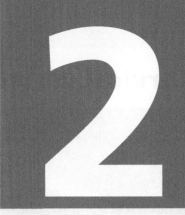

2

Cervical vertebrae

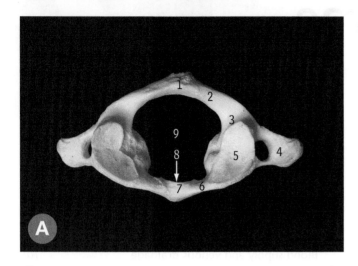

A from above

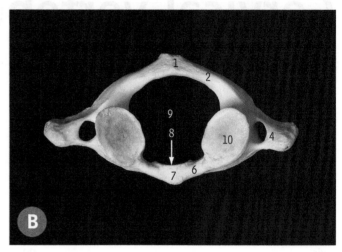

B from below

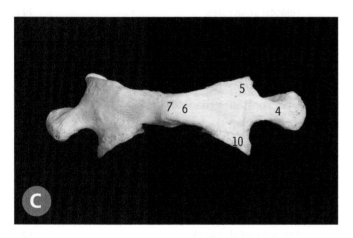

C from the front

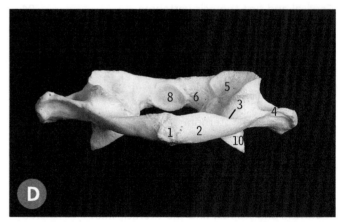

D from behind

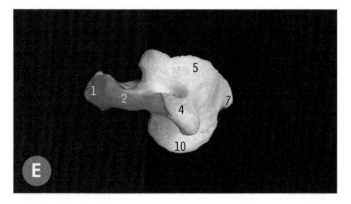

E from the right

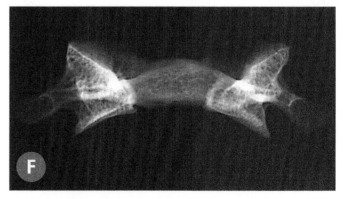

F radiograph of dried atlas, anteroposterior projection

Atlas *First cervical vertebra*

The atlas is unique in having no body; it consists of a lateral mass on each side with upper and lower articular facets (A5; B10), and anterior and posterior arches (A and B, 6 and 2).

1 Posterior tubercle
2 Posterior arch
3 Groove for vertebral artery
4 Transverse process and foramen transversarium
5 Lateral mass with superior articular facet
6 Anterior arch
7 Anterior tubercle
8 Facet for dens of axis
9 Vertebral foramen
10 Lateral mass with inferior articular facet

All seven cervical vertebrae have a foramen in their transverse processes, the **foramen transversarium**, (as at A4). This feature alone distinguishes them from the vertebrae of all other parts of the vertebral column.

The **foramen transversarium** of the 6th **cervical vertebra** is **important** to note because:
*   The **vertebral artery enters it**, ascends through the remaining five to pass into the foramen magnum (see 25 p. 206, 48 p. 246, 39 p. 248).
*   The **vertebral vein**, from a plexus surrounding the artery, **emerges from it**.
*   A small companion vein to the vertebral vein may descend to pass through the foramen transversarium of the 7th cervical vertebra, but this is variable.

The typical cervical vertebrae are the third to the sixth; as an example, the fifth is illustrated on page 92.

The first cervical vertebra (the atlas, this page), the second (the axis, page 90), and the seventh (page 92), have characteristic features.

The atlas is the only vertebra that has no body—it has been considered in the past to be represented by the dens of the axis (page 90, A1 and 3; page 90, F16), but see the note on page 91.

The atlas has no spinous process; instead there is a small posterior tubercle (A1).

The shapes of the articular facets on the lateral masses of the atlas enable the upper and lower surfaces to be identified:
*   the superior articular facets are concave and kidney-shaped (A5), for articulation with the occipital condyles of the skull (page 16, A33), forming the atlanto-occipital joints (page 248, B43).
*   the inferior facets are round and almost flat (B10), for articulation with the superior articular processes of the axis (page 90, C4), forming the lateral atlanto-axial joints (page 248, B41).

The anterior arch of the atlas (6) is straighter and shorter than the posterior arch (2), thus distinguishing the front and back of the bone. The anterior arch bears on its posterior surface the articular facet for the dens of the axis (A, B and D, 8), forming the median atlanto-axial joint (page 90, F17).

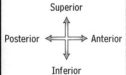

Superior

Posterior ⬌ Anterior

Inferior

G **Vertebral column overview, from the right**

Twenty-six (26) bones form the adult vertebral column
There are thirty-three (33) in the developing fetus.

*   **Seven (7)**   *Cervical vertebrae* - **Neck**
    The first cervical vertebra (C1), the atlas, supports the skull.

*   **Twelve (12)**   *Thoracic vertebrae* - **Thorax**
    Support twelve (12) pairs of ribs, the first seven pairs (T1-T7 the *true ribs*), unite via costal cartilage at their front ends with the sternum to form the bony thoracic cage.

*   **Five (5)**   *Lumbar vertebrae* - **Lower back, lumbar region**

*   **One (1)**   *Sacrum* - **Pelvis**
    Formed by the fusion of five (5) sacral vertebrae of the fetus. Unites with the left and right hip bones to form the pelvic girdle.

*   **One (1)**   *Coccyx* - **Pelvis (floor)**
    Formed by the fusion of four (4) coccygeal vertebrae of the fetus. Unites with the apex of the sacrum.

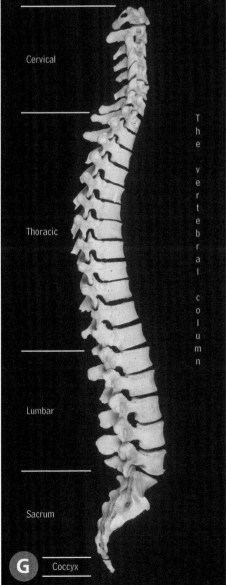

Cervical

The vertebral column

Thoracic

Lumbar

Sacrum

G Coccyx

Axis *Second cervical vertebra*

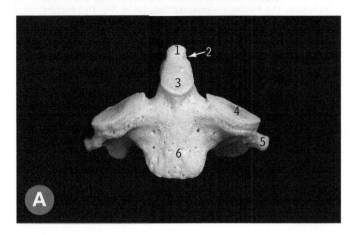

A from the front

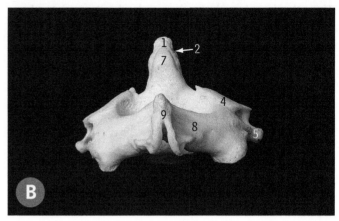

B from behind

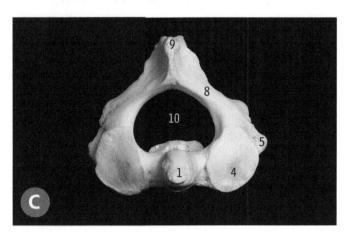

C from above

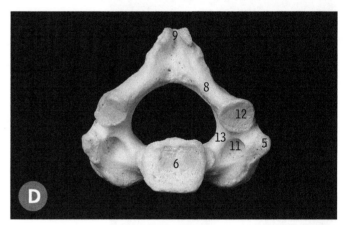

D from below

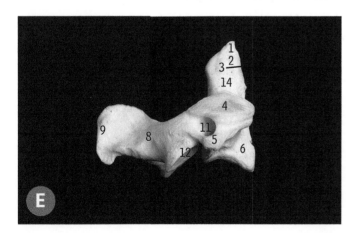

E from the right

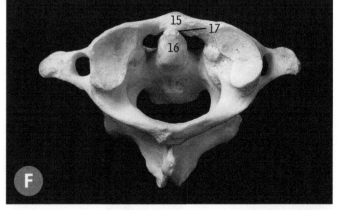

F articulated with the atlas, from above and behind

The axis is unique in having the dens (odontoid process, A and E, 1-3), which projects upwards from the body (6).

 1 Apex of dens
 2 Impression for alar ligament
 3 Anterior articular surface of dens
 4 Superior articular process
 5 Transverse process
 6 Body
 7 Posterior articular surface of dens
 8 Lamina
 9 Bifid spinous process
10 Vertebral foramen
11 Foramen transversarium
12 Inferior articular process
13 Pedicle
14 Dens
15 Anterior arch
16 Dens of axis
17 Median atlanto-axial joint

The dens has long been considered to represent the 'missing body' of the atlas, fused to the body of the axis, but studies in comparative anatomy suggest that it is a development in its own right.

The anterior articular surface of the dens (A and E, 3) forms a synovial joint (the median atlanto-axial joint, F17) with the facet on the posterior surface of the anterior arch of the atlas (page 88, D8).

The posterior articular surface of the dens (B7) forms a synovial joint (sometimes continuous with the joint cavity of one of the lateral atlanto-occipital joints) with the cartilage-covered anterior surface of the transverse ligament of the atlas.

The spinous process of the axis is large and often almost rectangular when viewed from the side (E9).

The surfaces of the superior articular processes are round and almost flat (C4), for articulation with the inferior articular facets of the atlas (page 88, B10), forming the lateral atlanto-axial joints.

Third to seventh cervical vertebrae

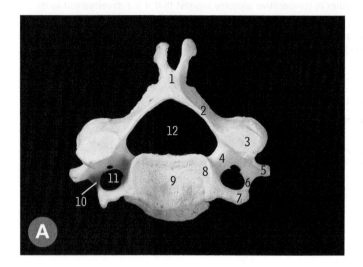

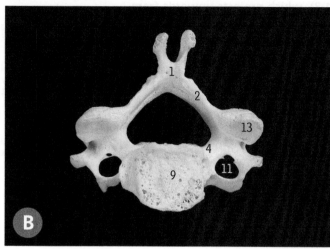

A fifth cervical vertebra, from above

B from below

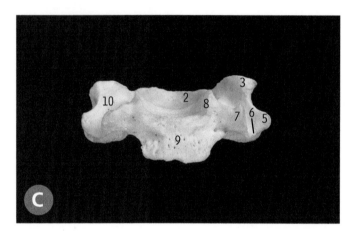

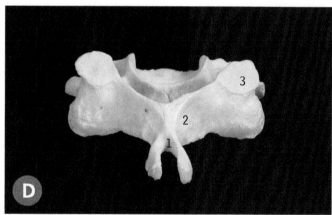

C from the front

D from behind

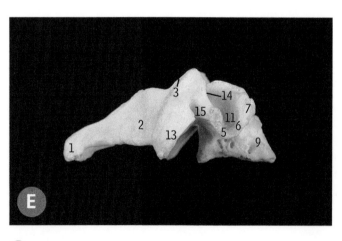

E from the right

1 Bifid spinous process
2 Lamina
3 Superior articular process
4 Pedicle
5 Posterior tubercle ⎫
6 Intertubercular lamella ⎬ of transverse process
7 Anterior tubercle ⎭
8 Uncus (posterolateral lip) of body
9 Body
10 Groove for spinal nerve (ventral ramus)
11 Foramen transversarium
12 Vertebral foramen
13 Inferior articular process
14 Superior ⎫
15 Inferior ⎬ vertebral notch

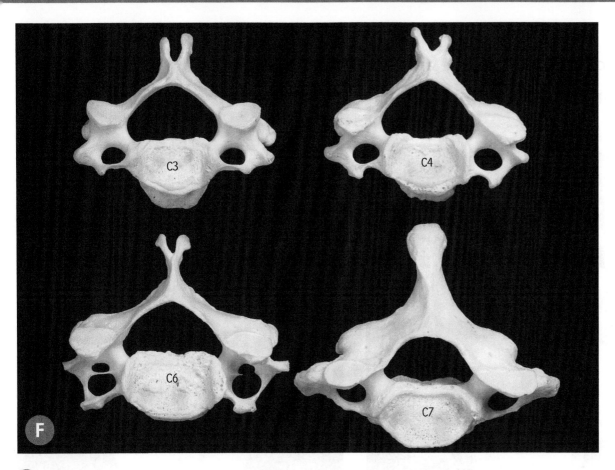

F **third, fourth, sixth and seventh vertebrae, from above and numbered C3, C4, C6 and C7, respectively**

The typical cervical vertebrae (third to sixth, exemplified here by the fifth, A-E) have superior articular processes (A and D, 3) that face upwards and backwards, an uncus (posterolateral lip, A and C, 8) at each side of the upper surface of the body, a triangular vertebral foramen (A12), and a bifid spinous process (A, B and D, 1).

The spinous process of any vertebra is commonly called the spine.

The vertebral arch is formed by the two pedicles (A4) and the two laminae (A2).

The vertebral *foramen* is the space between the arch and body. When vertebrae are articulated to form the vertebral column, the serial vertebral foramina constitute the vertebral *canal*. Do not confuse the vertebral foramen with the *intervertebral* foramen, which is the space between the pedicles of adjacent vertebrae through which the spinal nerves emerge—see the note on page 95 and page 94, D13.

The seventh cervical vertebra (vertebra prominens, F, C7) has a spinous process that ends in a single tubercle (instead of being bifid).

The costal (rib) element of a cervical vertebra is represented by the anterior root of the transverse process with the anterior tubercle (A7), the intertubercular lamella (A6) and the anterior part of the posterior tubercle (A5).

The intertubercular lamella (A and E, 6) is often but erroneously called the costotransverse bar.

The sixth cervical vertebra shown here (F, C6) has a small bony septum in the foramen of the right transverse process.

Cervical and first thoracic vertebrae

Articulated cervical vertebrae and first thoracic vertebra

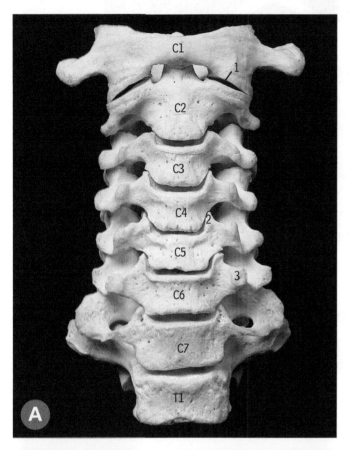

A

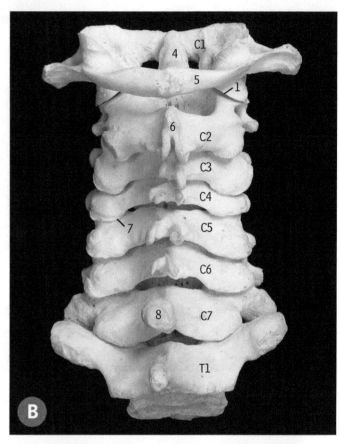

B

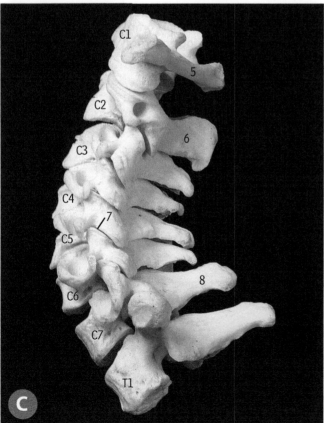

C

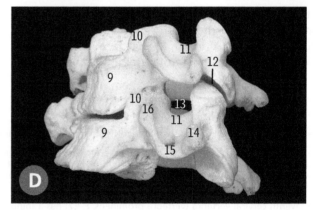

D

(A) articulated (but without intervertebral discs) and numbered C1-C7 and T1, from the front

(B) from behind

(C) from the left

(D) C4 and C5 vertebrae, from the left and slightly from the front

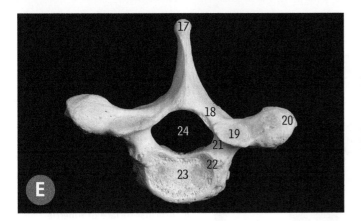

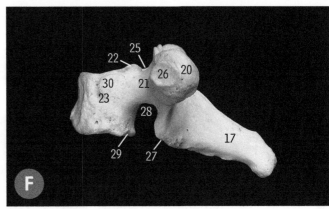

E first thoracic vertebra, from above

F from the left

The cervical part of the vertebral column with the first thoracic vertebra is illustrated in A-C. The side view in D is shown to emphasise the boundaries of an intervertebral foramen, while E and F give details of the first thoracic vertebra.

The cervical curvature of the vertebral column has an anterior convexity, as in C (like the lumbar curvature; the thoracic and sacral curvatures are concave anteriorly).

The spinous process of the seventh cervical vertebra is not bifid like that of typical cervical vertebrae but ends in a rounded tubercle (B and C, 8). Because of the extent of its backward projection it is usually the highest palpable spine in the median furrow at the back of the neck (hence the name vertebra prominens often given to this vertebra).

The intervertebral foramen (D13) is bounded above and below by the pedicles of adjacent vertebrae (D11), in front by the intervertebral disc and parts of the adjacent vertebral bodies (D9), and behind by the zygapophyseal joint (D12).

Typical thoracic vertebrae (the second to ninth, not illustrated) are characterised by upper and lower articular facets (demifacets) on the sides of the bodies (for joints with the heads of the ribs), an articular facet on the front of each transverse process (for joints with the tubercles of the ribs), a round vertebral foramen, a spinous process that points downwards and backwards, and superior articular processes that are vertical, flat, and face backwards and laterally.

The first thoracic vertebra differs from a typical thoracic vertebra in having an uncus on each side of the upper surface of the body (E22) and a triangular vertebral foramen (features like typical cervical vertebrae, although the foramen in E24 is rather oval), and a complete (round) superior costal facet (F30) on each side of the body (instead of just a demifacet, half-round).

 1 Lateral atlanto-axial joint
 2 Uncus of fifth cervical vertebra
 3 Carotid tubercle of sixth cervical vertebra
 4 Dens of axis
 5 Posterior arch of atlas
 6 Spinous process of axis
 7 Zygapophyseal joint
 8 Spinous process of seventh cervical vertebra
 9 Body
10 Uncus
11 Pedicle
12 Zygapophyseal joint between adjacent inferior
    and superior articular facets
13 Intervertebral foramen
14 Posterior tubercle
15 Intertubercular lamella
16 Anterior tubercle
} of transverse process

17 Spinous process
18 Lamina
19 Superior articular process
20 Transverse process
21 Pedicle
22 Uncus of body
23 Body
24 Vertebral foramen
25 Superior vertebral notch
26 Costal facet of transverse process
27 Inferior articular process
28 Inferior vertebral notch
29 Inferior
30 Superior
} costal facet of body

Other bones First rib, right

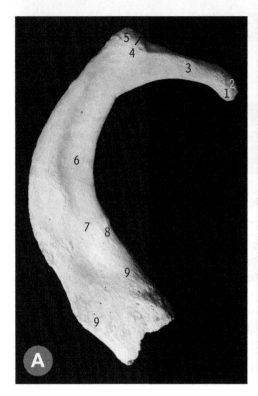

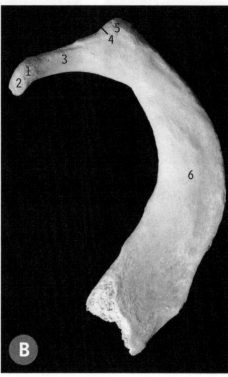

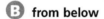

A from above

B from below

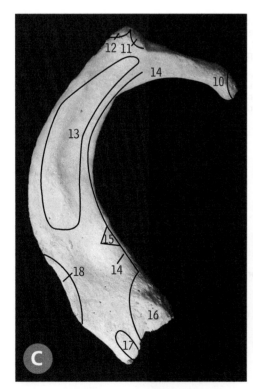

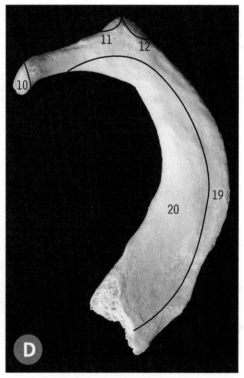

C from above, attachments

D from below, attachments

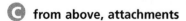

The 12 pairs of ribs form much of the bony framework of the thorax; only the first rib is shown here, since it is part of the thoracic inlet, at the junction of the neck and thorax (page 100).

1 Head
2 Articular surface of head
3 Neck
4 Articular surface of tubercle
5 Tubercle
6 Body
7 Groove for subclavian artery
8 Scalene tubercle
9 Groove for subclavian vein
10 Capsule of joint of head
11 Capsule of costotransverse joint
12 Lateral costotransverse ligament
13 Scalenus medius
14 Suprapleural membrane
15 Scalenus anterior
16 Costoclavicular ligament
17 Subclavius
18 Serratus anterior
19 Intercostal muscles
20 Area covered by pleura
21 Jugular notch
22 Clavicular notch
23 Notch for first costal cartilage
24 Notch for upper part of second costal cartilage
25 Surface for manubriosternal joint
26 Pectoralis major
27 Sternocleidomastoid
28 Capsule of sternoclavicular joint
29 Sternohyoid
30 Sternothyroid
31 Area covered by pleura
32 Transverse process and costal facet } forming costo-transverse joint
33 Tubercle and articular facet
34 Head and articular surface } forming joint of head of rib
35 Costal facet of body

Manubrium of the sternum

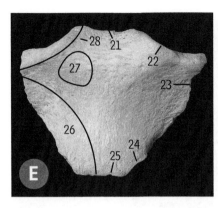

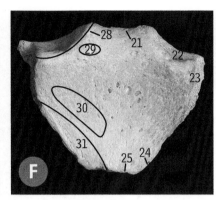

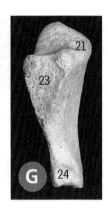

E from the front, with attachments

F from behind, with attachments

G from the right

The manubrium of the sternum is its upper part, joined to the body of the sternum at the manubriosternal joint (E25), and forming the front part of the thoracic inlet (page 100).

Costovertebral joints

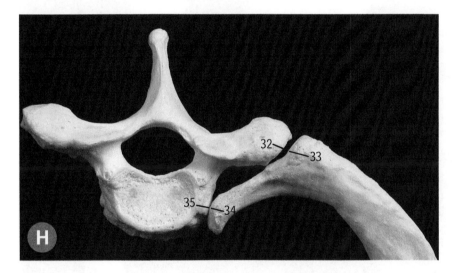

H left first rib and first thoracic vertebra, articulated, from above

The head of the rib (34) articulates with the upper costal facet on the body of the vertebra (35), forming the joint of the head of the rib. The tubercle of the rib (33) articulates with the costal facet of the transverse process of the vertebra (32), forming the costotransverse joint. These joints collectively form the costovertebral joints.

The main features of the *first rib* are:
- the head (A, 1 and 2)
- the neck (A3)
- the shaft or body (A6), with the scalene tubercle (A8) on the upper surface
- the tubercle (A, 4 and 5), at the back of the junction of the neck and body

The head of the first rib makes a synovial joint with the upper costal facet on the side of the body of T1 vertebra (H, 34 and 35).

The tubercle has articular and nonarticular parts. The articular part (A4) makes a synovial joint with the costal facet of the transverse process of T1 vertebra (H, 32 and 33).

The upper surface of the first rib is characterised by the scalene tubercle (A8), to which scalenus anterior is attached, with a slight groove behind it for the subclavian artery (A7) and a slight groove in front of it for the subclavian vein (A9). There is also a rough area for the attachment of scalenus medius.

The lower surface of the first rib is relatively smooth (B6) compared with the upper surface, and is largely covered by the pleura (D20).

The jugular notch at the top of the *manubrium of the sternum* (E21) is a readily visible and palpable landmark in the centre of the lowest part of the neck, and on either side the sternal end of the clavicle at the sternoclavicular joint (page 98, A11) is also easily seen and felt.

The anterior end of the first rib is joined to the side of the manubrium (E23) by the first costal cartilage (page 101, C23), to form the first sternocostal joint.

Bones of shoulder girdle *Clavicle and scapula, right*

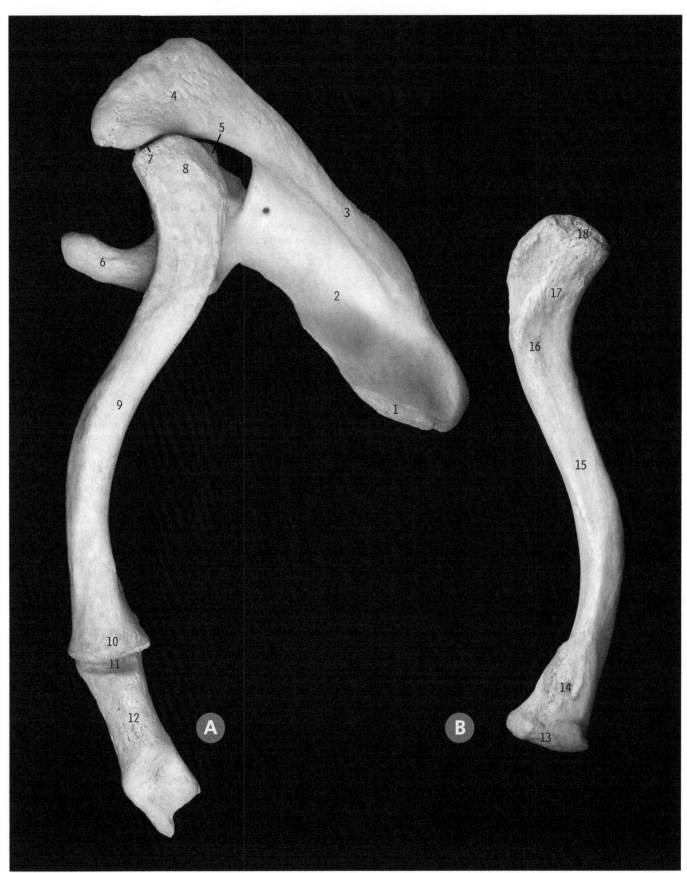

(A) from above, articulated, with the manubrium of the sternum

(B) clavicle, from below

The clavicle and scapula are the bones of the shoulder girdle (pectoral girdle) connecting the upper limb to the axial skeleton. The clavicle forms an obvious landmark at the root of the neck, and is easily palpable throughout its whole length.

 1 Superior angle
 2 Supraspinous fossa
 3 Spine
 4 Acromion
 5 Upper margin of glenoid cavity
 6 Coracoid process
 7 Acromioclavicular joint

} of scapula

 8 Acromial end
 9 Body
10 Sternal end

} of clavicle

11 Sternoclavicular joint
12 Jugular notch of manubrium of sternum
13 Sternal articular surface
14 Impression for costoclavicular ligament
15 Groove for subclavius muscle
16 Conoid tubercle
17 Trapezoid line
18 Acromial articular surface
19 Subscapularis
20 Head of humerus
21 Deltoid
22 Scapula
23 Infraspinatus

The main features of the *clavicle* are:
- the bulbous medial (sternal) end (A10)
- the flattened lateral (acromial) end (A8)
- the groove for the subclavius muscle on the middle of the inferior surface (B15)
- rough ligamentous markings near each end of the inferior surface (B, 14, 16 and 17)

The sternal end (A10) makes the sternoclavicular joint (A11) with the clavicular notch of the manubrium of the sternum (page 97, E22).

The acromial end (A8) makes the acromioclavicular joint (A7) with the acromion of the scapula (A4).

The rough marking on the inferior surface near the sternal end (B14) is for the costoclavicular ligament (page 100, B12).

The rough markings on the inferior surface near the acromial end (the conoid tubercle and the trapezoid line, B16 and 17) are for the conoid and trapezoid parts of the coracoclavicular ligament (page 100, B14 and 15).

The body of the clavicle is not straight but (when seen from above or below) is somewhat S-shaped; the medial part of the bone is curved forwards, to allow room for the subclavian vessels and the components of the brachial plexus to pass between the neck and arm. The formal description is that the bone has an anterior convexity in its medial two-thirds and an anterior concavity in its lateral one-third.

The acromion of the *scapula* (4), at the lateral end of the scapular spine (3), is palpable beyond the outer end of the clavicle (8).

For attachments to the clavicle and scapula see page 100.

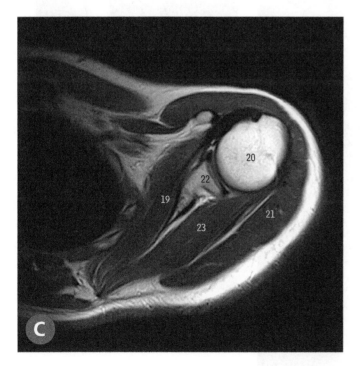

(C)

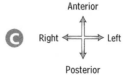

Anterior

Right ⬌ Left

Posterior

(C) axial magnetic resonance image (MRI) of the left shoulder

Shoulder girdle and upper thoracic skeleton
Clavicle and scapula and the thoracic inlet

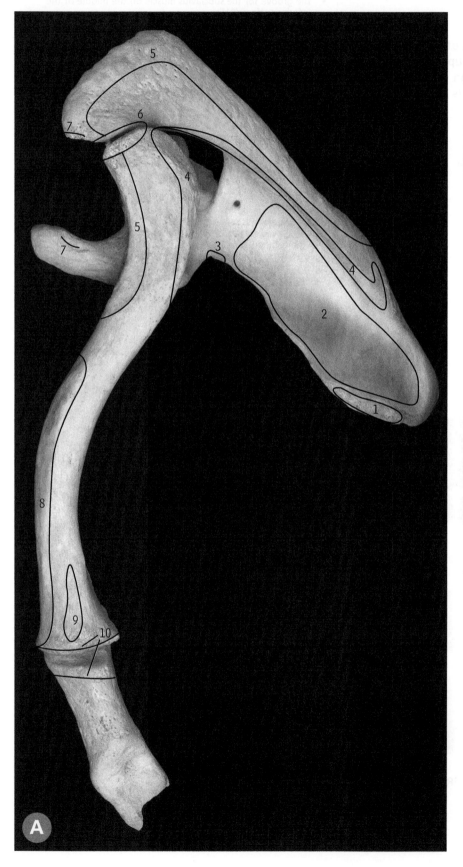

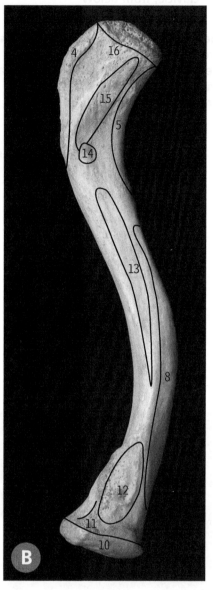

A right clavicle and scapula, from above, articulated and with the manubrium of the sternum. Attachments

B right clavicle, from below. Attachments

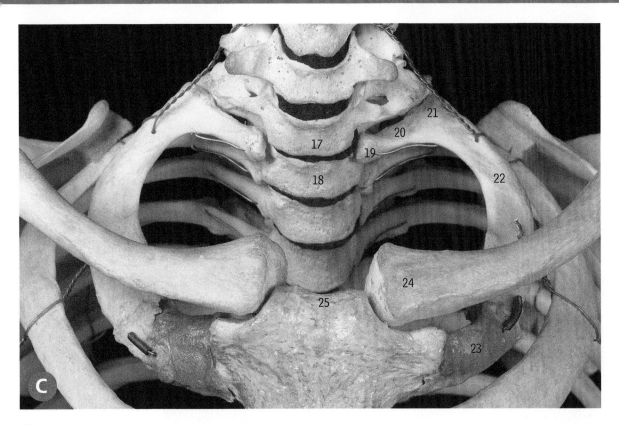

C thoracic inlet, in an articulated skeleton, from the front

Of the muscles whose attachments are shown here, deltoid (A5), supraspinatus (A2) and pectoralis major (A8) help to join the upper limb to the shoulder girdle (clavicle and scapula), while trapezius (A4) joins the girdle to the axial skeleton, together with the small subclavius (B13) and the much more important sternocleidomastoid (A9).

1 Levator scapulae	**14** Conoid ligament ⎫ coracoclavicular ligament
2 Supraspinatus	**15** Trapezoid ligament ⎭
3 Inferior belly of omohyoid	**16** Capsule of acromioclavicular joint
4 Trapezius	**17** Seventh cervical vertebra
5 Deltoid	**18** First thoracic vertebra
6 Capsule of acromioclavicular joint	**19** Head ⎫
7 Coraco-acromial ligament	**20** Neck ⎬ of first rib
8 Pectoralis major	**21** Tubercle ⎪
9 Sternocleidomastoid	**22** Body ⎭
10 Capsule of sternoclavicular joint	**23** First costal cartilage
11 Sternohyoid	**24** Sternal end of clavicle
12 Costoclavicular ligament	**25** Jugular notch of manubrium of sternum
13 Subclavius	

In C the bones forming the boundaries of the thoracic inlet are shown: T1 vertebra (C18); the first ribs and costal cartilages (C22 and 23); and the manubrium of the sternum (C25).

Clinically, the thoracic inlet is sometimes called the thoracic outlet.

Neck

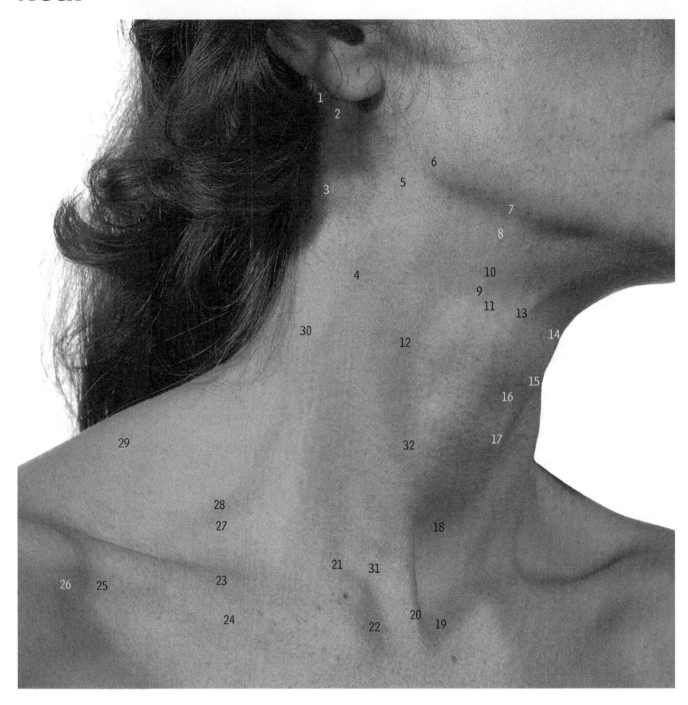

Neck *Surface markings on the front and right side of the neck*

Sternocleidomastoid (3) is the most obvious feature. The external jugular vein (4) courses obliquely downwards over its upper part. The accessory nerve (30) emerges from the posterior border of the junction of the upper and middle thirds of sternocleidomastoid (3). It runs down through the posterior triangle to pass under the anterior border of trapezius about 5 cm above the clavicle and enters the muscle on its deep surface. The upper trunk of the brachial plexus (28) can be felt in the angle between the clavicle (23) and the posterior border of sternocleidomastoid (21). The pulsation of the common carotid artery (carotid pulse, 32) can be felt in the angle between the side of the larynx (15) and the anterior border of sternocleidomastoid (3). The lower end of the internal jugular vein (31) lies behind the gap between the sternal and clavicular heads of the muscle (20 and 21). Compare with the dissections on pages 104-118.

1 Mastoid process
2 Tip of transverse process of atlas
3 Sternocleidomastoid
4 External jugular vein
5 Lowest part of parotid gland
6 Angle of mandible
7 Anterior border of masseter and facial artery
8 Submandibular gland
9 Tip of greater horn of hyoid bone
10 Hypoglossal nerve
11 Internal laryngeal nerve
12 Bifurcation of common carotid artery
13 Anterior jugular vein
14 Body of hyoid bone
15 Laryngeal prominence
16 Vocal fold
17 Arch of cricoid cartilage
18 Isthmus of thyroid gland
19 Jugular notch and trachea
20 Sternal head ⎫
21 Clavicular head ⎬ of sternocleidomastoid
22 Sternoclavicular joint and union of internal jugular and subclavian veins to form the brachiocephalic vein
23 Clavicle
24 Pectoralis major
25 Infraclavicular fossa and cephalic vein
26 Deltoid
27 Inferior belly of omohyoid
28 Upper trunk of brachial plexus
29 Trapezius and entry of accessory nerve
30 Accessory nerve emerging from sternocleidomastoid
31 Lower end of internal jugular vein
32 Position for palpation of common carotid pulse

The hyoid bone (14) is at the level of C3 vertebra.

The laryngeal prominence (15) is at the upper border of the central part of the thyroid cartilage (page 188, C22), which is at the level of C4 and 5 vertebrae.

The cricoid cartilage (17) is at the level of C6 vertebra. Confirm these levels in the sagittal section of the neck (page 168, 18, 20 and 11).

For surface markings on the face see page 132.

Ⓐ Head, neck and shoulder

Superficial muscles of the left side, from the left and front

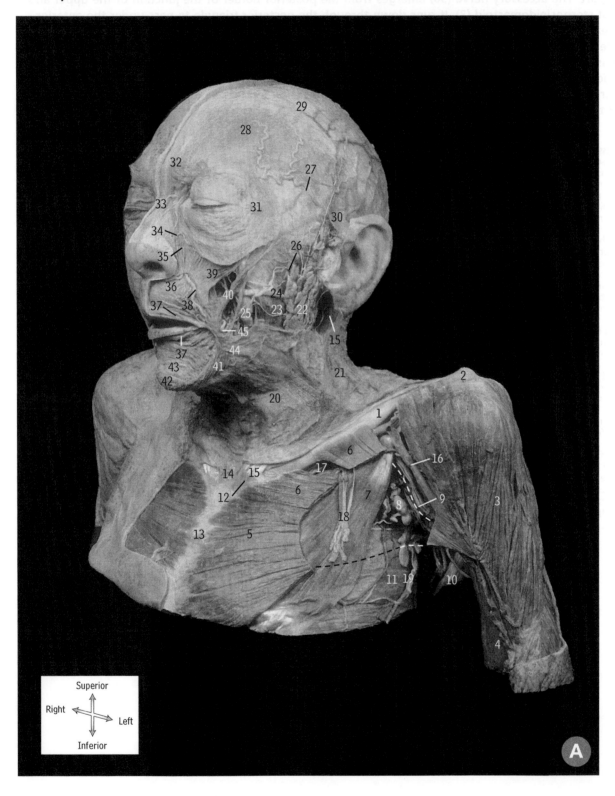

Superior

Right ← → Left

Inferior

Ⓐ

Skin and subcutaneous tissues have been removed to display the superficial structures of the face, neck and shoulder region. A central portion of pectoralis major (5-6), indicated by dotted lines, has been removed to display the underlying pectoralis minor (7), axillary lymph nodes (8) and median nerve (9) which is overlying the axillary artery.

1 Clavicle
2 Acromioclavicular joint
3 Deltoid
4 Biceps
5 Sternocostal part of pectoralis major
6 Clavicular part of pectoralis major
7 Pectoralis minor
8 Axillary lymph nodes
9 Median nerve overlying the axillary artery
10 Latissimus dorsi
11 Serratus anterior
12 Sternoclavicular joint
13 Body of sternum
14 Jugular notch
15 Sternocleidomastoid
16 Cephalic vein within deltopectoral groove
17 Subclavius
18 Thoraco-acromial vessels and lateral pectoral nerve
19 Thoracodorsal artery and nerve
20 Platysma
21 Prevertebral fascia
22 Parotid gland
23 Masseter
24 Parotid duct
25 Buccal fat pad
26 Branches of facial nerve
27 Superficial temporal artery
28 Frontal belly of occipitofrontalis
29 Epicranial aponeurosis (galea aponeurotica)
30 Temporoparietalis
31 Orbicularis oculi
32 Depressor supercilii
33 Procerus
34 Nasalis
35 Levator labii superioris alaeque nasi
36 Levator labii superioris
37 Orbicularis oris
38 Superior labial artery
39 Zygomaticus minor
40 Zygomaticus major
41 Depressor anguli oris
42 Mentalis
43 Depressor labii inferioris
44 Risorius
45 Facial artery
46 Lymphatic vessels
47 Vein
48 Artery

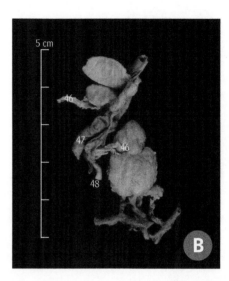

B a cluster of adult left axillary (lateral) lymph nodes with associated vessels, shown actual size as presented at dissection

- Grouped in defined clusters, there are approximately 400-450 lymph nodes present throughout the normal adult body, each group responsible for draining a specific region.

- Nodes are usually small, ovoid or kidney (reniform) shaped and vary between 0.1 and 2.5 cm in length.

- Some nodes may be palpable in their normal state, but particularly so when diseased.

- Between 20-30 nodes occur in the axillary group, which drains the upper limb and areas of the trunk; there are 60-70 nodes in the head and neck.

(See pages 114-115 for Lymphatic drainage of head and neck.)

Neck *Superficial dissection I*

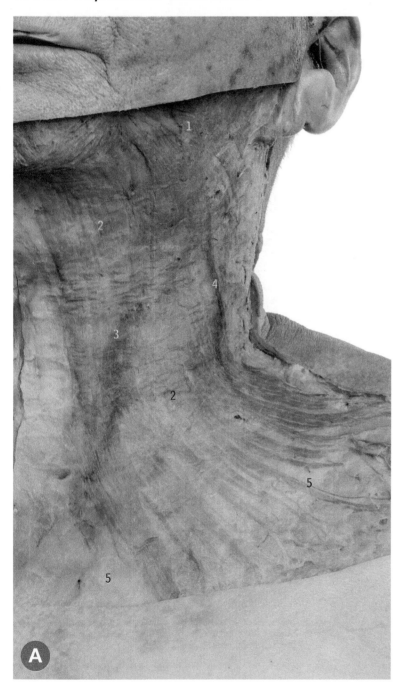

A

platysma, from the front

Superior ↑
Medial ←→ Lateral (left)
Inferior ↓

The left platysma and superficial veins

In A the skin has been removed and platysma has been dissected out from the subcutaneous tissue. In B platysma has been removed, to show that the larger superficial veins and nerves lie deep to the muscle but are superficial to the various parts of the deep cervical fascia (described in more detail in this same dissection on pages 110 and 111).

1 Lower border of body of mandible
2 Platysma
3 Anterior jugular vein
4 External jugular vein
5 Clavicle
6 Parotid gland
7 Great auricular nerve
8 Accessory nerve
9 Trapezius
10 Cervical nerves to trapezius
11 Superficial cervical vein
12 Supraclavicular nerves
13 Sternocleidomastoid
14 Transverse cervical nerve
15 Investing layer of deep cervical fascia
16 Submandibular gland

The lowest of the muscular strands that form platysma (2) are attached to the fascia overlying the upper part of pectoralis major and the medial part of deltoid.

The upper attachment of the muscle is to the lower border of the mandible (1), with some fibres blending with adjacent facial muscles and others (below the chin) interdigitating with their fellows of the opposite side.

The motor nerve supply of platysma is by the cervical branch of the facial nerve (page 112, 6). The muscle can be made to contract visibly by 'forcibly showing the teeth'.

The larger superficial veins (the anterior and external jugulars, 3 and 4), cutaneous branches of the cervical plexus (as at 7, 12 and 14), and the cervical branch of the facial nerve (page 112, 6) are all deep to the muscle, which is subcutaneous but superficial to the investing layer of the deep cervical fascia (see the notes on page 111).

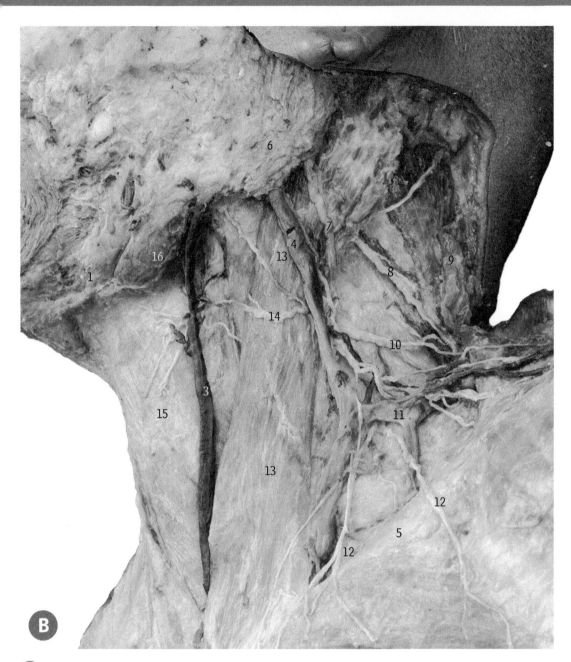

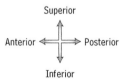

B superficial veins and nerves, from the left

Superior

Anterior ⟷ Posterior

Inferior

Neck *Blood supply and venous drainage*

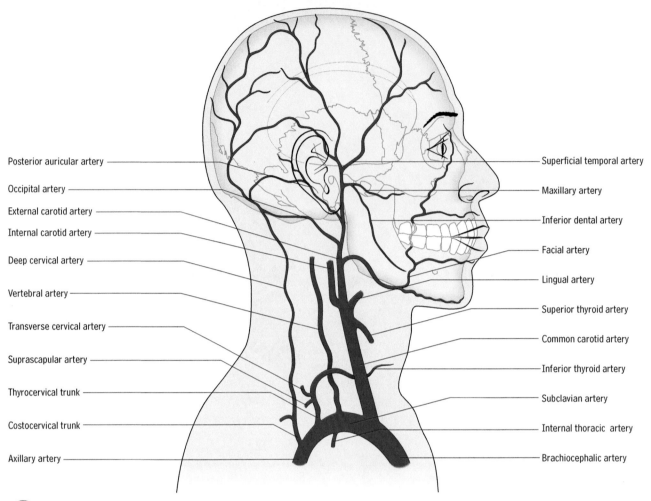

Posterior auricular artery

Occipital artery

External carotid artery

Internal carotid artery

Deep cervical artery

Vertebral artery

Transverse cervical artery

Suprascapular artery

Thyrocervical trunk

Costocervical trunk

Axillary artery

Superficial temporal artery

Maxillary artery

Inferior dental artery

Facial artery

Lingual artery

Superior thyroid artery

Common carotid artery

Inferior thyroid artery

Subclavian artery

Internal thoracic artery

Brachiocephalic artery

 main arterial supply to the head and neck

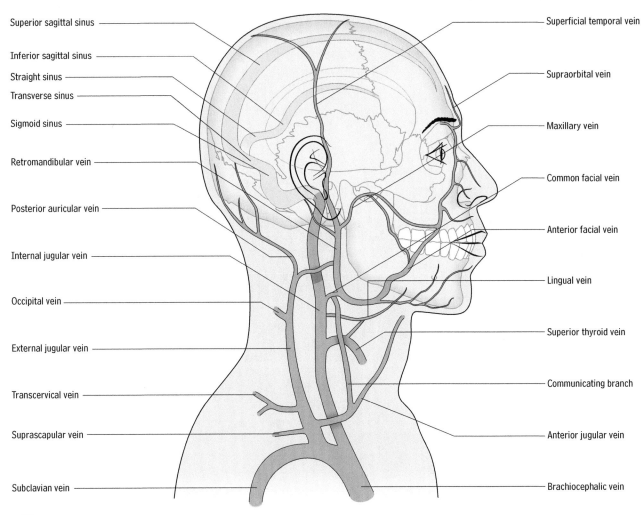

Superior sagittal sinus

Inferior sagittal sinus

Straight sinus

Transverse sinus

Sigmoid sinus

Retromandibular vein

Posterior auricular vein

Internal jugular vein

Occipital vein

External jugular vein

Transcervical vein

Suprascapular vein

Subclavian vein

Superficial temporal vein

Supraorbital vein

Maxillary vein

Common facial vein

Anterior facial vein

Lingual vein

Superior thyroid vein

Communicating branch

Anterior jugular vein

Brachiocephalic vein

B venous drainage from the head and neck

Neck *Superficial dissection II*

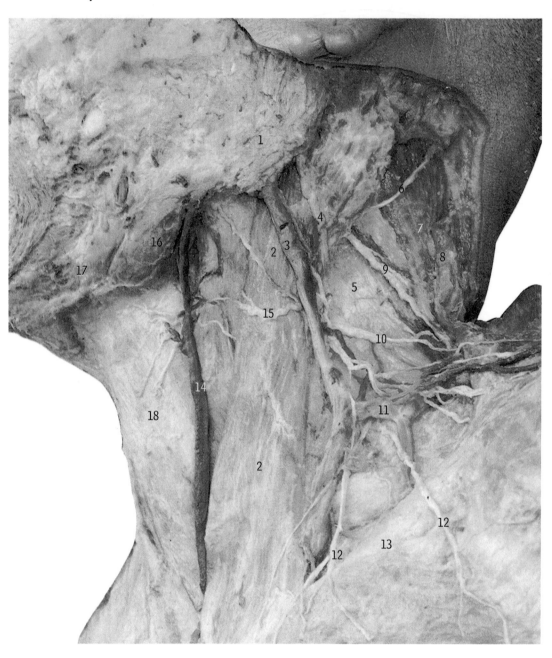

Superior

Anterior ←——→ Posterior

Inferior

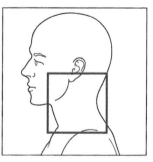

The left sternocleidomastoid and related structures

Platysma has been removed together with the investing layer of deep cervical fascia posterior to sternocleidomastoid (2), but the fascia (18) remains in place over the front part of the neck (deep to the anterior jugular vein, 14). Of the cutaneous branches of the cervical plexus which emerge behind the posterior border of sternocleidomastoid (2), the transverse cervical nerve (15) runs transversely forwards across the muscle; the great auricular nerve (4) passes upwards, crossing the muscle obliquely; the lesser occipital nerve (6) runs upwards and backwards at the posterior border of the muscle; and the branches of the supraclavicular nerve (12) pass downwards to fan out over the clavicle (13). The accessory nerve (9) leaves the posterior border of sternocleidomastoid (2) and runs down (embedded in the investing layer of deep cervical fascia that forms the roof of the posterior triangle—page 117) to pass under the anterior border of trapezius (8) about 5 cm above the clavicle (13). Branches of cervical nerves (10) also run into trapezius (and into sternocleidomastoid at a higher level, not shown).

The nerve commonly known in English as the accessory nerve or *spinal part* of the accessory nerve (9) is in official anatomical nomenclature the nervus externus of the truncus nervi accessorii. The cells of origin are in the upper five or six segments of the cervical part of the spinal cord, and the fibres are motor to sternocleidomastoid and trapezius. Both muscles receive some fibres from the cervical plexus (as at 10, and see the note on page 117), but these are usually afferent only. (The *cranial part* of the accessory nerve is derived from the nucleus ambiguus in the medulla oblongata of the brainstem and joins the vagus nerve to supply muscles of the larynx and soft palate (page 267).

The deep cervical fascia consists of:
- the investing layer
- the pretracheal layer
- the prevertebral layer
- the carotid sheath

The investing layer (18) surrounds the neck like a subcutaneous stocking. It forms the roof of the anterior and posterior triangles (page 113); it splits to enclose sternocleidomastoid and trapezius, and forms capsules for the parotid and submandibular glands.

The pretracheal layer forms a sheath for the thyroid gland (page 122).

The prevertebral layer forms the floor of the posterior triangle (5), lying in front of the vertebral column and prevertebral muscles (page 128).

The carotid sheath is formed by condensations of the prevertebral and pretracheal layers enclosing the internal jugular vein, common and internal carotid arteries, vagus nerve and the ansa cervicalis with its superior and inferior roots (page 118). Immediately below the base of the skull the last four cranial nerves (glossopharyngeal, vagus, accessory and hypoglossal) run a very short course through the uppermost part of the sheath.

---

1 Parotid gland
2 Sternocleidomastoid
3 External jugular vein
4 Great auricular nerve
5 Prevertebral fascia overlying levator scapulae
6 Lesser occipital nerve
7 Splenius capitis
8 Trapezius
9 Accessory nerve
10 Cervical nerves to trapezius
11 Superficial cervical vein
12 Supraclavicular nerves
13 Clavicle
14 Anterior jugular vein
15 Transverse cervical nerve
16 Submandibular gland
17 Lower border of mandible
18 Investing layer of deep cervical fascia

Neck *Superficial dissection III*

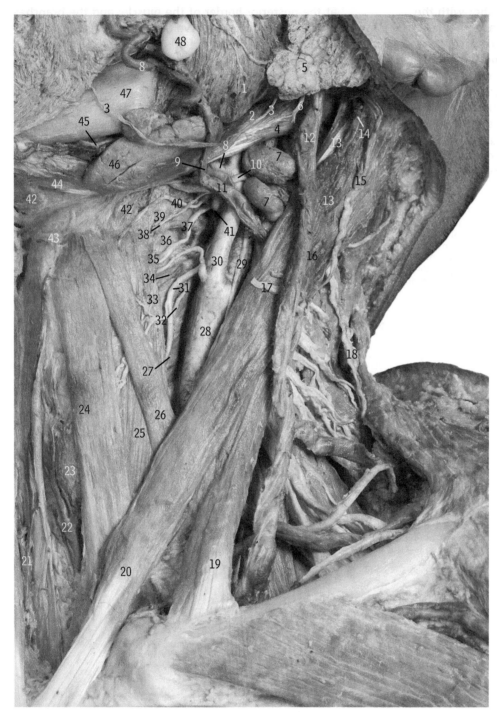

1   Masseter and angle of mandible
2   Stylohyoid
3   Marginal mandibular branch of facial nerve
4   Posterior belly of digastric
5   Parotid gland (lower pole)
6   Cervical branch of facial nerve
7   Jugulodigastric lymph nodes
8   Facial artery
9   Lingual vein
10 Hypoglossal nerve
11 Facial vein
12 Posterior branch of retromandibular vein
13 Sternocleidomastoid
14 Posterior auricular vein
15 Great auricular nerve
16 External jugular vein
17 Transverse cervical nerve
18 Accessory nerve
19 Clavicular head } of sternocleido-
20 Sternal head   } mastoid
21 Anterior jugular vein
22 Inferior thyroid vein
23 Isthmus of thyroid gland
24 Sternohyoid
25 Sternothyroid
26 Superior belly of omohyoid
27 Inferior constrictor of pharynx
28 Common carotid artery
29 Internal carotid artery and superior root of ansa cervicalis
30 External carotid artery
31 Superior thyroid artery
32 External laryngeal nerve
33 Thyrohyoid
34 Superior laryngeal artery
35 Internal laryngeal nerve
36 Thyrohyoid membrane
37 Greater horn of hyoid bone
38 Nerve to thyrohyoid
39 Hyoglossus
40 Suprahyoid artery
41 Lingual artery
42 Mylohyoid
43 Body of hyoid bone
44 Anterior belly of digastric
45 Submental artery and vein
46 Submandibular gland
47 Body of mandible
48 Buccal fat pad

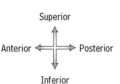

Superior

Anterior ⟷ Posterior

Inferior

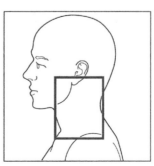

The left anterior triangle, from the left

All skin and fascia and contained superficial structures have been removed. The labelling in this illustration has largely concentrated on the structures in front of sternocleidomastoid (13); those behind it are shown on page 116, A. The upper part of the common carotid artery (28), and the lower parts of the internal and external carotid arteries (29 and 30), are seen at the anterior border of sternocleidomastoid (13). The submandibular gland (46) is below the body of the mandible (47), and the lower pole of the parotid gland (5) projects behind the angle of the mandible (1). The isthmus of the thyroid gland (23) is in the midline of the lower neck, with the lateral lobe under cover of sternohyoid (24) and sternothyroid (25).

The division of the neck into triangles (see the notes) is simply a descriptive means of sorting out a complicated region into a number of smaller 'packages', related to muscular landmarks that are easy to identify, and each containing specific structures.

While the bifurcation of the common carotid artery (28) is seen in the carotid triangle (see notes), the internal jugular vein is more posterior and covered by sternocleidomastoid (13); it is only seen when the muscle is displaced or removed (as on page 118, 14). The jugular venous pulse, which under certain conditions can be observed in the lower neck, is due to pulsation transmitted through the overlying muscle and not to direct vision of the vein itself.

Triangles of the neck
* Anterior triangle, subdivided into
  —Submental triangle
  —Digastric triangle
  —Muscular triangle
  —Carotid triangle

* Posterior triangle (see pages 116 and 117)

Anterior triangle
* *Boundaries:* anterior border of sternocleidomastoid (20), lower border of the mandible (47) and the midline.

Submental triangle
* *Boundaries:* anterior belly of digastric (44), body of hyoid bone (43) and the midline.
* *Floor:* mylohyoid (42, below 44).
* *Contents:* anterior jugular vein (page 110, 14) and submental lymph nodes.

Digastric triangle
* *Boundaries:* the two bellies of digastric (44 and 4) and the lower border of the mandible (47).
* *Floor:* mylohyoid, hyoglossus and middle constrictor (page 178, 23, 26 and 28).
* *Contents:* submandibular gland (46) and lymph nodes, and the lower part of the parotid gland posteriorly (5); facial artery (8) and vein (11) and submental vessels (45), and the carotid sheath posteriorly (under cover of 4); hypoglossal nerve (page 120, A14), mylohyoid nerve (page 120, A6) and vessels, stylopharyngeus and the glossopharyngeal nerve (page 140, C49).

Muscular triangle
* *Boundaries:* anterior border of sternocleidomastoid (20), superior belly of omohyoid (26) and the midline.
* *Floor:* sternohyoid (24) and sternothyroid (25).
* *Contents (beneath the floor):* thyroid gland, larynx, trachea, oesophagus.

Carotid triangle
* *Boundaries:* anterior border of sternocleidomastoid (20), posterior belly of digastric (4) and superior belly of omohyoid (26).
* *Floor:* thyrohyoid (33), hyoglossus (39), middle constrictor (unlabelled, above 37) and inferior constrictor (27).
* *Contents:* bifurcation of the common carotid artery (28); superior thyroid (31), lingual (41), facial (8), occipital and ascending pharyngeal branches (page 140, C52 and 50) of the external carotid artery (30); hypoglossal nerve (10) and its two branches— nerve to thyrohyoid (38) and superior root of ansa cervicalis (29); internal and external laryngeal nerves (35 and 32).

For notes on the submandibular gland see page 175.

Neck *Lymphatic system*

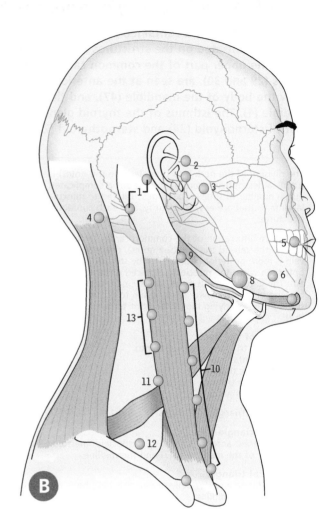

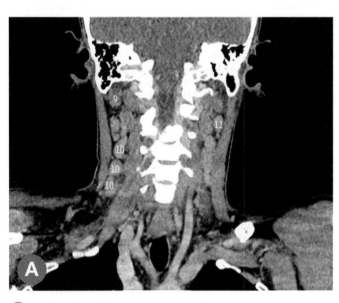

A Haematological malignancies such as lymphoma may present with widespread and dramatic lymphadenopathy, as seen in this coronal computed tomogram CT

1	Posterior auricular nodes	8	Submandibular nodes
2	Preauricular nodes	9	Jugulodigastric node
3	Parotid node	10	Deep cervical chain
4	Occipital node	11	Jugulo-omohyoid node
5	Buccal node	12	Anterior supraclavicular node
6	Facial node	13	Posterior deep cervical nodes
7	Submental nodes		

B lymphatic system of the head and neck

Lymphatic drainage of the head and neck is very important as it is involved in the spread of acute and chronic infections and malignancy from this region.

Lymphatic drainage of head and neck

Structure	Position	Nodes
Face and scalp	Anterior Lateral	Facial → Submandibular → Deep cervical Parotid → Deep cervical
Scalp	Posterior	Occipital → Deep cervical
Eyelids	Medial Lateral	Submandibular → Deep cervical Parotid → Deep cervical
Chin		Submental → Submandibular → Deep cervical
External ear	Anterior Posterior	Parotid → Deep cervical Post-aurical → Deep cervical
Middle ear		Parotid → Deep cervical
Neck	Superficial Deep	Superficial cervical (ant, lat and post) → Deep cervical Deep cervical
Floor of mouth	Anterior, Lower incisors Lateral, teeth except incisors	Submental → Submandibular → Deep cervical or Submental → Deep cervical
Palatine tonsil Pharyngeal tonsil Nasopharynx Paranasal sinuses Soft palate Nasal cavity	Anterior Posterior	Jugulodigastric → Deep cervical Retropharyngeal → Deep cervical Submandibular → Deep cervical Retropharyngeal → Deep cervical
Larynx	Above cords Below cords	Superior deep cervical Laryngeal and tracheal → Inferior deep cervical
Oropharynx		Deep cervical
Oesophagus		
Thyroid	Upper part Lower part	Laryngeal → Deep cervical Tracheal or superior mediastinal
Tongue	Tip Bilateral	Submental → Submandibular → Deep cervical and Jugulo-omohyoid
	Lateral borders	Submandibular → Deep cervical and Jugulo-omohyoid

C **Lymphatic drainage of head and neck**

Neck *Superficial dissection IV*

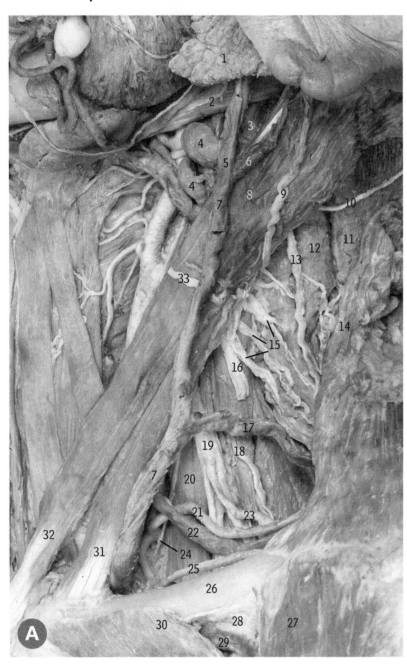

1 Parotid gland
2 Posterior belly of digastric
3 Internal jugular vein
4 Jugulodigastric lymph nodes
5 Posterior branch of retromandibular vein
6 Posterior auricular vein
7 External jugular vein
8 Sternocleidomastoid
9 Great auricular nerve
10 Lesser occipital nerve
11 Splenius capitis
12 Levator scapulae
13 Accessory nerve
14 Trapezius
15 Cervical nerves to trapezius
16 Supraclavicular nerve
17 Superficial cervical vein
18 Dorsal scapular nerve and scalenus medius
19 Upper trunk of brachial plexus
20 Scalenus anterior
21 Superficial cervical artery
22 Inferior belly of omohyoid
23 Suprascapular nerve
24 Phrenic nerve
25 Suprascapular artery
26 Clavicle
27 Deltoid
28 Clavipectoral fascia
29 Cephalic vein
30 Pectoralis major
31 Clavicular head ⎫
32 Sternal head   ⎬ of sternocleidomastoid
33 Transverse cervical nerve
34 Occipital vein
35 Occipital belly of occipitofrontalis
36 Greater occipital nerve
37 Occipital artery
38 Semispinalis capitis
39 Third occipital nerve

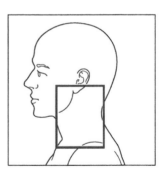

A from the left

Superior
Anterior ⟷ Posterior
Inferior

The left posterior triangle

The dissection in A is the labelled posterior part of the illustration shown on page 112. The most important structure near the middle of the triangle is the accessory nerve (13). In the lower part of the triangle the upper trunk of the brachial plexus (19) gives off the suprascapular nerve (23), with the superficial cervical and suprascapular arteries (21 and 25) running laterally below it. In B the apex of the posterior triangle is shown, with the occipital artery (37) at the very top of the triangle (see notes) and parts of semispinalis (38) and splenius (11) in the floor.

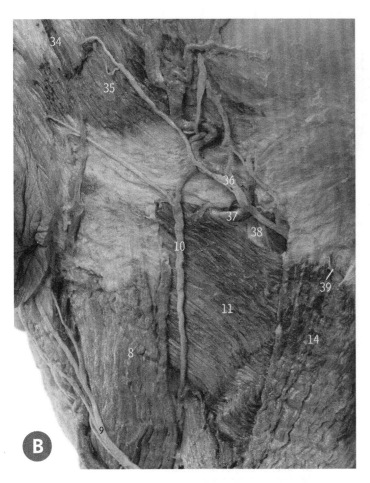

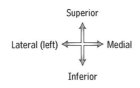

B the upper part of the triangle, from behind

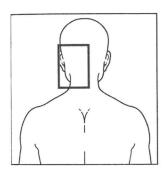

Superior

Lateral (left) ⟷ Medial

Inferior

The *posterior triangle:*

- *Boundaries:* posterior border of sternocleidomastoid (A8); anterior border of trapezius (A14); middle third of clavicle (A26).
- *Roof:* investing layer of deep cervical fascia (here removed), with accessory nerve (A13) embedded in it.
- *Contents:* arteries—occipital (B37); superficial cervical (A21); suprascapular (A25); subclavian (here just out of sight in A below origin of 21 and 25, behind tip of leaderline 24).
  —veins—external jugular (lower part of A7); superficial cervical (A17), suprascapular (removed)
  —nerves—branches of cervical plexus (great auricular, A9; lesser occipital, A10; transverse cervical, A33; supraclavicular, A16; muscular, A15); trunks of brachial plexus (as at A19; others hidden by sternocleidomastoid); branches of upper trunk—nerve to subclavius (removed) and suprascapular (A23); dorsal scapular nerve (A18, from uppermost root of plexus); accessory (A13, embedded in fascia of roof)
  —muscle—inferior belly of omohyoid (A22)
  —lymph nodes and fat (especially in lower part, removed)
- *Floor:* prevertebral layer of deep cervical fascia (page 110, 5), covering semispinalis capitis (B38); splenius capitis (A and B, 11); levator scapulae (A12); scalenus medius (A18); scalenus anterior (A20, easily seen here but usually hidden by sternocleidomastoid).

The highest structure in the posterior triangle is the occipital artery (B37), right up in the top corner on semispinalis capitis (38) and between sternocleidomastoid (8) and trapezius (14).

The subclavian artery is classified as one of the contents of the lower part of the triangle (in A it is unlabelled, behind the tip of the leaderline 24), but because of the downward slope of the first rib the subclavian vein is usually too low to be in the triangle (although it can just be seen on page 118, 42).

Do not confuse the accessory nerve (13) entering trapezius (14) with the branches of the cervical plexus to the muscle (15): the accessory nerve emerges from *within* sternocleidomastoid (8), whereas the cervical plexus branches emerge from *behind* the muscle.

In the lower part of the triangle, the suprascapular nerve (23), from the upper trunk of the brachial plexus (19), is a prominent nerve running just above the clavicle near the superficial cervical and suprascapular arteries (21 and 25). The dorsal scapular nerve (18) is smaller and emerges from scalenus medius.

The inferior belly of omohyoid (22) may be smaller than in this specimen and may be mistaken for a vessel or nerve.

The vessels commonly known as the superficial cervical artery (21) and vein (page 110, 11) are properly called transverse cervical, and are seen in the lower part of the posterior triangle. Note that the transverse cervical *nerve* (33) is at a much higher level and passes forwards over the anterior triangle.

Neck *Deep dissection I*

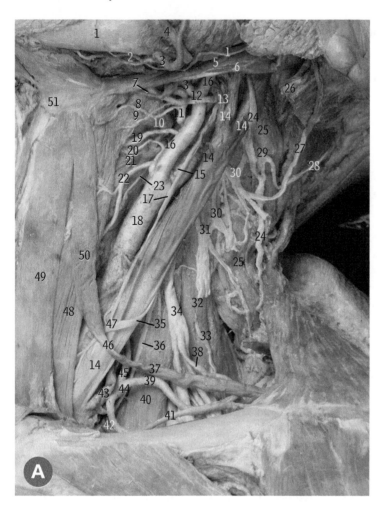

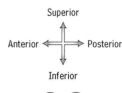

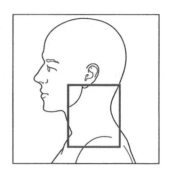

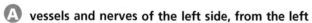

A   vessels and nerves of the left side, from the left

1   Marginal mandibular branch of facial nerve
2   Submental artery
3   Facial artery
4   Facial vein
5   Stylohyoid
6   Posterior belly of digastric
7   Vena comitans of hypoglossal nerve
8   Suprahyoid artery and hyoglossus
9   Thyrohyoid (and nerve in A)
10 Greater horn of hyoid bone
11 Lingual artery
12 Hypoglossal nerve
13 Lingual vein
14 Internal jugular vein (double at upper end in A)
15 Internal carotid artery and carotid sinus
16 External carotid artery
17 Superior root of ansa cervicalis
18 Common carotid artery
19 Internal laryngeal nerve and thyrohyoid membrane
20 Superior laryngeal artery
21 Inferior constrictor of pharynx
22 Superior thyroid artery
23 External laryngeal nerve
24 Accessory nerve
25 Levator scapulae
26 Sternocleidomastoid
27 Great auricular nerve
28 Lesser occipital nerve
29 Second ⎫
30 Third ⎬ cervical nerve ventral rami
31 Fourth ⎭
32 Scalenus medius
33 Dorsal scapular nerve
34 Upper trunk of brachial plexus
35 Inferior root of ansa cervicalis
36 Phrenic nerve
37 Inferior belly of omohyoid
38 Suprascapular nerve
39 Superficial cervical artery
40 Scalenus anterior
41 Suprascapular artery
42 Subclavian vein
43 Thoracic duct
44 Thyrocervical trunk
45 Inferior thyroid artery
46 Omohyoid tendon
47 Ansa cervicalis
48 Sternothyroid
49 Sternohyoid
50 Superior belly of omohyoid
51 Hyoid bone
52 Laryngeal prominence (Adam's apple)
53 Cricothyroid
54 Lateral lobe of thyroid gland
55 Middle thyroid vein
56 Trachea
57 Inferior thyroid vein
58 Isthmus of thyroid gland

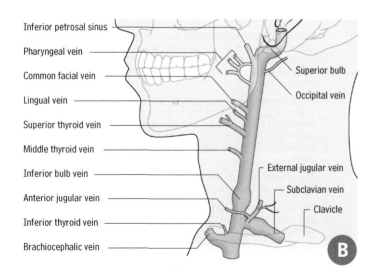

Inferior petrosal sinus

Pharyngeal vein

Common facial vein

Lingual vein

Superior thyroid vein

Middle thyroid vein

Inferior bulb vein

Anterior jugular vein

Inferior thyroid vein

Brachiocephalic vein

Superior bulb

Occipital vein

External jugular vein

Subclavian vein

Clavicle

B   main branches of the internal jugular vein

Great vessels and nerves and the thyroid gland

In A the removal of most of sternocleidomastoid (26) and its overlying cutaneous nerves displays the internal jugular vein (14) and adjacent structures. The vein lies posterolateral to the carotid vessels (18, 16 and 15); in this specimen the upper end of the vein is double, with the accessory nerve (24) passing between the two parts. The superior thyroid, lingual and facial arteries (22, 11 and 3) pass forward from the external carotid artery (16). The superior and inferior roots of the ansa cervicalis (17 and 35) embrace the lower part of the internal jugular vein (14) to form the ansa itself (47), which here lies just above the tendon of omohyoid (46). The phrenic nerve (36) runs obliquely down over the surface of scalenus anterior (40). The thyrocervical trunk (44) gives origin to the inferior thyroid, superficial cervical and suprascapular arteries (45, 39 and 41), and the thoracic duct (43) curls down to enter the junction of the internal jugular and subclavian veins (14 and 42).

In C parts of the left strap muscles (48 and 49) have been removed to display the left lateral lobe of the thyroid gland (54). The inferior thyroid vein (57) is here an unusually large single vessel whose upper end overlies the isthmus of the gland.

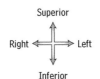

C thyroid gland, from the front

Superior
Right ⟷ Left
Inferior

The hypoglossal nerve (12) passes forwards *above* the tip of the greater horn of the hyoid bone (10), while the internal laryngeal nerve (19) passes downwards and forwards *below* the bone.

The common carotid artery (18) usually divides into the internal and external carotids (15 and 16) at about the level of the upper border of the thyroid cartilage (C4 vertebra).

The external carotid artery (16) can be distinguished easily from the internal carotid (15) because it gives off a number of branches. The internal carotid gives no branches in the neck.

The superior root (17) of the ansa cervicalis (47) runs down from the hypoglossal nerve (12) between the carotid and internal jugular vessels (18 and 14); the inferior root (35, from the cervical plexus) emerges from behind the posterior border of the vein.

The superior thyroid artery (22) runs downwards from the beginning of the external carotid artery (16), and has the external laryngeal nerve (23) immediately behind it.

The superior laryngeal artery (20, a branch of the superior thyroid, 22) runs forwards below the internal laryngeal nerve (19).

The tendon of omohyoid (46) lies over the internal jugular vein (14)—a guide to the position of the vein in operations on the lower neck.

The carotid *sinus* is a *baroreceptor* (pressure receptor) at the commencement of the internal carotid artery (within its wall); it receives nerve fibres from the glossopharyngeal and vagus nerves and is concerned with monitoring changes in blood pressure.

The carotid *body* is a *chemoreceptor* behind or between the bifurcation of the common carotid artery. An oval body a few millimetres long, it contains glomus cells within a connective tissue capsule; it receives nerve fibres from the glossopharyngeal and vagus nerves and is concerned with monitoring oxygen levels in the blood.

Neck *Deep dissection II*

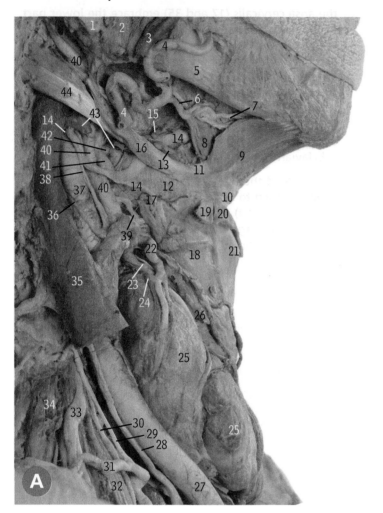
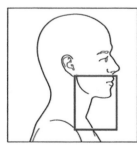
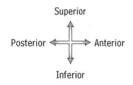
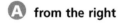
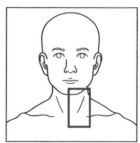

A **from the right**

Superior
Posterior ⬌ Anterior
Inferior

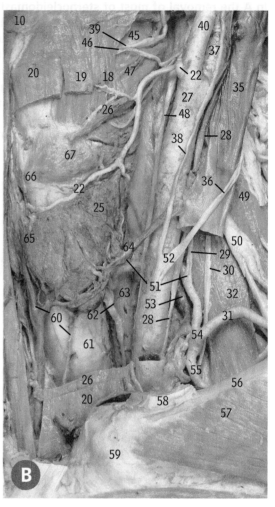
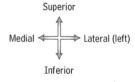

B **from the front and left**

Superior
Medial ⬌ Lateral (left)
Inferior

1 Parotid gland
2 Masseter
3 Facial vein
4 Facial artery
5 Body of mandible
6 Nerve to mylohyoid
7 Submental artery
8 Mylohyoid
9 Anterior belly of digastric
10 Body of hyoid bone
11 Digastric tendon
12 Hyoglossus
13 Vena comitans of hypoglossal nerve
14 Hypoglossal nerve
15 A tributary of 13
16 Stylohyoid
17 Nerve to thyrohyoid
18 Thyrohyoid

19 Superior belly of omohyoid
20 Sternohyoid
21 Laryngeal prominence
22 Superior thyroid artery
23 External laryngeal nerve
24 Superior thyroid vein
25 Lateral lobe of thyroid gland
26 Sternothyroid
27 Common carotid artery
28 Vagus nerve
29 Ascending cervical artery
30 Phrenic nerve
31 Superficial cervical artery
32 Scalenus anterior
33 Ventral ramus of fifth cervical nerve
34 Scalenus medius
35 Internal jugular vein
36 Inferior root of ansa cervicalis

37 Internal carotid artery
38 Superior root of ansa cervicalis
39 Internal laryngeal nerve
40 External carotid artery
41 Linguofacial trunk
42 Lingual artery
43 Lingual vein
44 Posterior belly of digastric
45 Thyrohyoid membrane
46 Superior laryngeal artery
47 Inferior constrictor of pharynx
48 Sympathetic trunk
49 Scalenus medius
50 Upper trunk of brachial plexus
51 Inferior thyroid artery
52 Ansa cervicalis
53 Thoracic duct

54 Thyrocervical trunk
55 Suprascapular artery
56 Clavicle
57 Pectoralis major
58 Sternocleidomastoid
59 Capsule of sternoclavicular joint
60 Inferior thyroid veins
61 Trachea
62 Recurrent laryngeal nerve
63 Oesophagus
64 Middle thyroid vein
65 Isthmus of thyroid gland
66 Arch of cricoid cartilage
67 Cricothyroid
68 Pyramidal lobe of thyroid gland and levator muscle
69 **Trachea**

The great vessels and the thyroid gland

In the upper part of A, the submandibular gland has been removed to show the facial artery (4) curling upwards over the body of the mandible (5) on to the face, with the facial vein (3, cut end) just behind it. Lower down, with the lower part of the internal jugular vein (35) removed, the vagus nerve (28) is revealed passing down between the vein and the common carotid artery (27). The thyroid gland (25) is here larger than normal, and is displayed by removing all but the uppermost ends of sternohyoid (20), omohyoid (19) and sternothyroid (26).

In contrast with A, the thyroid gland in B (25 and 65) is of normal size and has again been displayed by

removing most of the three 'strap' muscles (19, 20 and 26). The gap between the cut ends of the internal jugular vein (35) shows the phrenic nerve (30) running down over scalenus anterior (32); the thyrocervical trunk (54, from the underlying subclavian artery) giving rise to the three arteries—inferior thyroid (51), superficial cervical (31) and suprascapular (55); and the end of the thoracic duct (53), emerging from behind the common carotid artery (27) to run into the junction of the internal jugular and subclavian veins (see page 124, A14). In C the gland has a pyramidal lobe and levator muscle (68).

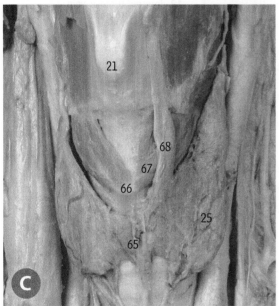

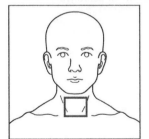

Superior

Right ⟷ Left

Inferior

C from the front

The **thyroid gland**, consisting of a central isthmus (B65) and two lateral lobes (B25), is enclosed in a connective tissue capsule derived from the pretracheal fascia, which attaches it to the larynx (hence the gland moves with the larynx during swallowing).

It extends from the level of C5 vertebra to T1 vertebra.

The isthmus of the gland (B and C, 65) overlies the second and third tracheal rings, with an anastomosis between the superior thyroid arteries of each side along its upper border (B22) and inferior thyroid veins leaving its lower border (B60).

The occasional pyramidal lobe (C68), usually on the left side, represents part of the remains of the embryonic thyroglossal duct (page 173).

Important relations of the lateral lobes include:
- laterally—sternothyroid (which limits upward extension of the gland), sternohyoid, omohyoid and sternocleidomastoid (page 118, C48, 49, 50 and 26).
- medially—lower larynx and upper trachea in front of the lower pharynx and upper oesophagus (page 120, B61 and 63),

cricothyroid (page 120, B67), inferior constrictor of the pharynx (page 190, A17), external and recurrent laryngeal nerves (page 190, A16 and 23).
- posterolaterally—common carotid artery within the carotid sheath (A27), parathyroid glands (page 123, B41, 44 and 47), inferior thyroid artery (B51), thoracic duct (on the left, page 120, B53).

The external laryngeal nerve lies just behind the superior thyroid artery as the artery approaches the upper pole of the lateral lobe (page 122, A5 and 4). Ligation of the artery during thyroidectomy is usually carried out at the very tip of the pole, to avoid damaging the nerve.

The recurrent laryngeal nerve (B62) (which enters the larynx by passing under the lower border of the inferior constrictor of the pharynx, immediately behind the cricothyroid joint, page 190, B23) lies either anterior or posterior to the inferior thyroid artery as the artery arches medially behind the lower part of the lateral lobe (B51). Ligation of the artery is usually carried out well away from the gland.

For laryngeal nerve injuries see page 193.

D Ultrasound of the thyroid. The isthmus overlies the second and third tracheal rings

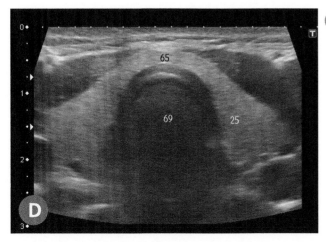

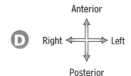

Anterior

Right ⟷ Left

Posterior

Neck *Deep dissection III*

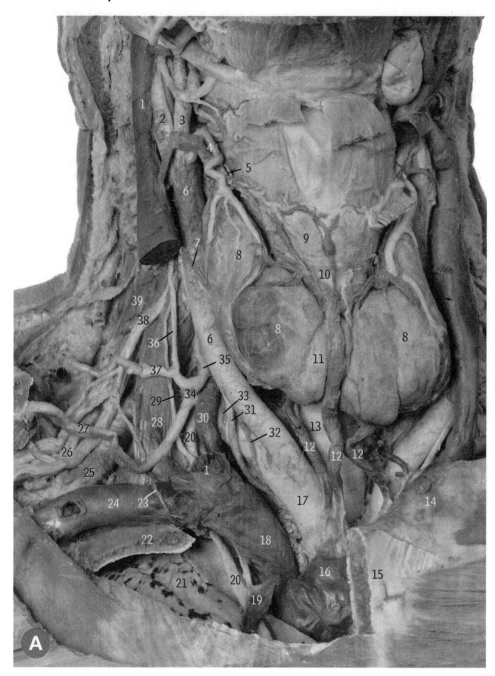

1	Internal jugular vein
2	Internal carotid artery
3	External carotid artery
4	Superior thyroid artery and vein
5	External laryngeal nerve
6	Common carotid artery
7	Middle thyroid vein
8	Lateral lobe of thyroid gland
9	Cricothyroid
10	Arch of cricoid cartilage
11	Isthmus of thyroid gland
12	Inferior thyroid veins
13	Trachea
14	Capsule of sternoclavicular joint
15	Manubrium of sternum
16	Left brachiocephalic vein
17	Brachiocephalic artery
18	Right brachiocephalic vein
19	Internal thoracic vein
20	Internal thoracic artery
21	Lung
22	First rib
23	Accessory phrenic nerve
24	Subclavian vein
25	Subclavian artery
26	Brachial plexus
27	Suprascapular artery
28	Scalenus anterior
29	Phrenic nerve
30	Vertebral vein
31	Vagus nerve
32	Jugular lymphatic trunk
33	Ansa subclavia
34	Thyrocervical trunk
35	Inferior thyroid artery
36	Ascending cervical artery
37	Superficial cervical artery
38	Ventral ramus of fifth cervical nerve
39	Scalenus medius
40	Superior thyroid artery and vein
41	Right superior parathyroid gland
42	Posterior border of right lateral lobe of thyroid gland
43	Branches of inferior thyroid artery
44	Right inferior parathyroid gland
45	Inferior thyroid veins
46	Isthmus of thyroid gland
47	Left superior parathyroid gland

Ⓐ the central and right side of the neck

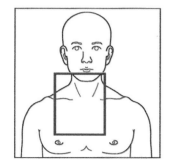

Superior
Right ⟷ Left
Inferior

The thyroid gland, parathyroid glands and the root of the neck

In A, part of the right clavicle, first rib (22) and manubrium of the sternum (15) have been removed, together with the lower part of the internal jugular vein (1) and infrahyoid muscles. In this specimen the thyroid gland is enlarged; compare with the normal size in B. The superior thyroid artery (4) approaches the front of the upper part of the lateral lobe (8), with the external laryngeal nerve (5) immediately behind it. The inferior thyroid artery (35) runs up behind the lower part of the lobe. The superior and middle thyroid veins (4 and 7) drain laterally to the internal jugular vein (1), but the inferior thyroid veins (12) run downwards in front of the trachea (13) to reach the left brachiocephalic vein (16). The subclavian vein (24) passes medially over the first rib (22) in front of scalenus anterior (28) to be joined by the internal jugular vein (1) to form the right brachiocephalic vein (18). The subclavian artery (25) is at a higher level behind scalenus anterior (28). The vertebral vein (30) and artery are deeply placed medial to scalenus anterior.

In B, the view of the thyroid gland from behind shows three visible parathyroid glands (41, 44 and 47).

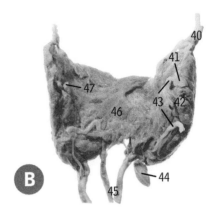

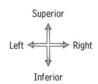

On the front of scalenus anterior (28), do not confuse the phrenic nerve (29) with the ascending cervical artery (36, here a branch of the superficial cervical artery, 37, but usually coming from the inferior thyroid, 35). Compare with page 124, A5 and 6.

The typical number of **parathyroid glands** is four (in 90% of individuals) but there may be more or less; in B, there are three (B41, 44 and 47).

The glands usually lie between the posterior surface of the lateral lobes of the thyroid gland and the thin capsule of the gland (which is inside the fascial sheath, derived from the pretracheal fascia).

The superior gland usually lies approximately level with the upper border of the thyroid isthmus (B41 and 47), and the inferior gland behind the lower pole of the lateral lobe (in B44 it is below the lower pole).

The blood supply of both superior and inferior parathyroid glands is from the inferior thyroid artery (A35). If the glands are difficult to identify, following small branches of this artery should lead to the glands.

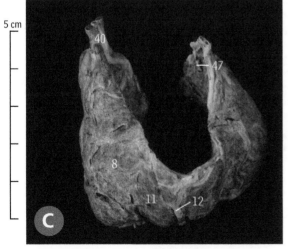

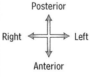

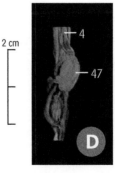

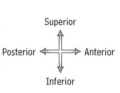

C an isolated thyroid gland shown actual size as presented at dissection, from above

D an isolated left superior parathyroid gland shown actual size as presented at dissection, from the right

Neck *Deep dissection IV*

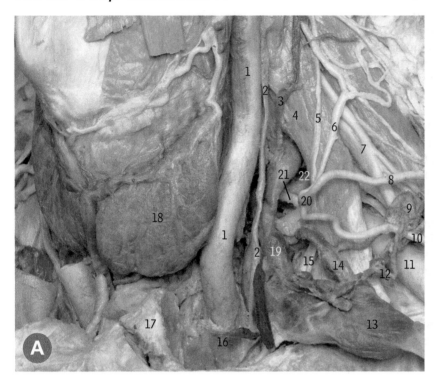

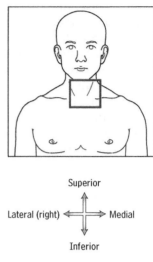

A left side, from the front and the left

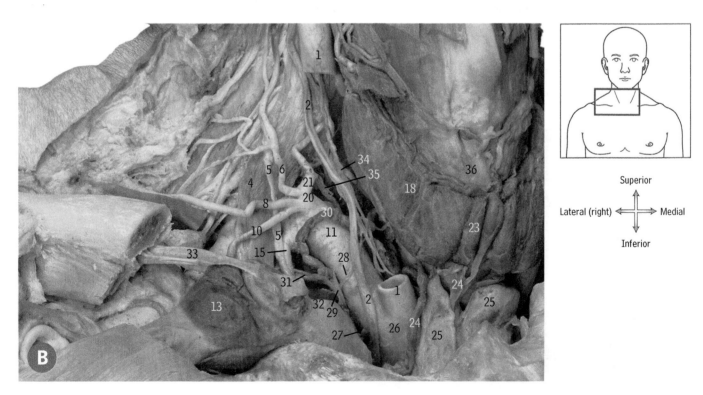

B right side, from the front and the right

The thyroid gland, thymus and the root of the neck

In A, on the left side, the clavicle has been removed at the sternoclavicular joint (17), and so has the internal jugular vein at its junction with the subclavian vein (13) to form the brachiocephalic vein (16). The vertebral vein (19) is seen joining the subclavian (13), and the thoracic duct (14) here runs into the subclavian vein, a little more laterally than usual (see page 118, 43). A lymph node (9) and a small lymphatic trunk (12) have been preserved.

In B, on the right side, the dissection is similar to that in A (and to page 122, A) but part of the common carotid artery (1) has been removed. The mediastinal lymphatic trunk (30) is seen curling over the subclavian artery (11) to join the subclavian lymphatic trunk (31) to form the right lymphatic duct (29) which (like the thoracic duct on the left side, page 128, 37) joins the junction of the internal jugular and subclavian veins (32 and 13). The recurrent laryngeal branch (27) of the vagus nerve (2) has just begun to hook underneath the subclavian artery (11).

1 Common carotid artery
2 Vagus nerve
3 Ascending cervical vein
4 Scalenus anterior
5 Phrenic nerve
6 Ascending cervical artery
7 Upper trunk of brachial plexus
8 Superficial cervical artery
9 A lower deep cervical lymph node
10 Suprascapular artery
11 Subclavian artery
12 A subclavian lymph trunk
13 Subclavian vein
14 Thoracic duct
15 Internal thoracic artery
16 Brachiocephalic vein
17 Disc of sternoclavicular joint
18 Lateral lobe of thyroid gland
19 Vertebral vein
20 Thyrocervical trunk
21 Inferior thyroid artery
22 Vertebral artery
23 Isthmus of thyroid gland
24 Inferior thyroid veins
25 Lobes of persistent thymus gland
26 Brachiocephalic artery
27 Recurrent laryngeal nerve
28 Ansa subclavia
29 Right lymphatic duct
30 Mediastinal lymphatic trunk
31 Subclavian lymphatic trunk
32 Cut end of internal jugular vein
33 Suprascapular vein
34 Sympathetic trunk and middle cervical ganglion
35 Tracheal branch of inferior thyroid artery
36 Cricoid cartilage

At the level of C6 vertebra:
- the cricoid cartilage (B36)
- the larynx continues as the trachea
- the pharynx continues as the oesophagus
- the middle cervical ganglion (B34)
- the vertebral artery (A and B, 22) enters the foramen transversarium of C6 vertebra
- the inferior thyroid artery (B21) arches medially

The sympathetic nervous system in the neck consists of the sympathetic trunk with the superior, middle and inferior cervical sympathetic ganglia and their branches.

The rather elongated *superior cervical ganglion* (page 128, 19) lies at the level of the second and third vertebrae between longus capitis (behind) and the internal carotid artery (page 128, 5), which is within the carotid sheath (in front). It gives off from its upper end the internal carotid nerve, which constitutes the cephalic part of the sympathetic nervous system and enters the cranial cavity with the internal carotid artery. Other branches include grey rami communicantes to the upper four cervical nerves, a cardiac branch and branches to cervical viscera and vessels and the carotid body.

The *middle cervical ganglion* (B34, the smallest of the three) is at the level of the sixth cervical vertebra, usually in front of the inferior thyroid artery and always in front of the vertebral artery. It gives grey rami communicantes to the fifth and sixth cervical nerves, forms the ansa subclavia (B28), and gives a cardiac branch and branches to cervical viscera and vessels.

The *inferior cervical ganglion* (page 128, 53) lies in front of the neck of the first rib and behind the vertebral artery; it is frequently fused with the first thoracic sympathetic ganglion to form the cervicothoracic (stellate) ganglion. It gives grey rami communicantes to the seventh and eighth cervical nerves (and to the first thoracic nerve if fused), a cardiac branch and branches to adjacent vessels.

The middle cervical ganglion (B34) lies in front of the vertebral artery; the inferior cervical ganglion lies behind it (page 128, 53 and 39).

Neck *Deep dissection V: Root of neck*

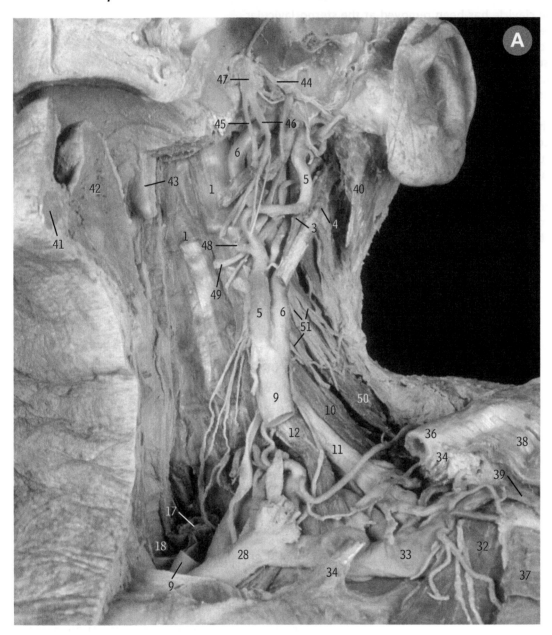

A left side, from the front left and slightly below

In A-B left side viscera has been removed by a paramedian incision just to the right of the midline, thus, the body of the mandible (41) genioglossus muscle of the tongue (42) and uvula (43) are seen in parasagittal section. A portion of the common carotid artery (9) has been removed to expose the underlying vagus nerve (15), vertebral vein (21) and deeper to it, the vertebral artery (13), middle cervical ganglion (22) and thyrocervical trunk (23).

In B the external (5) and internal (6) carotid arteries have been displaced laterally to expose the superior cervical ganglion (2) and commensurate nerve branches of the sympathetic trunk (8).

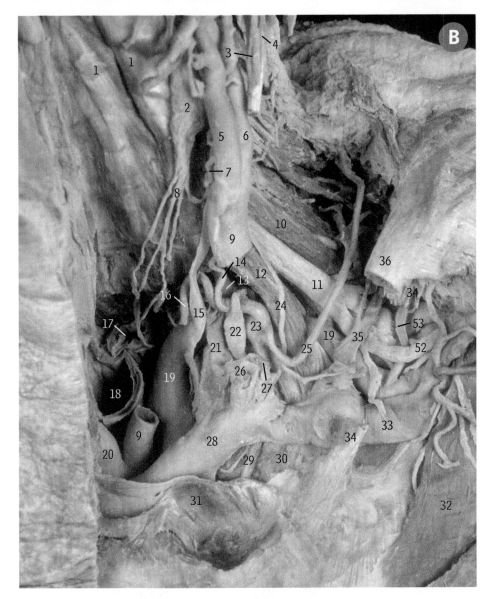

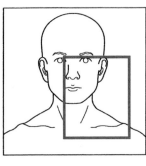

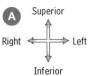

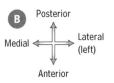

B Superior

Right ⟷ Left

Inferior

B Posterior

Medial ⟷ Lateral (left)

Anterior

B left side, from the front left and above

1	Longus capitis	**20**	Brachiocephalic artery	**38**	Deltoid
2	Superior cervical ganglion	**21**	Vertebral vein	**39**	Cephalic vein within deltopectoral groove
3	Stylohyoid	**22**	Middle cervical ganglion		
4	Posterior belly of digastric	**23**	Thyrocervical trunk	**40**	Sternocleidomastoid
5	External carotid artery	**24**	Phrenic nerve	**41**	Body of mandible
6	Internal carotid artery	**25**	Superficial cervical artery	**42**	Genioglossus
7	Superior thyroid artery	**26**	Internal jugular vein	**43**	Uvula
8	Sympathetic trunk	**27**	Thoracic duct	**44**	Auriculotemporal nerve
9	Common carotid artery	**28**	Left brachiocephalic vein	**45**	Lingual nerve
10	Scalenus medius	**29**	Internal thoracic artery	**46**	Inferior alveolar nerve
11	Upper trunk of brachial plexus	**30**	Pleura overlying apex of superior lobe left lung	**47**	Mandibular nerve
12	Scalenus anterior			**48**	Facial artery
13	Vertebral artery	**31**	Disc of sternoclavicular joint	**49**	Hypoglossal nerve
14	Ascending cervical artery	**32**	Pectoralis minor	**50**	Levator scapulae
15	Vagus nerve	**33**	Subclavian vein	**51**	Cervical nerves ventral rami
16	Inferior thyroid artery	**34**	Subclavius	**52**	Suprascapular nerve
17	Oesophagus	**35**	Suprascapular vein	**53**	Suprascapular artery
18	Trachea	**36**	Clavicle		
19	Left subclavian artery	**37**	Clavicular part of pectoralis major		

Neck *Deep dissection VI*

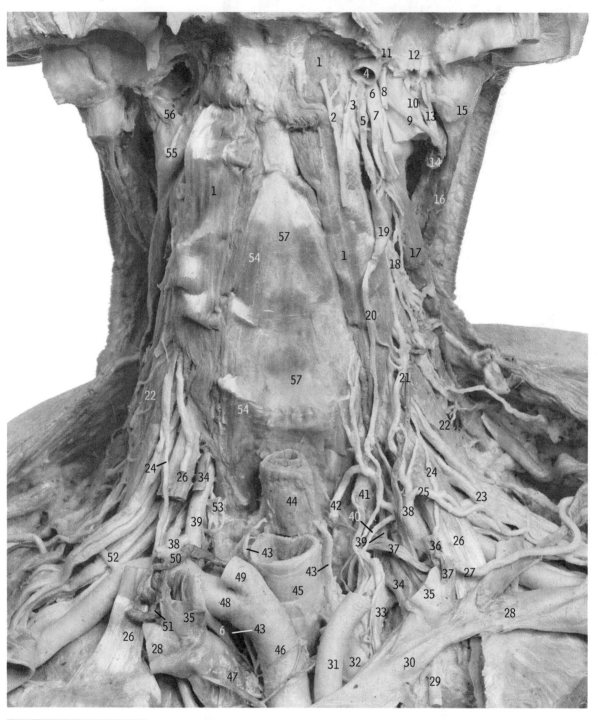

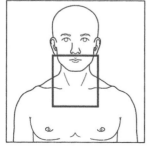

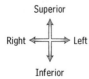

Superior

Right ⟷ Left

Inferior

The prevertebral muscles

All the viscera and some major vessels have been removed except for the lower ends of the trachea (45), oesophagus (44), internal jugular veins (35), and the left and right common carotid arteries (31 and 49). Longus capitis (1) and longus colli (54) are the more medial prevertebral muscles, with levator scapulae (17), scalenus medius (22) and scalenus anterior (26) more laterally. The internal carotid nerve (5) extends up from the superior cervical ganglion (19), which is joined by a long length of sympathetic trunk (20) to the middle cervical ganglion (41). The inferior thyroid artery (42) arches medially from the thyrocervical trunk (38), and at a lower level the thoracic duct (37) arches laterally in front of the vertebral vessels (34 and 39). The origin of the right recurrent laryngeal nerve (43) from the vagus (6) is seen just below the right subclavian artery (48).

1 Longus capitis	**30** Left brachiocephalic vein
2 Ascending pharyngeal artery	**31** Left common carotid artery
3 Meningeal branch of ascending pharyngeal artery	**32** Left subclavian artery
4 Internal carotid artery	**33** Vagus nerve
5 Internal carotid nerve	**34** Vertebral vein
6 Vagus nerve	**35** Internal jugular vein
7 Inferior vagal ganglion	**36** Jugular lymphatic trunk
8 Glossopharyngeal nerve	**37** Thoracic duct
9 Accessory nerve (spinal root)	**38** Thyrocervical trunk
10 Internal jugular vein	**39** Vertebral artery
11 Spine of sphenoid bone	**40** A large oesophageal branch
12 Tympanic part of temporal bone	of inferior thyroid artery
13 Occipital artery	**41** Middle cervical ganglion
14 Posterior belly of digastric	**42** Inferior thyroid artery
15 Mastoid process	**43** Recurrent laryngeal nerve
16 Sternocleidomastoid	**44** Oesophagus
17 Levator scapulae	**45** Trachea
18 Ventral ramus of third cervical nerve	**46** Brachiocephalic artery
19 Superior cervical ganglion	**47** Right brachiocephalic vein
20 Sympathetic trunk	**48** Right subclavian artery
21 Ascending cervical artery and vein	**49** Right common carotid artery
22 Scalenus medius	**50** Mediastinal lymphatic trunk
23 Upper trunk of brachial plexus	**51** Right lymphatic duct
24 Phrenic nerve	**52** Dorsal scapular artery
25 Superficial cervical artery	**53** Inferior cervical ganglion
26 Scalenus anterior	**54** Longus colli
27 Suprascapular artery	**55** Transverse process of atlas
28 Subclavian vein	**56** Rectus capitis lateralis
29 Internal thoracic artery	**57** Anterior longitudinal ligament

In the lowest part of the neck the thoracic duct lies behind the left margin of the oesophagus. It ascends to arch laterally (37) at the level of C7 vertebra, passing behind the common carotid artery and internal jugular vein (31 and 35, here cut just below the duct) and in front of the vertebral artery and vein (39 and 34), and enters the junction of the internal jugular and subclavian veins (35 and 28). The right lymphatic duct (51) pursues a similar course on the right side.

The recurrent laryngeal nerves (43) run up on each side in the groove between the trachea and oesophagus. The right nerve arises in the lower part of the neck from the vagus (6) and hooks under the right subclavian artery (48); the left nerve arises in the thorax and hooks under the arch of the aorta.

Face, orbit and eye

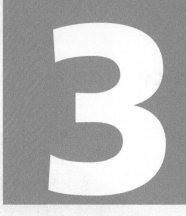

Face Surface markings

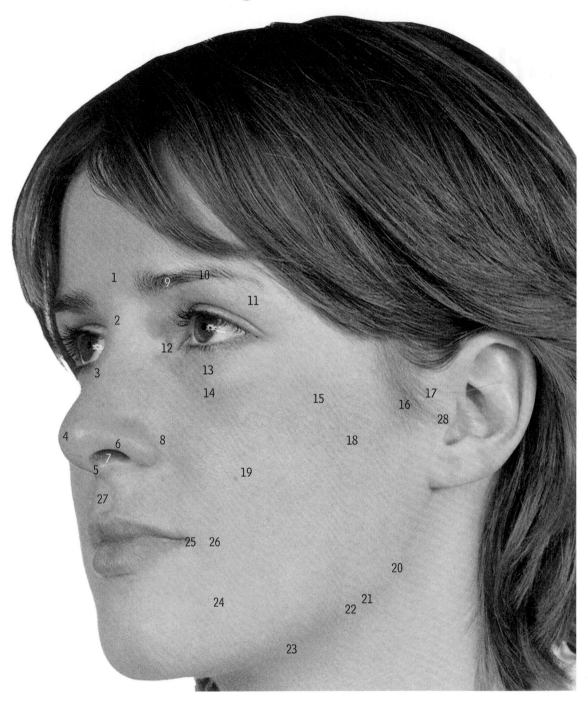

Some surface markings of the front and left side

Among the more important surface markings on the face are those for the pulses of the superficial temporal artery (17), in front of the tragus of the ear (28) and behind the head of the mandible (16), and the facial artery (22), where it passes on to the face from the neck at the anterior border of the masseter muscle and 2.5 cm in front of the angle of the mandible (20). The parotid duct (18 and 19) lies under the middle third of a line drawn between the tragus of the ear (28) and the midpoint of the philtrum (27), the rectangular area between the two ridges below the nose and above the upper lip.

1 Glabella
2 Root
3 Dorsum
4 Apex
5 Septum   } of nose
6 Ala
7 Anterior naris
8 Alar groove
9 Frontal notch and supratrochlear nerve and artery
10 Supra-orbital notch (or foramen), nerve and artery
11 Lateral part of supra-orbital margin
12 Medial palpebral ligament and lacrimal sac
13 Infra-orbital margin
14 Infra-orbital foramen, nerve and vessels
15 Zygomatic arch
16 Head of mandible
17 Auriculotemporal nerve and superficial temporal artery
18 Parotid duct emerging from gland
19 Parotid duct turning medially at anterior border of masseter
20 Angle of mandible
21 Lower border of ramus
22 Anterior border of masseter and facial artery and vein
23 Lower border of body of mandible
24 Mental foramen, nerve and artery
25 Lateral angle of mouth
26 Modiolus
27 Philtrum
28 Tragus of ear

The supra-orbital, infra-orbital and mental foramina (10, 14 and 24) lie in approximately the same vertical plane, in line with the pupil when looking straight ahead and viewed from the front. Compare with page 2, 6, 12 and 16.

The medial end of the eyebrow is level with the supra-orbital margin (as at 9), but the lateral end is above the margin (above 11).

For further details of the eye see page 144, and of the ear see page 182.

The anterior naris (7) is commonly called the nostril.

The muscles of the face (including buccinator) and platysma are all supplied by the facial nerve (page 134).

Facial nerve paralysis (Bell's palsy):
• The lower eyelid droops (but not the upper lid, which is supplied by the oculomotor nerve), and the cornea may become damaged by dryness because the eye cannot be closed properly
• The angle of the mouth droops, with dribbling of saliva, and it is not possible to 'show the teeth' on the affected side
• Whistling is not possible, and food collects between the teeth and the cheek (due to paralysis of the buccinator)

The facial paralysis may be accompanied by the following additional features depending on the site of the damage. If the damage:
• is in the pons (where the facial nerve fibres overlie the abducent nucleus) there may be paralysis of the lateral rectus
• is in the cerebellopontine angle or internal acoustic meatus where the facial and vestibulocochlear nerves lie close together, there may be deafness
• involves the nerve to stapedius, there may be hyperacusis (extreme sensitivity to sound) due to loss of the dampening effect on the vibration of the stapes
• involves the chorda tympani, there may be loss of taste sensation from the anterior two-thirds of the tongue (the unilateral loss of submandibular and sublingual secretion will not be noticed)

The above notes on facial nerve paralysis refer to 'infranuclear paralysis', i.e. damage to the axons derived from the facial nerve nucleus in the pons.

Supranuclear paralysis refers to paralysis due to interruption of the pathway from the cerebral cortex to the facial nerve nucleus, i.e. damage to corticonuclear fibres. The axons from the cell bodies of the upper part of the facial nerve nucleus (in the pons) supply the forehead muscle (frontal belly of occipitofrontalis) and receive corticonuclear fibres from the cerebral cortex of both sides, i.e. there are two sources of corticonuclear supply. The lower part of the facial nerve nucleus supplying the lower facial muscles and platysma receives corticonuclear fibres from the opposite cerebral cortex only, i.e. only one source of corticonuclear supply. Therefore, unilateral supranuclear lesions (e.g. from haemorrhage in the internal capsule involving corticonuclear fibres) causes paralysis of the lower facial muscles of the opposite (contralateral) side but does not affect movement of the forehead on that side, because the neurons supplying the forehead muscle still have an intact corticonuclear supply from the same (ipsilateral) side.

Face *Superficial dissection*

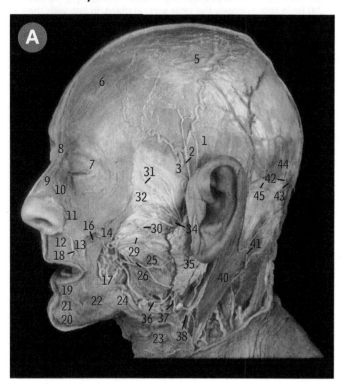

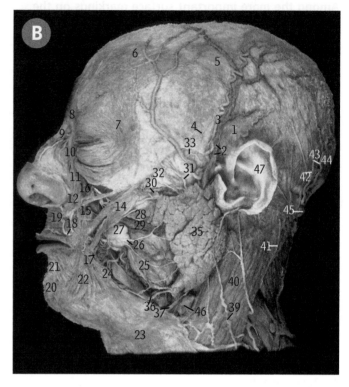

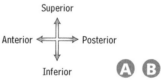

Superior

Anterior ⟷ Posterior

Inferior   **A B**

The left parotid gland, facial nerve and muscles

Two examples are given to display variations that often exist in the shape and size of the parotid gland and facial muscles of expression, distribution of the fine branches of the facial nerve and superficial veins.

Skin and subcutaneous tissues have been removed to display the superficial structures of the face. Five groups of branches of the facial nerve fan out from below the anterior border of the parotid gland (35): temporal (33), zygomatic (31), buccal (26), marginal mandibular (36) and cervical (37). The facial artery and vein (17 and 16) lie deep to platysma (23), risorius (24), and zygomaticus major and minor (14 and 13).

The marginal mandibular branch of the facial nerve (36) usually runs near the lower border of the mandible (to supply facial muscles near the mouth), but it may dip below the mandible (as on page 112, 3) and overlie the submandibular gland. The nerve may be at risk in incisions to expose the gland unless the cut is made 2 cm below the mandible.

The **parotid gland** (35) spills over into the irregular space bounded in front by the ramus of the mandible (page 8, 30, with the attachments of masseter laterally and the medial pterygoid medially), behind by the mastoid process (page 8, 13, with the attachments of sternocleidomastoid laterally and the posterior belly of digastric medially), and medially by the styloid process (page 8,

18, with its three attached muscles—stylohyoid, styloglossus and stylopharyngeus). It is enclosed in a capsule derived from the investing layer of the deep cervical fascia.

Embedded within the gland are:
- the various facial branches of the facial nerve (33, 31, 26, 36 and 37)
- the retromandibular vein (page 174, C64 and 65)
- the upper end of the external carotid artery (page 174, C62) and the beginning of its two terminal branches (superficial temporal, 3, and maxillary, page 174, 62)
- lymph nodes
- filaments from the auriculotemporal nerve (2)

A B

1 Temporoparietalis	**26** Buccal branches of facial nerve
2 Auriculotemporal nerve	**27** Buccal fat pad
3 Superficial temporal artery	**28** Accessory parotid gland
4 Zygomaticotemporal nerve piercing temporalis fascia	**29** Parotid duct
5 Epicranial aponeurosis (galea aponeurotica)	**30** Transverse facial artery
6 Frontal belly of occipitofrontalis	**31** Zygomatic branch of facial nerve
7 Orbicularis oculi	**32** Zygomatic arch
8 Depressor supercilii	**33** Temporal branches of facial nerve
9 Procerus	**34** Deep part of parotid gland
10 Nasalis	**35** Superficial part of parotid gland
11 Levator labii superioris alaeque nasi	**36** Marginal mandibular branch of facial nerve
12 Levator labii superioris	**37** Cervical branch of facial nerve
13 Zygomaticus minor	**38** External jugular vein
14 Zygomaticus major	**39** Great auricular nerve
15 Levator anguli oris	**40** Sternocleidomastoid
16 Facial vein	**41** Lesser occipital nerve
17 Facial artery	**42** Greater occipital nerve
18 Superior labial artery	**43** Occipital artery
19 Orbicularis oris	**44** Occipital belly of occipitofrontalis
20 Mentalis	**45** Occipital vein
21 Depressor labii inferioris	**46** Cervical lymph node
22 Depressor anguli oris	**47** Cartilage of pinna
23 Platysma	
24 Risorius	
25 Masseter	

The pathway for parotid gland secretion: from the inferior salivary nucleus in the pons by the glossopharyngeal nerve and its tympanic branch, the tympanic plexus and the lesser petrosal nerve to the otic ganglion (synapse), and then to the gland by filaments of the auriculotemporal nerve.

For the parotid gland in transverse section and a medial view, see page 174.

The main part of the epicranius muscle (a term rarely used) consists of the frontal and occipital bellies of occipitofrontalis (6 and 44, commonly called occipitalis and frontalis), united centrally by the epicranial aponeurosis (galea aponeurotica, 5). Temporoparietalis (1), which is also classified as part of epicranius, is the name given to muscle fibres (if present) at the side of the scalp between frontalis and the auricular muscles (usually small and unimportant and not illustrated here).

The occipital belly of occipitofrontalis (see also page 117) has a bony attachment to the supreme nuchal line (page 12, A11) and the mastoid process; the frontal belly has no bony attachment.

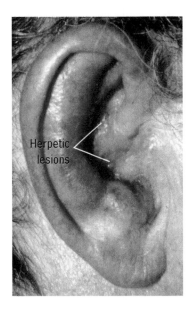

Herpetic lesions

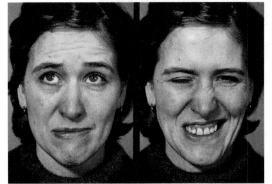

D lower motor neurone palsy of the facial nerve following inflammation of the facial nerve in the stylomastoid canal

C Herpes zoster (shingles) of the facial nerve may present as vesicles on the pinna together with a facial palsy

Face *Deep dissection I*

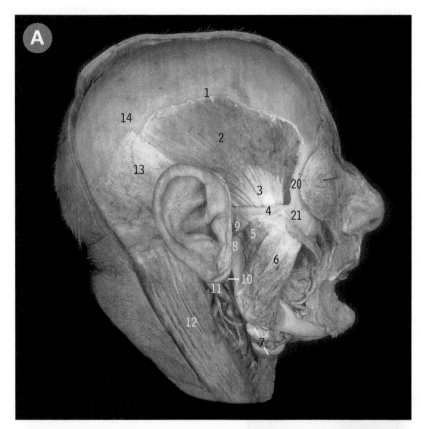

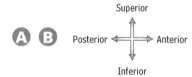

The right temporalis and masseter muscles and the temporomandibular joint

A muscles and joint, from the right

B temporalis muscle and tendon, from the right

C temporalis insertion, from the right and front

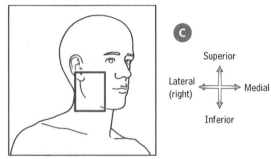

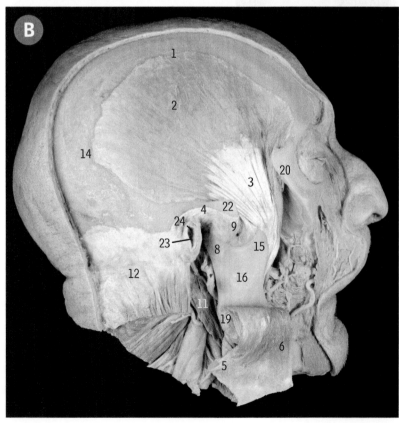

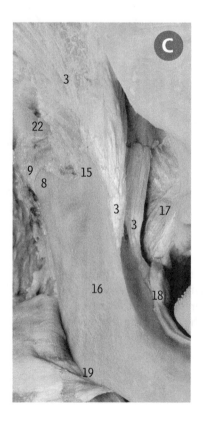

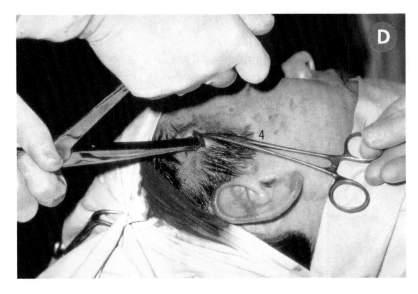

D

Using a Rowe's elevator the fractured and displaced body of the zygoma is reduced through a temporal incision above the hairline and through the temporal fascia—the 'Gillies' approach'

In A, the parotid gland, facial muscles and all vessels and nerves have been removed, together with part of the temporalis fascia (13). The capsule of the temporomandibular joint is displayed (9), below the zygomatic arch (4) and in front of the external acoustic meatus. The posterior belly of digastric is seen between the ramus of the mandible (16) and sternocleidomastoid (12), and the styloid process (10) is more deeply placed.

In B, masseter (5, 6) has been reflected inferiorly from its attachments. Most of the zygomatic arch (4) has been removed by cutting through anteriorly, the zygomatic bone (temporal margin (20) and temporal process (21)), and posteriorly, the temporal bone zygomatic process (22) just anterior to the temporomandibular joint (9). Fibres of the 'fan shaped' temporalis muscle (2) become tendinous (3) as they converge towards the medial surface of the coronoid process (15) of the mandible.

Although superficially placed, temporalis and masseter are classified (with the medial and lateral pterygoids) as muscles of mastication, not muscles of the face.

Temporalis (2) arises from the floor of the temporal fossa and from the overlying temporalis fascia (13), which passes from the superior temporal line to the zygomatic arch. The attachment of the muscle is limited above by the inferior temporal line.

The insertion of temporalis is to the apex, anterior and posterior borders and medial surface of the coronoid process (15), and extends down the anterior border of the ramus (16) almost as far as the third molar tooth.

Masseter consists of three overlapping layers:
• superficial (6), arising from the maxillary process of the zygomatic bone and the anterior two-thirds of the lower border of the zygomatic process (arch) of the temporal bone
• middle, arising from the deep surface of the anterior two-thirds of the arch and the lower border of the posterior third
• deep, from the deep surface of the arch

The layers fuse anteriorly and are inserted into the lateral surface of the angle, ramus and coronoid process of the mandible (19, 16 and 15).

Both temporalis and masseter, together with the medial and lateral pterygoid muscles (the 'muscles of mastication' group), are supplied by the mandibular branch of the trigeminal nerve.

In trigeminal nerve paralysis, there is paralysis of the muscles of mastication with eventual hollowing above and below the zygomatic arch due to wasting of temporalis and masseter.

In C, part of the zygomatic arch (22) and the whole of the masseter have been removed to show the extensive attachment of the tendon of temporalis (3) to the front of the ramus of the mandible (16).

1 Inferior temporal line	
2 Temporalis muscle	
3 Temporalis tendon	
4 Zygomatic arch	
5 Middle layer	} of masseter
6 Superficial layer	
7 Submandibular gland	
8 Neck of mandible	
9 Lateral ligament of temporomandibular joint	

10 Styloid process	
11 Posterior belly of digastric	
12 Sternocleidomastoid	
13 Temporalis fascia	
14 Superior temporal line	
15 Coronoid process	} of mandible
16 Ramus	
17 Medial pterygoid	
18 Cut edge of mucous membrane of mouth	

19 Angle of mandible	
20 Temporal margin	} of zygomatic bone
21 Maxillary process	
22 Zygomatic process of temporal bone	
23 External acoustic meatus	
24 Auricular cartilage	

Face *Deep dissection II*

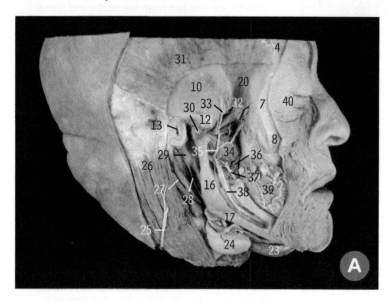

A after removal of temporalis, the zygomatic arch, masseter, auricle and part of the mandible. (see also E, F page 37)

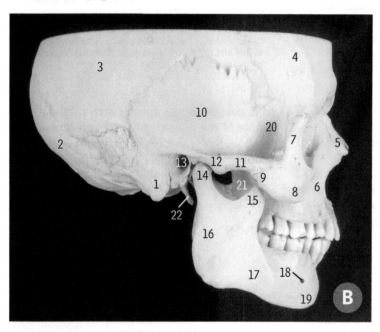

B skull from the right

F The right infratemporal fossa and temporomandibular joint

A B E

F

Superior ↕ Inferior
Posterior ↔ Anterior

C

Posterior ↕ Anterior
Lateral (right) ↔ Medial

D

Anterior ↕ Posterior
Lateral (right) ↔ Medial

A B

1	Mastoid process	
2	Occipital bone	
3	Parietal bone	
4	Frontal bone	
5	Nasal bone	
6	Maxilla	
7	Temporal margin	
8	Maxillary margin	of zygomatic bone
9	Temporal process	
10	Squamous part of temporal bone	
11	Zygomatic arch	
12	Zygomatic process of temporal bone	
13	External acoustic meatus	

14	Condylar process	
15	Coronoid process	of mandible
16	Ramus	
17	Body	
18	Mental foramen	
19	Mental protuberance	
20	Greater wing of sphenoid bone	
21	Lateral pterygoid plate	
22	Styloid process	
23	Anterior belly of digastric	
24	Submandibular gland	
25	Great auricular nerve	
26	Sternocleidomastoid	
27	Posterior belly of digastric	

28	Stylohyoid ligament
29	Styloid process
30	Capsule of temporomandibular joint
31	Temporalis muscle
32	Upper head of lateral pterygoid
33	Deep temporal artery
34	Lower head of lateral pterygoid
35	Maxillary artery
36	Medial pterygoid
37	Lingual nerve
38	Inferior alveolar artery and nerve within mandibular canal
39	Buccinator
40	Orbicularis oculi

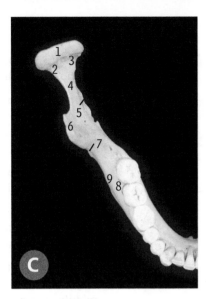

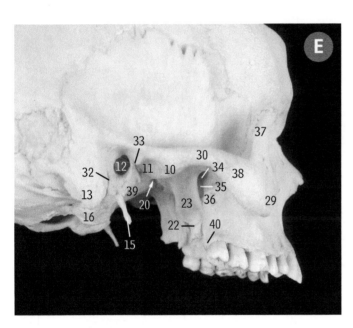

C right side of mandible, from above

D right side of base of skull, from below

E skull, without mandible, from the right and slightly below (see also A, page 20)

Infratemporal fossa and temporomandibular joint
● The temporomandibular joint is a synovial joint formed by the articulation between the head of the mandible and the mandibular fossa and articular tubercle of the temporal bone at the base of the skull. Both bone surfaces are covered by fibrocartilage.
● The fibrous joint capsule that surrounds the temporomandibular joint is attached to the articular area of the temporal bone and around the neck of the mandible.
● The fibrocartilaginous disc divides the joint cavity into a superior and inferior compartment; the disc fuses with the joint capsule.
See page 138, figure F

1 Head	forming condylar
2 Neck	process of mandible
3 Pterygoid fovea	
4 Mandibular notch	
5 Angle	
6 Coronoid process	
7 Anterior border of ramus and coronoid notch	
8 Body	
9 Alveolar part	
10 Articular tubercle	
11 Mandibular fossa	
12 External acoustic meatus	
13 Mastoid process	

14 Stylomastoid foramen
15 Styloid process
16 Occipital condyle
17 Jugular foramen
18 Carotid canal
19 Apex of petrous part of temporal bone
20 Foramen ovale
21 Foramen spinosum
22 Medial pterygoid plate
23 Lateral pterygoid plate
24 Pterygoid hamulus
25 Pyramidal process of maxilla
26 Horizontal plate of palatine bone
27 Greater palatine foramen

28 Palatine process of maxilla
29 Maxillary margin of zygomatic bone
30 Zygomatic arch
31 Zygomatic process of temporal bone
32 Tympanomastoid fissure
33 Squamotympanic fissure
34 Pterygomaxillary fissure
35 Sphenopalatine foramen
36 Infratemporal surface of maxilla
37 Temporal margin ⎫ of zygomatic bone
38 Temporal process ⎭
39 Pharyngeal tubercle of occipital bone
40 Tuberosity of maxilla

Face *Deep dissection III*

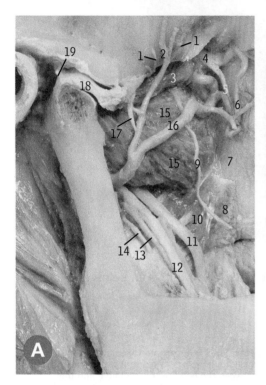

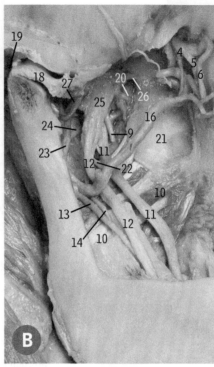

The right infratemporal fossa and temporomandibular joint

A after removal of temporalis, the zygomatic arch, masseter and part of the mandible

B after removal of the lateral pterygoid

C after removal of the mandible and some adjacent neck structures

D from above, after removal of part of the floor of the middle cranial fossa

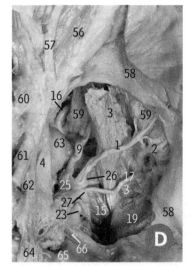

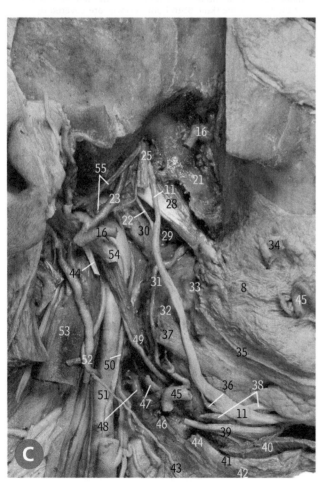

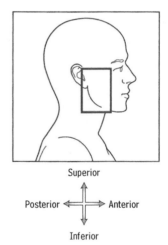

Superior

Posterior ⟷ Anterior

Inferior

A **B** **C**

Anterior

Medial ⟷ Lateral (right)

D Posterior

In A the removal of much of the ramus of the mandible displays the two pterygoid muscles and associated structures. The maxillary artery (16) runs obliquely upwards across the lateral pterygoid (15), and the lingual and inferior alveolar nerves (11 and 12) pass obliquely downwards over the medial pterygoid (10). Farther forward the buccal nerve (9) emerges between the two heads of the lateral pterygoid (3 and 15).

In B after removing the lateral pterygoid, the mandibular nerve (25) is seen just after emerging from the foramen ovale, with the chorda tympani (22) joining the back of the lingual nerve (11), as also seen more clearly in C, after removal of the whole mandible and the medial pterygoid.

The view in D looks down on the temporomandibular joint (19) from above after removing the floor of the lateral part of the middle cranial fossa. It shows temporal and masseteric nerves (1 and 17), running laterally above the upper head of the lateral pterygoid (3), with the buccal nerve (9) and the nerve to the lateral pterygoid (26) passing below this head; i.e. between the two heads (3 and 15).

The boundaries of the infratemporal fossa (see pages 16, A and 32):
- roof—the infratemporal surface of the greater wing of the sphenoid bone (bounded laterally by the infratemporal crest, page 16, A15), containing the foramen ovale and spinosum (page 16, A44 and 43), a small part of the squamous part of the temporal bone in front of the articular tubercle (page 16, A17), and laterally the gap between the zygomatic arch (page 16, A16) and the side of the skull (forming the communication between the temporal and infratemporal fossae)
- medially—the lateral pterygoid plate (pages 16, A14 and 20, A2)
- laterally—the ramus of the mandible (page 8, 30)
- in front—the infratemporal (posterior) surface of the maxilla (page 20, A5)
- behind—the styloid process and tympanic part of the temporal bone (page 8, 18 and 14)

The contents of the infratemporal fossa:
- the temporalis muscle and its insertion into the coronoid process (page 136, C3 and 16)
- the medial and lateral pterygoid muscles (A10 and 15)
- the pterygoid plexus of veins
- the maxillary artery and its branches (B16)
- the mandibular nerve and its branches (B25)
- the chorda tympani (C22)

In C the maxillary artery (upper 16) is seen passing through the pterygomaxillary fissure (page 20, A4) in front of the lateral pterygoid plate (21) to enter the pterygopalatine fossa. For the boundaries of the fossa, see page 75.

The contents of the pterygopalatine fossa:
- the maxillary artery (C, upper 16)
- the maxillary nerve (page 176, A2)
- the pterygopalatine ganglion (page 176, A4)

The medial and lateral pterygoid muscles both have an origin from the respective sides of the lateral pterygoid plate (page 18, 3, 4 and 6).

The lateral pterygoid helps to open the mouth by pulling the head of the mandible forwards on to the articular tubercle in front of the mandibular fossa (page 16, A17). The other muscles of the mastication group (medial pterygoid, temporalis and masseter) help to close it.

---

1 Deep temporal nerve
2 Deep temporal artery
3 Upper head of lateral pterygoid
4 Maxillary nerve
5 Posterior superior alveolar nerve
6 Posterior superior alveolar artery
7 Infratemporal surface of maxilla
8 Buccinator
9 Buccal nerve
10 Medial pterygoid
11 Lingual nerve
12 Inferior alveolar nerve
13 Inferior alveolar artery
14 Nerve to mylohyoid
15 Lower head of lateral pterygoid
16 Maxillary artery
17 Masseteric nerve
18 Articular disc and head of mandible ⎫ of temporomandibular joint
19 Capsule ⎭
20 Nerve to medial pterygoid
21 Lateral pterygoid plate
22 Chorda tympani
23 Middle meningeal artery
24 Accessory meningeal artery
25 Mandibular nerve
26 Nerve to lateral pterygoid
27 Auriculotemporal nerve
28 Tensor veli palatini
29 Levator veli palatini
30 Pharyngobasilar fascia
31 Ascending palatine artery
32 Superior constrictor of pharynx
33 Pterygomandibular raphe
34 Parotid duct
35 Mucoperiosteum of mandible
36 Submandibular ganglion
37 Styloglossus
38 Submandibular duct
39 Hypoglossal nerve
40 Mylohyoid
41 Tendon of digastric
42 Hyoid bone
43 Thyrohyoid and nerve
44 Stylohyoid
45 Facial artery
46 Hyoglossus
47 Stylohyoid ligament
48 Lingual artery
49 Stylopharyngeus and glossopharyngeal nerve
50 Ascending pharyngeal artery
51 Internal carotid artery
52 Hypoglossal nerve hooking round occipital artery and sternocleidomastoid branch
53 Internal jugular vein
54 Styloid process
55 Roots of auriculotemporal nerve
56 Posterior part of orbit
57 Frontal nerve
58 Floor of lateral part of middle cranial fossa
59 Temporalis
60 Optic nerve
61 Oculomotor nerve
62 Ophthalmic nerve
63 Sphenoidal sinus
64 Trigeminal nerve and ganglion
65 Petrous part of temporal bone
66 Greater petrosal nerve

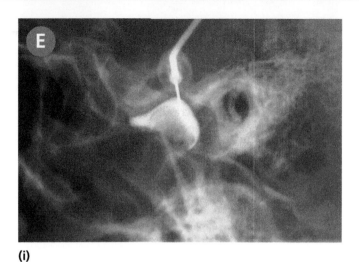

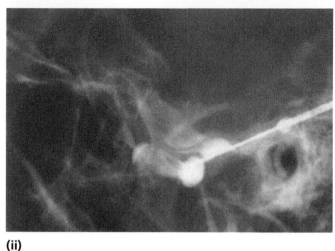

(i)   (ii)

E A radio-opaque dye has been injected into the lower joint space of the temporomandibular joint (TMJ), and these fluroscopic images show the (i) closed and (ii) dislocated position of the condyle. Note the dye ultimately escaping into the upper joint space

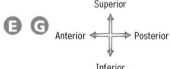

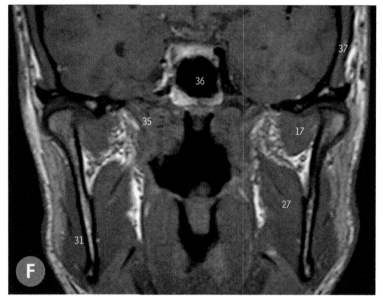

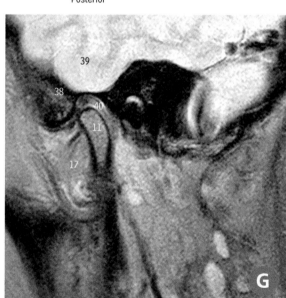

F Coronal T1-weighted magnetic resonance image (MRI) obtained in the closed-mouth position showing the normal TMJ

G Morphological appearances of the normal TMJ articular disc Sagittal oblique magnetic resonance image (MRI) (closed-mouth)

1 Auricular cartilage of ear	**14** Zygomatic process of temporal bone	**27** Medial pterygoid
2 External acoustic meatus	**15** Zygomatic bone	**28** Lateral pterygoid plate of sphenoid
3 Mastoid air cells	**16** Temporalis and tendon	**29** Tendon of temporalis
4 Cerebellar hemisphere	**17** Lateral pterygoid	**30** Coronoid process of mandible
5 Sigmoid sinus	**18** Trigeminal nerve V	**31** Masseter
6 Medulla	**19** Maxillary artery	**32** Lingual nerve
7 Basi-occiput	**20** Maxillary sinus	**33** Inferior alveolar nerve
8 Longus capitis	**21** Base of occipital condyle	**34** Styloid process
9 Internal carotid artery	**22** Tonsil of cerebellum	**35** Tensor veli palatini
10 Glossopharyngeal nerve IX, vagus nerve X and accessory nerve XI	**23** Spinal cord	**36** Sphenoid sinus
11 Condylar process of mandible	**24** Vertebral artery	**37** Temporalis
12 Articular disc of temporomandibular joint	**25** Opening of auditory (Eustachian) tube (arrowed)	**38** Articular disc
13 Superficial temporal artery and vein	**26** Nasal septum	**39** Temporal lobe of brain
		40 Posterior attachment of articular disc

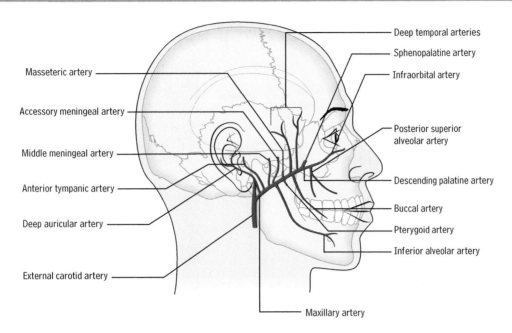

Deep temporal arteries

Sphenopalatine artery

Infraorbital artery

Masseteric artery

Accessory meningeal artery

Posterior superior alveolar artery

Middle meningeal artery

Anterior tympanic artery

Descending palatine artery

Deep auricular artery

Buccal artery

Pterygoid artery

Inferior alveolar artery

External carotid artery

Maxillary artery

H Diagram of the branches of the maxillary artery showing the blood supply to the maxillae; there are three portions—the mandibular, the pterygoid and the pterygopalatine

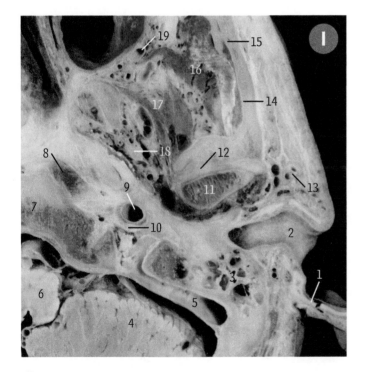

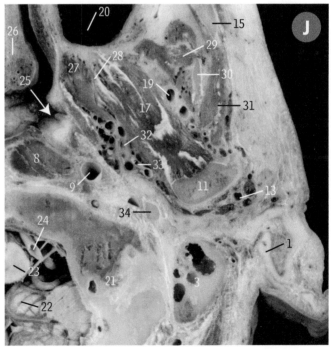

I axial section through the left temporomandibular joint, from below

J axial section through the left head of mandible, 1 cm below section I, from below

Orbit and eye Eye and lacrimal apparatus

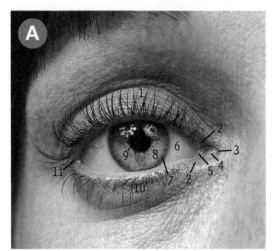

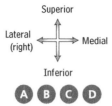

Superior

Lateral
(right) ⟷ Medial

Inferior

A B C D

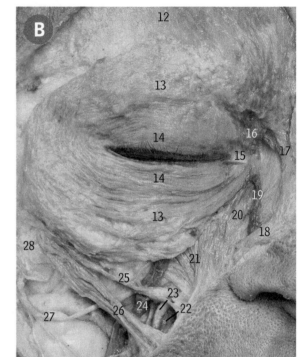

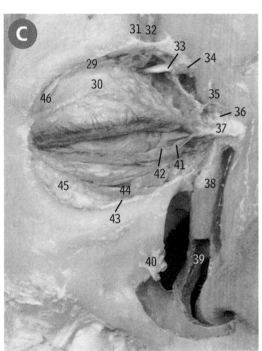

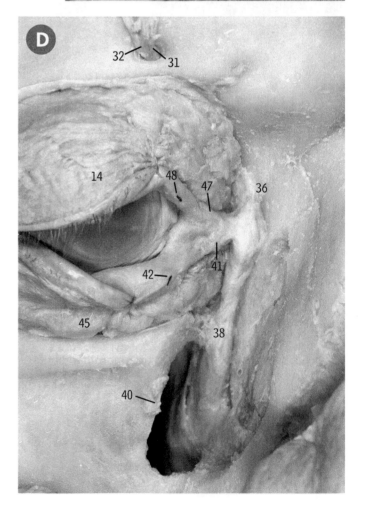

The eye

A surface features

B the orbicularis oculi muscle

C **D** the nasolacrimal duct

When looking straight ahead, as in A, the lower eyelid (10) is approximately level with the sclerocorneal junction (7), but the upper eyelid (1) is below the junction.

In B, skin and subcutaneous tissue have been removed to show orbicularis oculi (13 and 14), with the angular vein (19) beginning near the medial palpebral ligament (15).

In C, the facial muscles and part of the skull have been dissected away to display the nasolacrimal duct (38) opening into the inferior meatus of the nose (39; compare with page 160, B17).

In D (magnified), fine black bristles have been placed in the openings of the upper (48) and lower (42) lacrimal puncta.

The lacrimal apparatus consists of:
- the lacrimal gland (C46; page 148, A1)
- the upper and lower lacrimal puncta (C and D, 42, 48) opening into the lacrimal canaliculi (C and D, 41, 47)
- the lacrimal sac (C and D, 36) into which the canaliculi drain
- the nasolacrimal duct (C and D, 38), continuing downwards from the lacrimal sac and opening into the inferior meatus of the nose (page 160, B17)

Some connective tissues of the eye and orbit:
- Orbital septum—a thin sheet of tissue continuous with the periosteum at the orbital margin (C43), blending in the upper eyelid with the superficial lamella of the aponeurosis of levator palpebrae superioris (C30), and in the lower eyelid with the anterior surface of the tarsus.
- Lacrimal fascia—stretches between the anterior and posterior lacrimal crests, behind the medial palpebral ligament (C37) and covering the lacrimal sac (C36), being pierced by the lacrimal canaliculi (C41).
- Fascial sheath of the eyeball (Tenon's capsule)—envelops the eyeball from the optic nerve to the sclerocorneal junction. It is pierced by the ciliary vessels and nerves and the tendons of the eyeball muscles, being reflected on to each muscle as a sheath.
- Medial and lateral check ligaments—expansions of the sheath of the medial and lateral rectus muscles, attached to the posterior lacrimal crest (medial) and marginal tubercle (lateral) (page 34, A26 and 9).
- Suspensory ligament of the eyeball—the lower part of the sheath of the eyeball, between the medial and lateral check ligaments.
- Medial palpebral ligament (B15; C37)—from the medial ends of the two tarsi to the anterior lacrimal crest (page 34, A23) and the adjoining part of the frontal process of the maxilla. It lies in front of the lacrimal sac (C36) with the lacrimal fascia intervening.
- Lateral palpebral ligament—from the lateral ends of the two tarsi to the marginal tubercle (page 34, A9) where it is attached in front of the lateral check ligament and behind the lateral palpebral raphe. It is a less well-defined structure than the medial palpebral ligament.
- Lateral palpebral raphe—formed by the interlacing fibres of the palpebral part of orbicularis oculi (B14).

The angular vein (19, the name given to the uppermost end of the facial vein) lies in front of the medial palpebral ligament (B15, C37), and may cause haemorrhage during incisions to divide the ligament to expose the lacrimal sac (C36) which is behind the ligament.

1 Upper eyelid	**26** Zygomaticus major
2 Lacrimal papilla	**27** Buccal ⎫ branches of facial nerve
3 Medial angle (inner canthus)	**28** Zygomatic ⎭
4 Lacrimal caruncle	**29** Muscle fibres ⎫ of levator palpebrae superioris
5 Plica semilunaris	**30** Aponeurosis ⎭
6 Sclera with overlying conjunctiva	**31** Supra-orbital nerve
7 Sclerocorneal junction (limbus)	**32** Supra-orbital artery
8 Iris	**33** Tendon of superior oblique
9 Pupil	**34** Trochlea
10 Lower eyelid	**35** Dorsal nasal artery
11 Lateral angle (outer canthus)	**36** Lacrimal sac (upper extremity)
12 Frontal belly of occipitofrontalis	**37** Medial palpebral ligament
13 Orbital part ⎫ of orbicularis oculi	**38** Nasolacrimal duct
14 Palpebral part ⎭	**39** Opening of nasolacrimal duct (anterior wall removed) in inferior meatus of nose
15 Medial palpebral ligament	**40** Infra-orbital nerve
16 Depressor supercilii	**41** Lower lacrimal canaliculus
17 Procerus	**42** Lower lacrimal papilla and punctum
18 Nasalis	**43** Cut edge of orbital septum and periosteum
19 Angular vein	**44** Inferior oblique
20 Levator labii superioris alaeque nasi	**45** Orbital fat pad
21 Levator labii superioris	**46** Lacrimal gland
22 Levator anguli oris	**47** Upper lacrimal canaliculus
23 Facial artery	**48** Upper lacrimal papilla and punctum
24 Facial vein	
25 Zygomaticus minor	

Eye and lacrimal apparatus

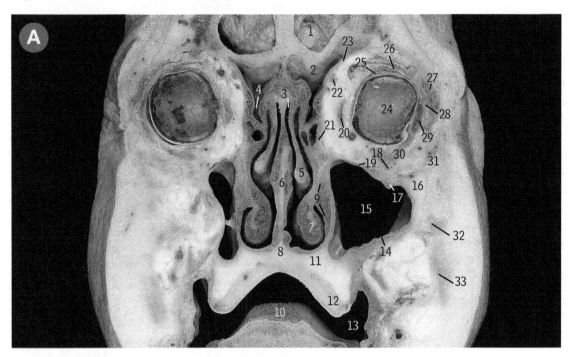

A   coronal section of head, at the level of the eyes, from the front

B   the same surface of section A (enlarged central area)

C   the surface of the opposing section (enlarged central area)

D **E**   diagrams of the right lacrimal passages

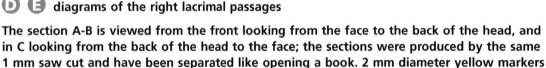

The section A-B is viewed from the front looking from the face to the back of the head, and in C looking from the back of the head to the face; the sections were produced by the same 1 mm saw cut and have been separated like opening a book. 2 mm diameter yellow markers have been placed in the opening tract of the nasolacrimal duct.

1 Frontal lobe of brain	**23** Orbital part of frontal bone
2 Frontal sinus	**24** Vitreous humour
3 Roof of nasal cavity	**25** Superior rectus
4 Infundibulum draining frontal sinus	**26** Levator palpebrae superioris
5 Middle nasal concha	**27** Lacrimal gland (orbital part)
6 Nasal septum	**28** Lacrimal gland (palpebral part)
7 Inferior nasal concha	**29** Lateral rectus
8 Hard palate	**30** Inferior oblique
9 Nasolacrimal duct—lower part opening into the inferior meatus	**31** Orbicularis oculi
10 Dorsum of tongue	**32** Zygomaticus minor
11 Palatine process of maxilla	**33** Zygomaticus major
12 Alveolar process of maxilla	**34** Middle meatus
13 Vestibule of mouth	**35** Inferior meatus
14 Maxilla	**36** Opening of nasolacrimal duct
15 Maxillary sinus	**37** Ethmoid air cells
16 Orbital margin of zygomatic bone	**38** Lacrimal sac
17 Infra-orbital artery and nerve within infra-orbital canal of maxilla	**39** Upper lacrimal canuliculus
	40 Upper lacrimal papilla and punctum
18 Inferior rectus	**41** Lower lacrimal papilla and punctum
19 Orbital surface of maxilla	**42** Lower lacrimal canuliculus
20 Medial rectus	**43** Lacrimal duct
21 Lacrimal bone	**44** Nasolacrimal duct—upper part merging with the lacrimal sac within the lacrimal canal
22 Tendon of superior oblique	

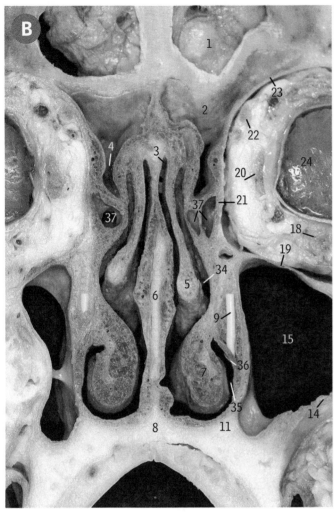

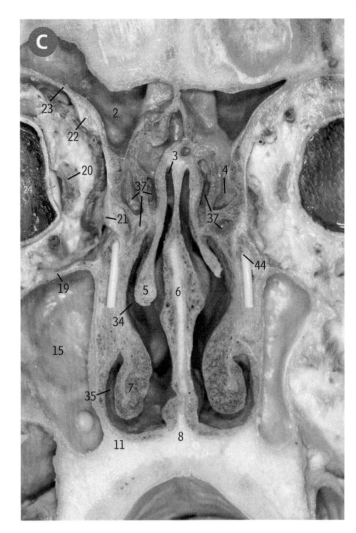

B

Superior

Right ⟷ Left

Inferior

C

Superior

Left ⟷ Right

Inferior

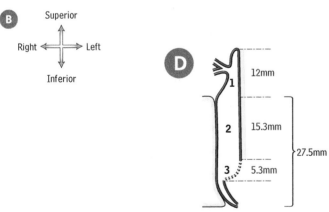

D

1 12mm

2 15.3mm

27.5mm

3 5.3mm

Diagram of the nasolacrimal duct divided into three parts according to external relations; with measurements (after Power and Aubaret)

1 Lacrimal sac
2 Nasolacrimal duct (interosseous part)
3 Nasolacrimal duct (meatal part)

The rare condition of prolongation of the passage below the opening is indicated by a dotted line.

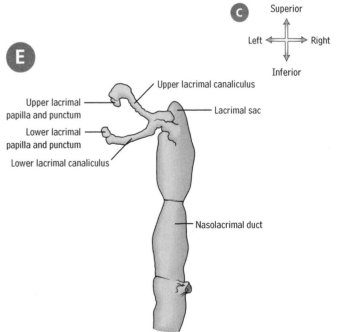

E

Upper lacrimal canaliculus

Upper lacrimal papilla and punctum

Lacrimal sac

Lower lacrimal papilla and punctum

Lower lacrimal canaliculus

Nasolacrimal duct

Orbit and eye *Orbital contents I*

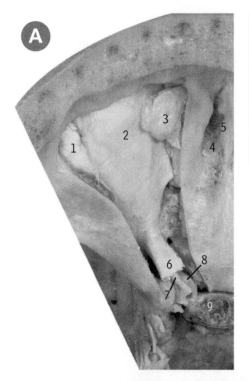

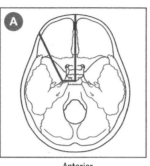

Anterior

Lateral
(left) ⟷ Medial

Posterior

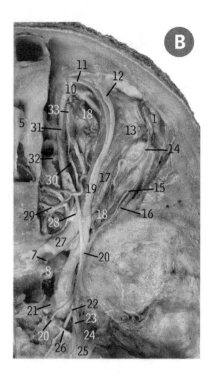

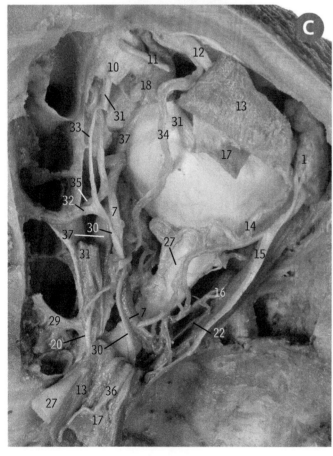

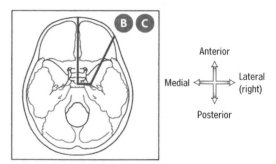

B C

Anterior

Medial ⟷ Lateral
(right)

Posterior

The orbits from above, and the extraocular muscles

Ⓐ the left orbit, after removal of the roof

Ⓑ superficial dissection of the right orbit

Ⓒ dissection of the right orbit (enlarged)

A is the view looking down from the anterior cranial fossa after removing bone of part of the floor of the fossa, i.e. the roof of the orbit. The orbital contents are embedded in a mass of orbital fat (2), with the lacrimal gland (1) at the anterolateral corner.

In B the contents of the orbit are shown from above after removal of the orbital fat. The frontal nerve (19) lies on top of levator palpebrae superioris (13), which in turn overlaps most of the superior rectus (17). The superior oblique (31), high on the medial wall with its nerve, the trochlear (20), and its tendon hooking through the trochlea (10), obscures the medial rectus, which is lower down and only seen when the superior oblique is removed (as in C37). The lateral rectus (16)

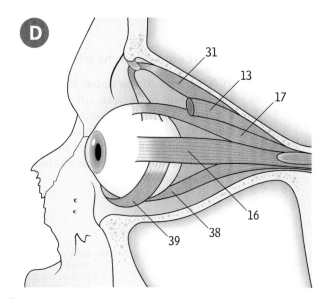

D diagram of the left extraocular muscles, from the left

lies along the lateral wall with the lacrimal nerve (15) above it, running to the gland (1) with the lacrimal artery (14).

In C (magnified), parts of levator palpebrae superioris (13) and the superior rectus (17) have been removed and reflected to show the optic nerve (27) being crossed superficially by the nasociliary nerve (30) and the ophthalmic artery (7). About halfway along the medial side of the orbit, the nasociliary nerve (30) gives off the anterior ethmoidal nerve (32) and then continues forwards as the infratrochlear nerve (33). At the bottom of the picture, the superior branch of the oculomotor nerve (36) is on the under surface of the proximal reflected part of the superior rectus (17), and on the lateral side the abducent nerve (22) enters the deep surface of the lateral rectus (16).

The diagram in D shows the extraocular muscles from the left side (the medial rectus is obscured by the eye and the lateral rectus).

1	Lacrimal gland	**21**	Oculomotor nerve
2	Orbital fat	**22**	Abducent nerve
3	Ethmoidal air cell	**23**	Ophthalmic nerve
4	Cribriform plate of ethmoid bone	**24**	Trigeminal ganglion
5	Crista galli	**25**	Trigeminal nerve
6	Dural sheath of optic nerve	**26**	Petrosphenoidal ligament
7	Ophthalmic artery	**27**	Optic nerve
8	Internal carotid artery	**28**	Common tendinous ring
9	Pituitary gland	**29**	Posterior ethmoidal artery
10	Trochlea	**30**	Nasociliary nerve
11	Supratrochlear nerve	**31**	Superior oblique
12	Supra-orbital nerve	**32**	Anterior ethmoidal nerve
13	Levator palpebrae superioris	**33**	Infratrochlear nerve
14	Lacrimal artery	**34**	Supra-orbital artery
15	Lacrimal nerve	**35**	Anterior ethmoidal artery
16	Lateral rectus	**36**	Superior branch of oculomotor nerve
17	Superior rectus		
18	Superior ophthalmic vein	**37**	Medial rectus
19	Frontal nerve	**38**	Inferior rectus
20	Trochlear nerve	**39**	Inferior oblique

The supra-orbital artery, which normally arises from the ophthalmic artery near the back of the orbit, as in C34, was absent in B.

Nerve supplies of the eye and eye muscles:

Motor to eye muscles:
- Lateral rectus (C16) by the abducent nerve (C22)
- Superior oblique (B31) by the trochlear nerve (B20)
- All other muscles by the oculomotor nerve: superior rectus (B and C, 17) by the superior branch (C36, which also supplies levator palpebrae superioris, B and C, 13), and inferior rectus, inferior oblique and medial rectus by the inferior branch (page 152, A19, 17, 18 and 15)

Sensory:
- To the cornea: long and short ciliary nerves (page 152, A28)
- To the conjunctiva: lacrimal, supra-orbital, supratrochlear, infratrochlear and infra-orbital (the same nerves that supply the skin of the eyelids)

Individual eye muscles turn the eye as follows:
- Lateral rectus: out
- Medial rectus: in
- Superior rectus: up and in
- Inferior rectus: down and in
- Superior oblique: out, and down when turned in
- Inferior oblique: out, and up when turned in

The superior and inferior recti not only turn the eye upwards or downwards, respectively, but also assist the medial rectus in turning it inwards. This is because the insertions of the superior and inferior recti on the eye lie medial to the vertical axis.

The superior and inferior oblique muscles not only turn the eye downwards or upwards, respectively, but also outwards. This is because their insertions lie lateral to the vertical axis. However, it must be noted that the *depressor* action of the *superior* oblique and the *elevator* action of the *inferior* oblique can only occur when the eye is turned in.

Levator palpebrae superioris contains some smooth muscle fibres which receive a sympathetic nerve supply.

Apart from the six muscles that move the eye (the four recti and two obliques) and the levator palpebrae superioris, there is an eighth muscle within the orbit, the orbitalis. It consists of smooth muscle that bridges over the infra-orbital groove and inferior orbital fissure (page 34, A15 and 11), and although large in some animals it is an unimportant vestigial structure in the human orbit.

Lesions of the motor nerves to the eye muscles all give varying degrees of diplopia (double vision) and strabismus (squint).

Oculomotor nerve paralysis:
- The upper eyelid droops (ptosis), closing the eye, due to paralysis of levator labii superioris (the part of the levator supplied by sympathetic fibres is not sufficient to keep the eye open).
- When the upper eyelid is lifted up, the eye is seen to be looking outwards and slightly downwards, due to the unopposed action of the lateral rectus (abducent nerve) and superior oblique (trochlear nerve).
- The eye cannot look straight upwards or downwards or inwards, due to paralysis of the superior, inferior and medial recti.
- The pupil is dilated and does not react to light or on accommodation, due to interruption of the parasympathetic fibres from the Edinger-Westphal nucleus that run in the oculomotor nerve to the ciliary ganglion and which normally act to constrict the pupil.

Trochlear nerve paralysis:
- There is a weakness when looking downwards with the eye turned in, due to paralysis of the superior oblique.

Abducent nerve paralysis:
- The eye cannot look outwards, due to paralysis of the lateral rectus, and is deviated inwards by the unopposed action of the medial, superior and inferior recti (oculomotor nerve).

Orbit and eye *Orbital contents II*

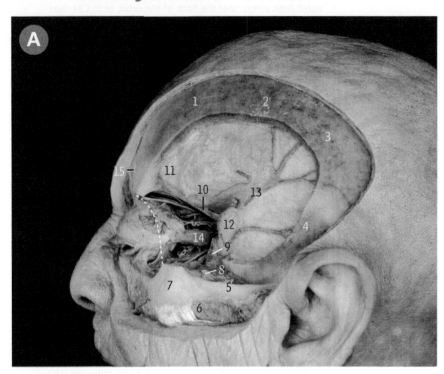

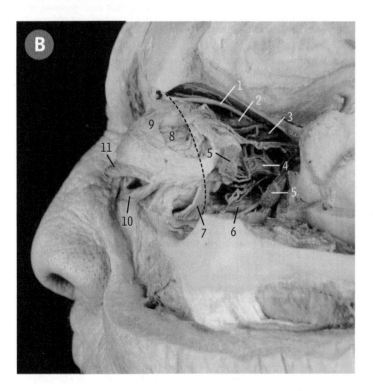

The left orbit, from the left

In A-B bones of the upper left front side of skull have been cut away to expose the dural covering of the cerebral hemisphere, as have part of the roof and lateral wall of the orbit to display the eyeball and associated structures in situ.

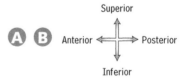

A

1 Frontal bone
2 Coronal suture
3 Parietal bone
4 Temporal bone
5 Zygomatic arch
6 Masseter
7 Zygomatic bone
8 Temporalis
9 Greater wing of sphenoid bone
10 Orbital part of frontal bone
11 Dura mater overlying frontal pole of cerebral hemisphere
12 Dura mater overlying temporal pole of cerebral hemisphere
13 Frontal branch of middle meningeal artery
14 Lateral rectus
15 Supra-orbital nerve emerging from supra-orbital notch

A   B   Anterior ⟷ Posterior / Superior ↕ Inferior

B

1 Supra-orbital nerve
2 Levator palpebrae superioris
3 Superior rectus
4 Optic nerve
5 Lateral rectus (divided and reflected laterally)
6 Inferior rectus
7 Inferior oblique
8 Lacrimal gland
9 Aponeurosis of levator palpebrae superioris
10 Lower eyelid
11 Upper eyelid

Orbit and eye *Orbital contents II*

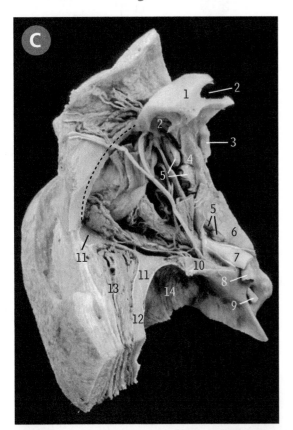

The left orbit, optic nerve and ciliary ganglion, from the left and above

In C-D bones that form the roof and lateral wall of the orbit have been cut away to expose the eyeball and associated structures within the orbit; levator palpebrae superioris and superior rectus have been cut and reflected superiorly to expose the optic nerve and on its lateral outer surface the ciliary ganglion which is approximately 2 mm in diameter.

C

1	Frontal bone	8	Internal carotid artery
2	Frontal sinus	9	Oculomotor nerve
3	Crista galli of ethmoid bone	10	Lesser wing of sphenoid bone
4	Cribriform plate of ethmoid bone	11	Greater wing of sphenoid bone
5	Ethmoidal air cells	12	Temporal bone
6	Jugum of sphenoid bone	13	Temporalis
7	Optic nerve	14	Anterior part of middle cranial fossa

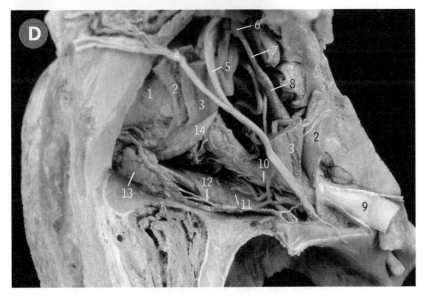

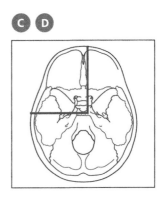

Anterior   Medial

Lateral
(left)   Posterior

D

1	Superior outer surface of eyeball	8	Superior oblique
2	Levator palpebrae superioris	9	Optic nerve
3	Superior rectus	10	Ciliary ganglion
4	Supra-orbital nerve	11	Lateral rectus
5	Supratrochlear nerve	12	Lacrimal nerve
6	Trochlea	13	Lacrimal gland
7	Tendon of superior oblique	14	Posterior outer surface of eyeball

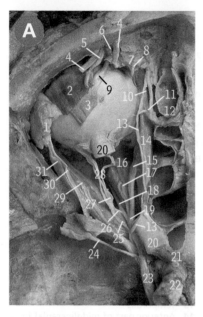

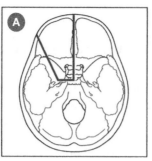

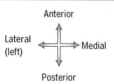

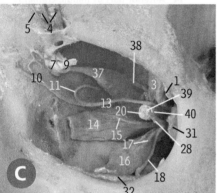

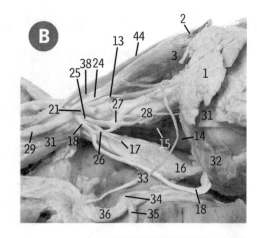

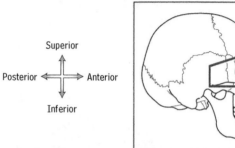

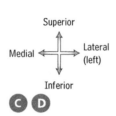

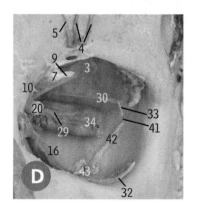

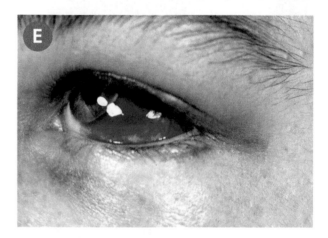

The ciliary ganglion and dissection from the front

A the left orbit and ciliary ganglion, from above

B the right orbit and ciliary ganglion, from the right

C the left orbit, from the front and the left

D the left orbit, from the front and the right

E following fracture of the orbital rim and breach of the periosteum, a subconjunctival haemorrhage may result which extends posteriorly around the globe. It appears red as oxygen diffuses through the conjunctiva

In **A** removal of the superior oblique (seen high on the lateral wall; C37) enables the lateral rectus to be seen (31), with its nerve, the abducent (29). Removal of much of the optic nerve (20) displays the inferior rectus (16) with its nerve (17) and the nerves to the medial rectus (15) and inferior oblique (18); these three nerves are all branches of the inferior branch of the oculomotor nerve (19).

In **B** with the lateral wall of the orbit removed, the ciliary ganglion (27) is shown, lying lateral to the optic nerve (20) near the back of the orbit.

The views in **C** and **D** show muscles and nerves in relation to the orbital walls after removal of the eye. In **C** note the extension of the subarachnoid space (39) and the dural sheath (40) round the optic nerve (20). In **B** the zygomatic branch of the maxillary nerve has been removed, and the communicating branch (33) with the lacrimal nerve (30) has arisen directly from the maxillary nerve (36).

1 Lacrimal gland
2 Levator palpebrae superioris
3 Superior rectus
4 Supra-orbital nerve
5 Supra-orbital artery
6 Superior ophthalmic vein
7 Trochlea
8 Supratrochlear nerve
9 Tendon of superior oblique
10 Infratrochlear nerve
11 Anterior ethmoidal nerve
12 Ethmoidal air cell
13 Nasociliary nerve
14 Medial rectus
15 Nerve to medial rectus
16 Inferior rectus
17 Nerve to inferior rectus
18 Nerve to inferior oblique
19 Inferior branch of oculomotor nerve
20 Optic nerve
21 Ophthalmic artery
22 Internal carotid artery
23 Oculomotor nerve
24 Superior branch of oculomotor nerve
25 Nasociliary root of ciliary ganglion
26 Oculomotor (parasympathetic) root of ciliary ganglion
27 Ciliary ganglion
28 Short ciliary nerves
29 Abducent nerve
30 Lacrimal nerve
31 Lateral rectus
32 Inferior oblique
33 Communication between **30** and **36** (in **B**) or **42** (in **D**)
34 Infra-orbital nerve
35 Infra-orbital artery
36 Maxillary nerve
37 Superior oblique
38 Trochlear nerve
39 Subarachnoid space
40 Dural sheath of optic nerve
41 Zygomatico-orbital foramen
42 Zygomatic nerve
43 Inferior orbital fissure
44 Frontal nerve

Ciliary nerves:
- The short ciliary nerves (A and B, 28, eight to ten in number) are branches from the ciliary ganglion (B27) that contain postganglionic parasympathetic fibres for the pupillary and ciliary muscles. They also contain afferent fibres from the eye, including the cornea.
- The long ciliary nerves (two or three in number, here removed) are branches of the nasociliary nerve (A and B, 13) and contain afferent fibres from the eye, including the cornea.

Ciliary arteries (here removed to display the more important nerves):
- The *anterior* ciliary arteries (variable in number) are so named because they arise near the front of the orbit from muscular branches of the ophthalmic artery, and run to the front of the eyeball along the tendon of the rectus muscles.
- The *posterior* ciliary arteries are so named because they arise near the back of the orbit.
- The *short posterior* ciliary arteries (about seven in number) run from the ophthalmic artery along the outside of the dural sheath of the optic nerve and divide into further branches before piercing the sclera near the nerve.
- The *long posterior* ciliary arteries (usually two) pass from the ophthalmic artery to pierce the sclera on either side of the optic nerve.

The four parasympathetic ganglia in the head and neck:
- The ciliary ganglion (B27), lying at the back of the orbit on the lateral side of the optic nerve about 8 mm in front of the opening of the optic canal;
- The pterygopalatine ganglion (page 176, A4) in the pterygopalatine fossa below the maxillary nerve;
- The otic ganglion (page 176, A11) on the medial side of the mandibular nerve just below the foramen ovale.
- The submandibular ganglion (page 176, A40) below the lingual nerve on the outer surface of hyoglossus.

The pupillary light reflexes:
- The direct pupillary light reflex—shining a light into one eye causes the pupil of that eye to constrict.
- The indirect (consensual) pupillary light reflex—shining a light into one eye causes the pupil of the opposite eye to constrict.
- The pathway for the pupillary light reflexes: from the retina by the optic nerve, chiasma and tract to the pretectal nucleus (synapse) at the level of the superior colliculus, then to the Edinger-Westphal part of the oculomotor nucleus and by the inferior division of the oculomotor nerve and the branch to the inferior oblique to reach the ciliary ganglion (synapse), and then by short ciliary nerves to the sphincter pupillae. The pupils of both eyes constrict because (a) some fibres cross in the optic chiasma, and (b) fibres from the pretectal nucleus pass to the Edinger-Westphal nuclei of both sides.

The accommodation-convergence (near) reflex: for looking at near objects the eye is focused by adjustment of the lens by the ciliary muscles (accommodation), the pupil constricts, and the eyes converge by contraction of both medial rectus muscles. These combined reflexes are sometimes collectively called the near reflex.

The probable pathways for the near reflex:
- For accommodation: from the visual cortex by the posterior limb of the internal capsule to the Edinger-Westphal nucleus (*not* via the pretectal nucleus) and so to the ciliary ganglion, sphincter pupillae and ciliary muscle as for the pupillary light reflexes.
- For convergence: from the visual cortex by association fibres to the frontal eye field (middle frontal gyrus) (synapse), then by the anterior limb of the internal capsule to those cell bodies of the oculomotor nucleus that supply the medial rectus.

Orbit and eye *Orbital contents III*

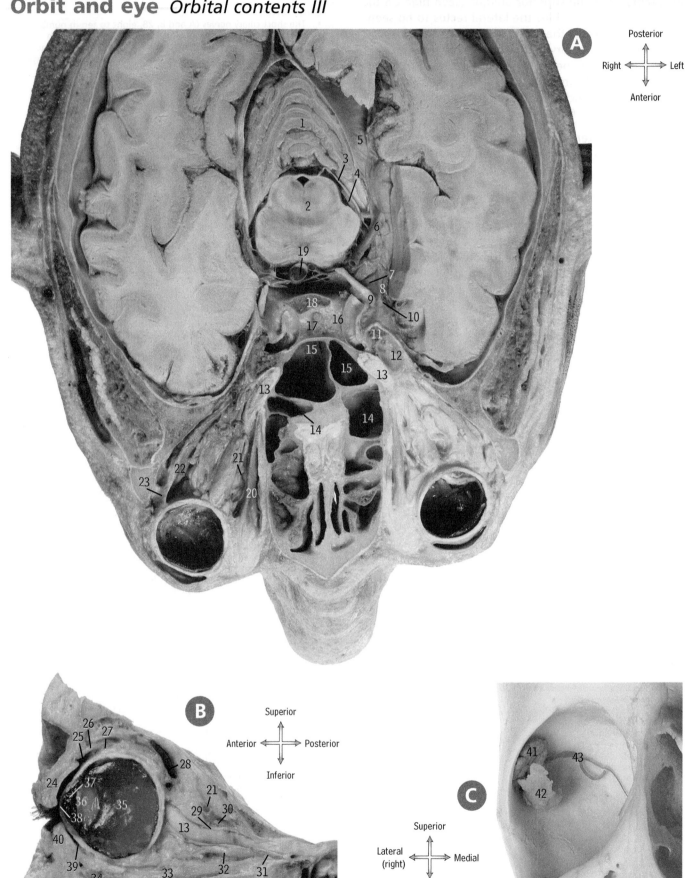

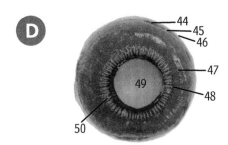

The eyes in section and the lacrimal gland

A transverse section through the orbits and the nasal and cranial cavities, from above

B sagittal section through the right orbit, from the left

C an isolated right lacrimal gland, replaced within the orbit, from the left and below

D the anterior half of an eye sectioned through the equator, from behind (enlarged)

E the section in D with the lens removed and placed at the side (enlarged)

In A the section has passed through the eyes just above the optic nerves (13) which, at the back of the orbits, lie immediately adjacent to the sphenoidal sinuses (15) and the most posterior ethmoidal air cells (14).

In B the vertically sectioned eye shows the extent of the conjunctival fornices (25 and 39) with the lids almost closed (24 and 40).

In C the right lacrimal gland has been dissected free from all other structures apart from the lacrimal artery and nerve (43), to emphasise its position in the upper outer corner of the front of the orbit.

In D and E (enlarged) the eye has been sectioned through the equator, i.e. in the coronal plane, and the front half is viewed from behind. In D the lens (49) is in place, and in E it has been removed and placed at one side to show the margin of the pupil (51) and the posterior surface of the cornea (52).

The *lacrimal gland* has an upper (larger) orbital part (C41) and a lower (smaller) palpebral part (C42), continuous with each other round the lateral (concave) border of the aponeurosis of levator palpebrae superioris.
- The orbital part lies in the lacrimal fossa of the frontal bone (page 34, B13), above the levator (page 148, A1).
- The palpebral part lies below the levator and extends into the lateral part of the upper eyelid (page 144, C46).
- About 12 small ducts open into the superior conjunctival fornix (B25)—those from the orbital part passing through the palpebral part.

The pathway for lacrimal gland secretion: from the superior salivary nucleus by the nervus intermedius part of the facial nerve, greater petrosal nerve and nerve of the pterygoid canal to the pterygopalatine ganglion (synapse), and then to the gland by the maxillary nerve, its zygomatic branch and the communication with the lacrimal nerve.

The tarsi are plates of dense fibrous tissue within each eyelid.

1	Cerebellum	
2	Junction of pons and midbrain	
3	Trochlear nerve	
4	Superior cerebellar artery	
5	Tentorium cerebelli	
6	Posterior cerebral artery	
7	Attached margin of tentorium cerebelli	
8	Roof of cavernous sinus	
9	Oculomotor nerve	
10	Free margin of tentorium cerebelli	
11	Anterior clinoid process	
12	Extension of posterior ethmoidal air cell into lesser wing of sphenoid bone	
13	Optic nerve	
14	Posterior ethmoidal air cell	
15	Sphenoidal sinus	
16	Diaphragma sellae	
17	Pituitary stalk	
18	Dorsum sellae	
19	Basilar artery	
20	Medial rectus	
21	Ophthalmic artery	
22	Lateral rectus	
23	Lateral check ligament	
24	Superior tarsus in upper eyelid	
25	Superior conjunctival fornix	
26	Levator palpebrae superioris	
27	Tendon of superior rectus	
28	Superior ophthalmic vein	
29	Dural sheath of optic nerve	
30	Nasociliary nerve	
31	Central artery of retina	
32	Inferior ophthalmic vein	
33	Inferior rectus	
34	Inferior oblique	
35	Vitreous humour	
36	Lens	
37	Anterior chamber	
38	Cornea	
39	Inferior conjunctival fornix	
40	Inferior tarsus in lower eyelid	
41	Orbital part } of lacrimal gland	
42	Palpebral part }	
43	Lacrimal artery and nerve	
44	Retina (optic part)	
45	Choroid	
46	Sclera	
47	Ora serrata	
48	Ciliary part of retina	
49	Posterior surface of lens	
50	Ciliary processes	
51	Margin of pupil	
52	Posterior surface of cornea	
53	Aponeurosis of levator palpebrae superioris	

F an isolated right lacrimal gland shown actual size as presented at dissection, from above

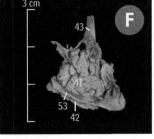

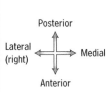

Nose, oral cavity, pharynx, ear and larynx

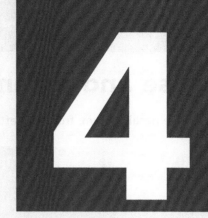

Nose and paranasal sinuses

A the nasal septum, from the left

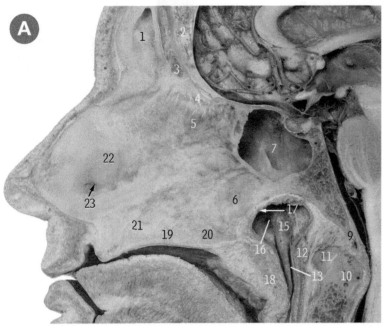

B the skeleton of the external nose, from the left

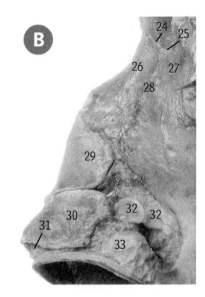

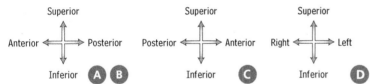

Superior	Superior	Superior
Anterior ⟷ Posterior	Posterior ⟷ Anterior	Right ⟷ Left
Inferior **A** **B**	Inferior **C**	Inferior **D**

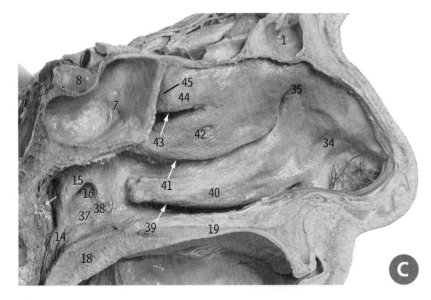

C the lateral wall of the left nasal cavity and nasopharynx

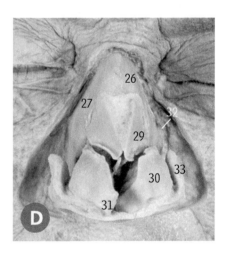

D the skeleton of the external nose, from the front

Nasal cavity *The nasal cartilages and the nasal cavity*

In A the nasal septum is intact, while in C it has been removed to show the lateral wall of the nasal cavity with the conchae (44, 42 and 40), each with an underlying meatus (43, 41 and 39). The specimen in E shows the occasional supreme concha and meatus (46 and 47). The upper bony and lower cartilaginous parts of the external nose are illustrated in B and D.

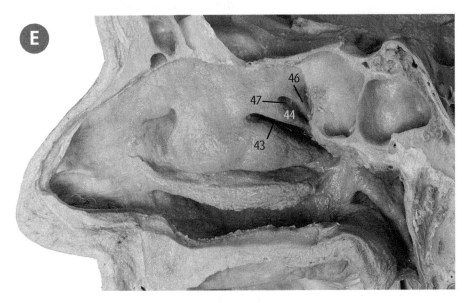

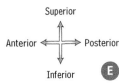

Superior

Anterior ⟷ Posterior

Inferior **E**

E **as C, with a supreme nasal concha**

The nose consists of the external nose (on the face) and the nasal cavity. The cavity is divided into right and left halves by the nasal septum, and each half contains olfactory, vestibular and respiratory parts, depending on the type of mucous membrane present. The olfactory part occupies the area over the superior concha on the lateral wall, and the adjacent parts of the roof and of the septum level with the superior concha; it contains olfactory nerve endings as well as fibres for ordinary sensation. The vestibular part is the small area just inside the nostril, and is lined by hairy skin. The large remaining area is the respiratory part, lined by respiratory mucous membrane with pseudostratified columnar ciliated epithelium and mucous glands.

The main parts of the skeleton of the external nose are the nasal bone (B26), and the lateral, greater and lesser nasal cartilages (B29, 30 and 32).

The main parts of the nasal septum are the vomer (A6) and the perpendicular plate of the ethmoid (A5), both of bone, and the septal cartilage (A22).

The nasal conchae are on the lateral wall of the cavity. The superior and middle nasal conchae are part of the ethmoid bone (page 44, C12 and 10); the inferior nasal concha is a separate bone (page 53, G-J).

1 Frontal sinus	**17** Right choana (posterior nasal aperture)	**33** Fibrofatty tissue
2 Falx cerebri	**18** Soft palate	**34** Atrium
3 Crista galli	**19** Hard palate	**35** Agger nasi
4 Cribriform plate of ethmoid bone and filaments of olfactory nerve	**20** Nasal crest of palatine bone	**36** Vestibule
5 Perpendicular plate of ethmoid bone	**21** Nasal crest of maxilla	**37** Levator elevation
6 Vomer	**22** Septal cartilage	**38** Salpingopalatal fold
7 Sphenoidal sinus	**23** Vomeronasal organ	**39** Inferior meatus
8 Pituitary gland	**24** Frontonasal suture	**40** Inferior nasal concha
9 Anterior margin of foramen magnum	**25** Frontomaxillary suture	**41** Middle meatus
10 Dens of axis	**26** Nasal bone	**42** Middle nasal concha
11 Anterior arch of atlas	**27** Frontal process of maxilla	**43** Superior meatus
12 Pharyngeal tonsil	**28** Nasomaxillary suture	**44** Superior nasal concha
13 Pharyngeal recess	**29** Lateral nasal cartilage	**45** Spheno-ethmoidal recess
14 Salpingopharyngeal fold	**30** Greater nasal cartilage	**46** Supreme nasal concha
15 Tubal elevation	**31** Septal process (medial crus) of greater nasal cartilage	**47** Supreme meatus
16 Opening of auditory tube	**32** Lesser alar cartilages	

Nasal cavity *The walls of the nasal cavity*

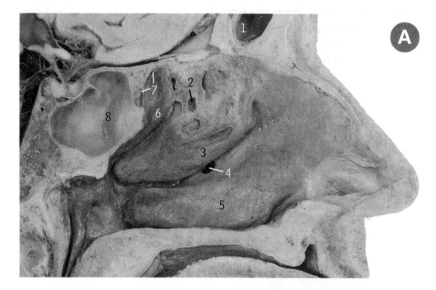

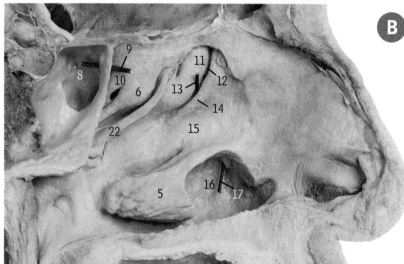

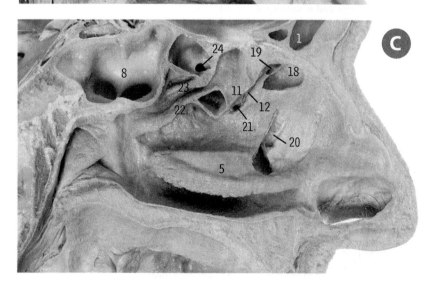

A the left lateral wall

B the left lateral wall and semilunar hiatus

C the left lateral wall and apertures of sinuses

D the right lateral wall and nasal nerves

1 Frontal sinus
2 A middle ethmoidal air cell
3 Middle nasal concha
4 Unusually low aperture of maxillary sinus
5 Inferior nasal concha
6 Superior nasal concha
7 Spheno-ethmoidal recess
8 Sphenoidal sinus
9 Bristle in aperture of sphenoidal sinus
10 Supreme nasal concha
11 Ethmoidal bulla
12 Semilunar hiatus
13 Bristle in aperture of maxillary sinus
14 Mucous membrane overlying uncinate process of ethmoid bone
15 Middle meatus
16 Inferior meatus
17 Bristle in opening of nasolacrimal duct
18 An anterior ethmoidal air cell
19 Frontonasal duct
20 Lower end of nasolacrimal duct
21 Aperture of maxillary sinus
22 Base of middle nasal concha
23 Base of superior nasal concha
24 Aperture of a posterior ethmoidal air cell
25 Olfactory nerve filaments
26 Sphenopalatine artery and foramen
27 Pterygopalatine ganglion
28 A lateral posterior superior nasal nerve
29 Greater palatine nerve and canal
30 A posterior inferior nasal nerve
31 Vestibule of nose
32 Anterior ethmoidal nerve

Superior

Posterior ⟷ Anterior

Inferior

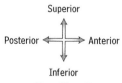

In cutting the section in A the superior nasal concha and the upper part of the middle concha have been shaved off. The opening of the maxillary sinus (4) is unusually low and large.

In B the middle concha has been removed to show the semilunar hiatus (12) bounded above by the ethmoidal bulla (11) and below by the ridge caused by the uncinate process of the ethmoid bone (14) (compare with page 34, D61 and 46). Removal of the front part of the inferior concha (5) reveals the opening of the nasolacrimal duct (17).

In C parts of all three nasal conchae have been removed to show an ethmoidal air cell aperture (24), the frontonasal duct (19) and the nasolacrimal duct (20).

In D mucous membrane high on the lateral wall has been dissected away to show filaments of the olfactory nerve (25) and the anterior ethmoidal nerve (32). Some bone at the back of the lateral wall has been removed to display the pterygopalatine ganglion (27), seen in the pterygopalatine fossa by looking through the sphenopalatine foramen (26), with the greater palatine nerve (29) running down from the ganglion, and other nasal nerves passing forwards (28 and 30).

For details of the sinuses see pages 162–165.

Drainage of the sinuses:
- Frontal sinus—into the middle meatus by the frontonasal duct (C19)
- Ethmoidal sinus—anterior ethmoidal air cells into the frontonasal duct or the infundibulum (the upward anterior continuation of the semilunar hiatus, B12); middle ethmoidal air cells on or above the ethmoidal bulla in the middle meatus (B11); and posterior ethmoidal air cells into the superior meatus (C24)
- Sphenoidal sinus—into the spheno-ethmoidal recess (B9 and A7)
- Maxillary sinus—into the semilunar hiatus in the middle meatus (B13 and C21)

Drainage into the meatuses:
- Superior meatus—posterior ethmoidal air cells (C24)
- Middle meatus—frontal sinus (C1 and 19), anterior and middle ethmoidal air cells (A2), and the maxillary sinus (C21)
- Inferior meatus—nasolacrimal duct (C20)
- Spheno-ethmoidal recess—sphenoidal sinus (B8)

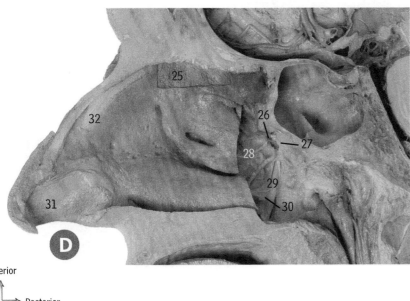

Superior

Anterior ⟵⟶ Posterior

Inferior

Paranasal sinuses

The frontal and ethmoidal sinuses, in sections of parts of the skull

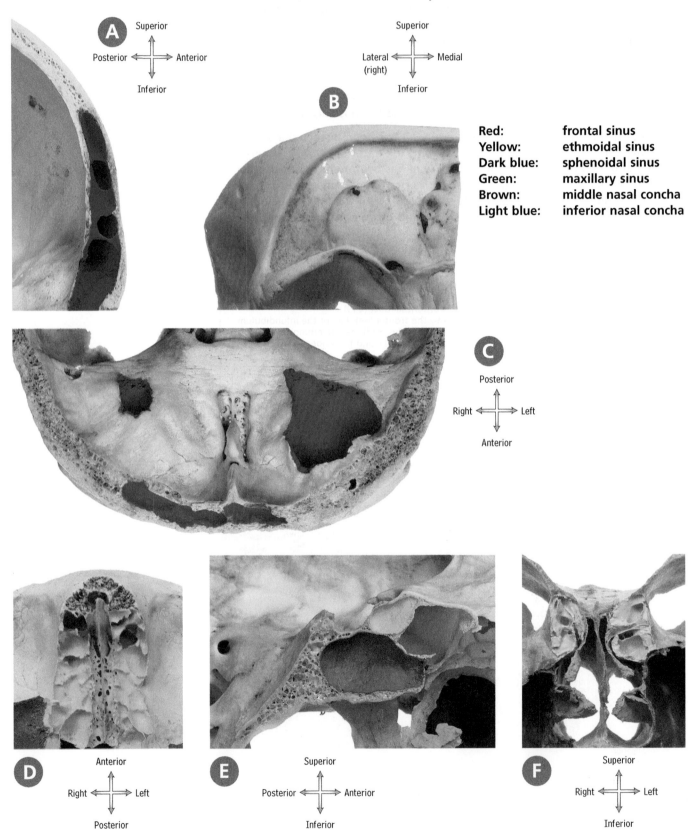

A

Superior

Posterior ←→ Anterior

Inferior

B

Superior

Lateral (right) ←→ Medial

Inferior

Red:	frontal sinus
Yellow:	ethmoidal sinus
Dark blue:	sphenoidal sinus
Green:	maxillary sinus
Brown:	middle nasal concha
Light blue:	inferior nasal concha

C

Posterior

Right ←→ Left

Anterior

D

Anterior

Right ←→ Left

Posterior

E

Superior

Posterior ←→ Anterior

Inferior

F

Superior

Right ←→ Left

Inferior

In A the frontal sinus has extended far up into the squamous part of the frontal bone.

In B the front of the skull and diploë have been dissected away to show the bony wall of a sinus.

In C parts of the floor of the anterior cranial fossa have been removed to show frontal sinuses extending far back in the orbital part of the frontal bone (over the roof of the orbit).

In D the cribriform plates of the ethmoid bone (in the roof of the nose, with many foramina) are seen adjacent to air cells of the ethmoidal sinuses, whose roofs are formed by the orbital parts of the frontal

bone (compare with page 42, B19). In the left sinus some anterior ethmoidal air cells lie in front of the lowest part of the frontal sinus (red).

In E, a midline sagittal section, two large posterior ethmoidal air cells overlap the left sphenoidal sinus (blue).

In F, a coronal section through the centre of the nasal and orbital cavities and looking from the front towards the back of the skull, the middle nasal conchae (brown) on each side overlaps the bulging ethmoidal air cell that forms the ethmoidal bulla (compare with page 44, F13).

(A) a large left frontal sinus in sagittal section, from the right

(B) a right frontal sinus dissected out of the diploë, from the front

(C) large frontal sinuses opened from above

(D) the roof of the ethmoidal sinuses, from below

(E) a midline sagittal section through the base of the skull, with unusually large left posterior ethmoidal air cells

(F) the ethmoidal sinuses in coronal section, from the front

(G) coronal computed tomogram (CT) through the nose and paranasal sinuses

---

There are four pairs of *paranasal air sinuses:* frontal, ethmoidal, sphenoidal and maxillary. The two of each pair (left and right) are rarely symmetrical and vary greatly in size and shape.

The *frontal sinus* lies in the lower part of the squamous part of the frontal bone (as in B), and may extend higher into the squamous part (as in A) and back into the orbital part of the bone (as in C). It drains into the middle meatus by the frontonasal duct (page 160, C19).

The *ethmoidal sinus* occupies the body of the ethmoid bone (ethmoidal labyrinth, page 44, A1). It is divided by bony septa into a number of ethmoidal air cells (3 to 18). The posterior ethmoidal air cells drain into the superior meatus (page 160, C24), and the middle and anterior air cells into the middle meatus (see notes on page 161). The thin lateral wall of the ethmoidal labyrinth (page 44, E8) forms part of the medial wall of the orbit (page 63, D and E, 20). The medial wall of the labyrinth has the superior and middle nasal conchae projecting from it (page 44, C and D, 10 and 12).

For the *sphenoidal* and *maxillary sinuses* see pages 164 and 165.

For a summary of the drainage of the sinuses see page 161.

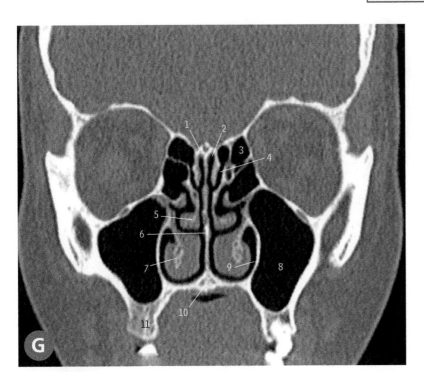

1 Cribiform plate of ethmoid
2 Roof of nasal cavity
3 Ethmoidal air cells
4 Infundibulum draining frontal sinus
5 Middle nasal concha
6 Nasal septum
7 Inferior nasal concha
8 Maxillary sinus
9 Inferior nasal meatus
10 Hard palate
11 Alveolar process of maxilla

Superior
Right ⟵ ⟶ Left
Inferior

Paranasal sinuses

The sphenoidal and maxillary sinuses, in sections of parts of the skull

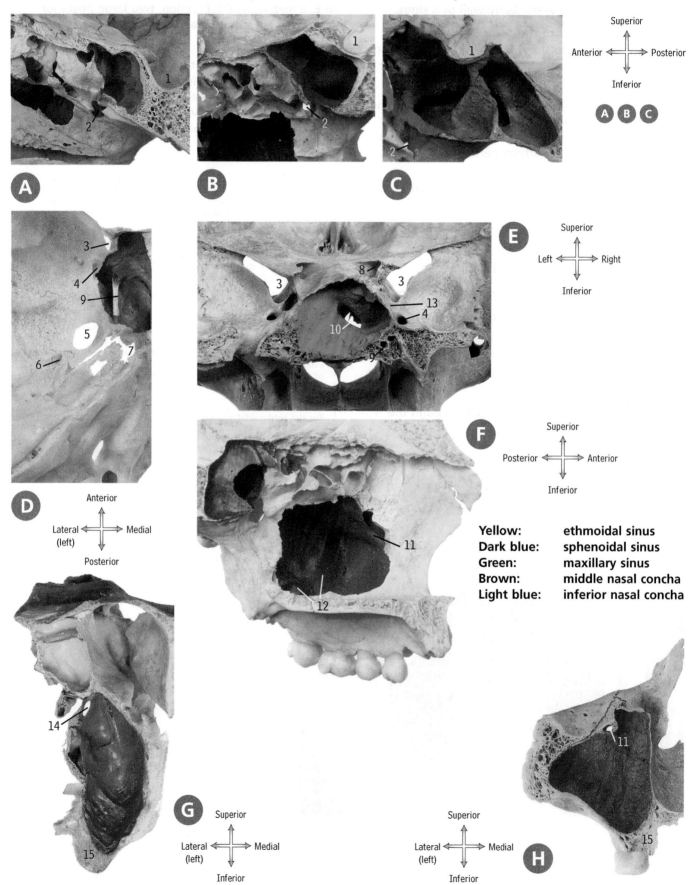

Yellow: ethmoidal sinus
Dark blue: sphenoidal sinus
Green: maxillary sinus
Brown: middle nasal concha
Light blue: inferior nasal concha

Small sphenoidal sinuses (as in A) usually lie in front of the pituitary fossa (1), with larger ones extending below the fossa (as in B) and even backwards into the basisphenoid (as in C). In D a large left sinus has been opened up from above and part of the floor dissected away to show the pterygoid canal (9), which lies below the floor; compare with the section of the right sinus in E. In the coronal section in E there is a large right sinus with its aperture visible at the front (10), and a very small left sinus, seen level with the medial

end of the superior orbital fissure (3). In F the maxillary sinus shows indentations of the bony wall produced by the roots of molar teeth (12), and by the infra-orbital canal (11) whose relation to the roof of the sinus is shown in the coronal section H. In G and H the sinus extends into the alveolar process of the maxilla (15), but the smaller sinus in J has not done so. The section in G shows the aperture of the sinus, high up on the medial wall (14).

A a small right sphenoidal sinus, in a midline sagittal section, from the left

B a medium-sized right sphenoidal sinus, sectioned as in A

C a large right sphenoidal sinus, sectioned as in A

D the floor of the left sphenoidal sinus, from above

E sphenoidal sinuses in coronal section, from behind

F a left maxillary sinus, from the right with the medial wall removed

G a left maxillary sinus in coronal section, from the front

H a left maxillary sinus in coronal section, from behind

J a small right maxillary sinus in coronal section, from the front

K if there are polyps in the maxillary antrum and the patient has a patent oro-antral fistula, the polyps may prolapse into the oral cavity through the fistula

1	Pituitary fossa
2	Sphenopalatine foramen
3	Superior orbital fissure
4	Foramen rotundum
5	Foramen ovale
6	Foramen spinosum
7	Foramen lacerum
8	Optic canal
9	Pterygoid canal
10	Aperture of sphenoidal sinus
11	Projection of infra-orbital canal
12	Elevation over molar tooth
13	Carotid groove
14	Aperture of maxillary sinus
15	Alveolar process of maxilla

The *sphenoidal sinuses* (left and right) occupy the body of the sphenoid bone (page 46, A14). Although adjacent they do not normally communicate with one another. Large sinuses may be indented by the pituitary gland in the pituitary fossa (C1; page 30, A14; page 196, 50); by the optic nerve in the optic canal (E8; page 30, A19; page 206, 4); by the internal carotid artery in the carotid groove (E8; page 30, A17; page 204, C38); by the maxillary nerve in the foramen rotundum (E4; page 31, B50; page 176, A2); and by the pterygoid canal with its nerve (D9; page 46, A18; page 176, A6). Each sinus drains into the sphenoethmoidal recess of its own side (page 160, B9).

The *maxillary sinus* occupies the body of the maxilla (page 50, C25); a large sinus may extend into the zygomatic and alveolar processes. Its medial wall forms much of the lateral wall of the nasal cavity (page 66). The roof is indented by the infra-orbital canal (F and H, 11), and the floor by some molar tooth roots (F12), and even by premolar or canine roots, especially if the sinus invades the alveolar process (as in G and H). The sinus drains into the semilunar hiatus of the middle meatus (page 66, C21), by an aperture which is high in the medial wall of the sinus (G14).

Infection in the frontal or ethmoidal sinuses may become transferred to the maxillary sinus, because they all drain into the semilunar hiatus (page 160, C12) and infected fluid from the first two can gravitate into the maxillary aperture (page 160, C21).

For a summary of the drainage of the sinuses see page 161.

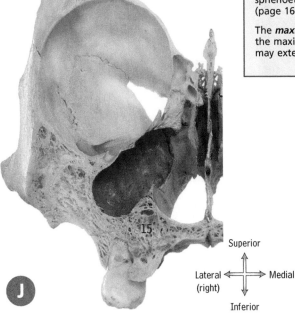

Superior

Lateral ⟷ Medial
(right)

Inferior

J

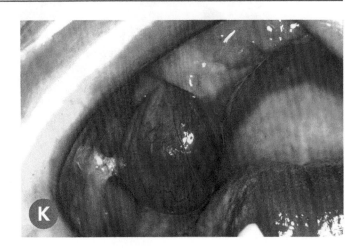

K

Paranasal sinuses and nasal septum

Transverse and coronal sections and nerves of the nasal septum

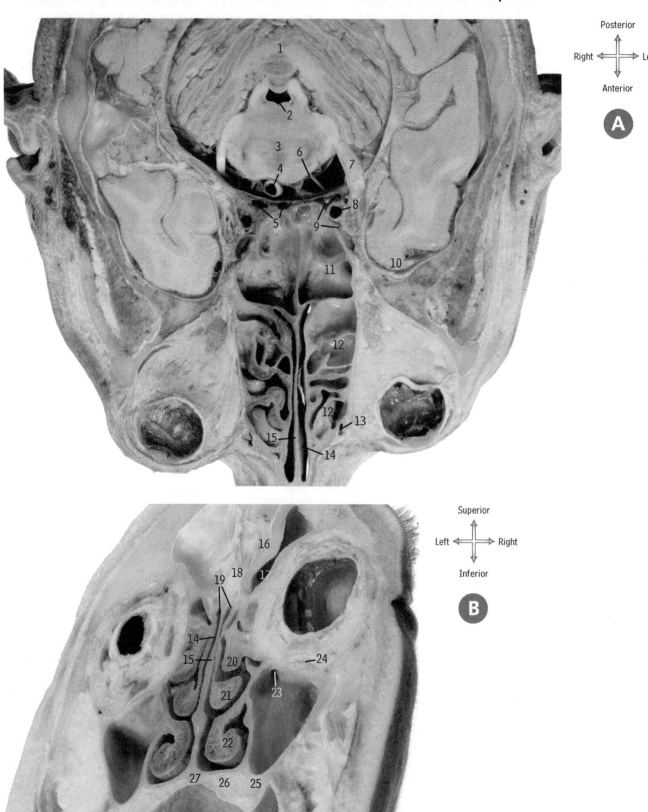

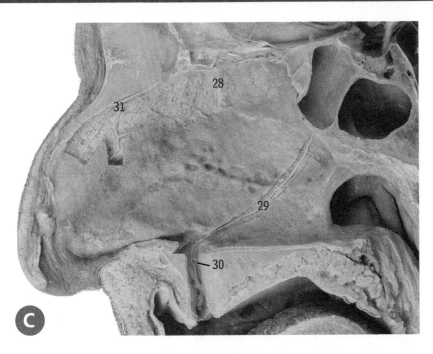

Ⓐ transverse section of the head, at the level of the palpebral fissures, from above

Ⓑ oblique coronal section of the head, at the level of the eyes, from the right, behind and below

Ⓒ nerves of the left side of the nasal septum

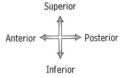

Superior

Anterior ⟷ Posterior

Inferior

Ⓒ

The sections in A and B illustrate the narrowness of the roof (B19) and upper parts of the nasal cavities on either side of the septum (A and B, 14 and 15). The slightly oblique coronal section in B has been orientated so that, looking forwards from below and behind, the aperture of the right maxillary sinus (23) can be seen high up on the medial wall of the sinus.

In C parts of the mucous membrane of the septum have been removed to show the principal nerves: olfactory (28), anterior ethmoidal (31) and nasopalatine (29).

1 Cerebellum
2 Upper part of fourth ventricle
3 Pons
4 Basilar artery
5 Basilar sinus
6 Abducent nerve
7 Trigeminal nerve
8 Internal carotid artery
9 Cavernous sinus
10 Temporal pole
11 Sphenoidal sinus
12 Ethmoidal air cells
13 Nasolacrimal duct
14 Nasal cavity
15 Nasal septum
16 Dura mater of anterior wall of anterior cranial fossa
17 Frontal sinus
18 Crista galli
19 Roof of nasal cavity
20 Superior ⎤
21 Middle ⎬ nasal concha
22 Inferior ⎦
23 Aperture of maxillary sinus
24 Infra-orbital nerve
25 Alveolar process ⎤
26 Palatine process ⎦ of maxilla
27 Hard palate
28 Olfactory nerve filaments
29 Nasopalatine nerve
30 Incisive canal
31 Anterior ethmoidal nerve

The narrowness of the roof and upper part of the nasal cavity (A14; B14 and 19), only a millimetre or two wide, should be compared with the floor (B26) which is over a centimetre wide.

Nerves of the nasal septum:
• Olfactory—over an area opposite the superior nasal concha (C28)
• Anterior ethmoidal—to the anterior part (C31)
• Medial posterior superior nasal—to a small area of the posterior part
• Nasopalatine—to the posterior part (C29)

Nerves of the lateral wall of the nose:
• Olfactory—over the superior nasal concha (and the narrow roof also) (page 161, D25)
• Infra-orbital—to the skin of the vestibule (page 161, D31)
• Anterior ethmoidal—to the anterior part (page 161, D32)
• Nasal branch of the anterior superior nasal—to a small part of the inferior meatus
• Lateral posterior superior nasal—to the upper posterior part (page 161, D28)
• Posterior inferior nasal—to the lower posterior part (page 161, D30)

Oral cavity

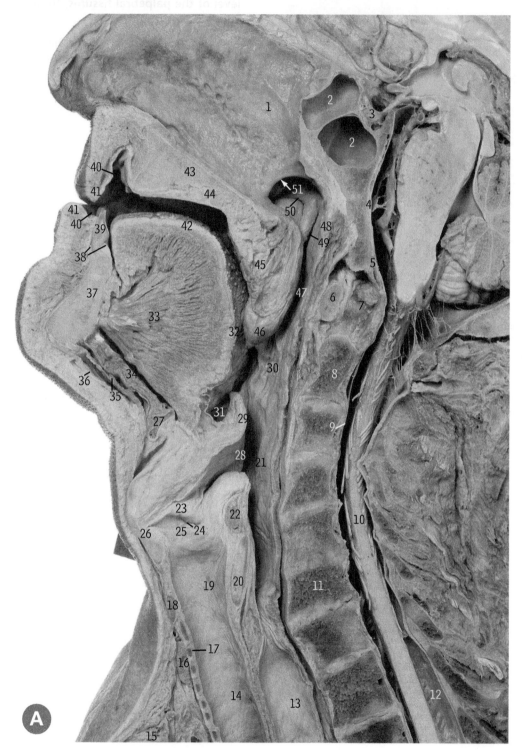

1	Nasal septum
2	Sphenoidal sinus
3	Pituitary gland
4	Clivus
5	Anterior margin of foramen magnum
6	Anterior arch of atlas
7	Dens of axis
8	Body of axis
9	Spinal subarachnoid space
10	Spinal cord
11	Body of sixth cervical vertebra
12	Subarachnoid septum
13	Oesophagus
14	Trachea
15	Jugular notch of manubrium of sternum
16	Isthmus of thyroid gland
17	Second tracheal ring
18	Arch of cricoid cartilage
19	Lower part of larynx
20	Lamina of cricoid cartilage
21	Laryngeal part of pharynx
22	Transverse arytenoid muscle
23	Vestibular fold
24	Ventricle of larynx
25	Vocal fold (vocal cord)
26	Lamina of thyroid cartilage
27	Body of hyoid bone
28	Aryepiglottic fold and inlet of larynx
29	Epiglottis and epiglottic cartilage
30	Oral part of pharynx
31	Vallecula
32	Postsulcal part of dorsum of tongue
33	Genioglossus
34	Geniohyoid
35	Mylohyoid
36	Platysma
37	Body of mandible
38	Gingiva
39	Left lower central incisor tooth
40	Vestibule of mouth
41	Lip
42	Presulcal part of dorsum of tongue
43	Hard palate
44	Palatal glands in mucoperiosteum
45	Soft palate
46	Uvula
47	Nasal part of pharynx
48	Pharyngeal tonsil
49	Pharyngeal recess
50	Opening of auditory tube
51	Posterior nasal aperture (choana)

A sagittal section through the head and neck, from the left

B Sagittal Magnetic Resonance Image (MRI) of the nasopharynx and oropharynx

C This postmortem specimen demonstrates the fatal consequences of inhaling a partial denture

Mouth, palate, pharynx and larynx

The section is just to the left of the midline (showing the whole of the dens of the axis, 7), and the head is tilted slightly backwards (extended). The hard palate (43) forms the floor of the nose and roof of the mouth, and is on approximately the same level as the foramen magnum (5). The soft palate (45) with the uvula at its lower end (46) hangs down from the back of the hard palate (43). The geniohyoid and mylohyoid muscles (34 and 35) form the floor of the mouth. The opening of the auditory tube (50) is in the nasal part of the pharynx, behind the choana (51), with the pharyngeal tonsil (48) on the posterior wall. Behind the tongue (32) the mouth opens into the oral part of the pharynx (30). Below and behind the epiglottis (29) the larynx opens into the laryngeal part of the pharynx (28 and 21).

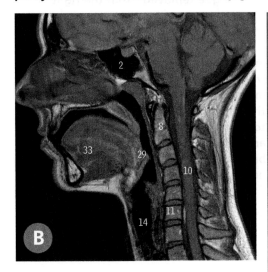

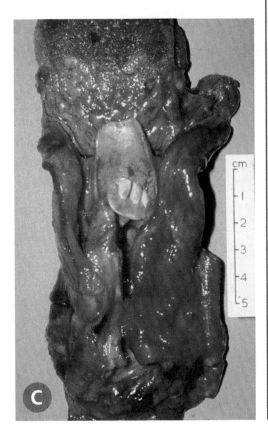

The *mouth* or oral cavity consists of the vestibule (40) and the oral cavity proper.

The vestibule of the mouth is the narrow space bounded on the outer side by the lips and cheeks, and inside by the gingivae (gums) and teeth.

The oral cavity proper is bounded at each side and in front by the alveolar arches with the teeth and gingivae; at the back it communicates with the oral part of the pharynx (30) by the oropharyngeal isthmus which lies between the palatoglossal arches (page 170, B22). The (palatine) tonsils, which lie behind the palatoglossal arches (page 170, B21), are therefore in the oral part of the pharynx, not in the mouth.

The *pharynx* extends from the base of the skull (5) to the level of C6 vertebra (11), a distance of about 12 cm.

The nasal part (nasopharynx, 47) extends as far down as the lower border of the soft palate (45 and 46). It contains the opening of the auditory tube and the pharyngeal recess laterally (50 and 49), the pharyngeal tonsil on the posterior wall (48), and opens anteriorly into the nasal cavity through the posterior nasal apertures (choanae, 51).

The oral part (oropharynx, 30), between the soft palate (45 and 46) and the upper border of the epiglottis (29), contains the palatine tonsil and the palatopharyngeal arch in its lateral wall (here obscured by 46), and opens anteriorly into the mouth through the oropharyngeal isthmus (palatoglossal arches).

The laryngeal part (laryngopharynx, 21) extends from the upper border of the epiglottis (29) to the lower border of the cricoid cartilage (20, level with C6 vertebra, 11), and is continuous below with the oesophagus (13). The larynx projects backwards into the laryngopharynx, with a piriform recess on either side (page 192, A4).

Muscles of the tongue
- Extrinsic muscles (attached to structures outside the tongue): genioglossus (the largest), hyoglossus, styloglossus, and palatoglossus. They can alter the shape of the tongue and move it bodily.
- Intrinsic muscles (within the tongue): longitudinal (superior and inferior), transverse and vertical. They can alter the shape of the tongue without moving it bodily.

Muscles of the soft palate
- Palatoglossus, palatopharyngeus, tensor veli palatini, levator veli palatini and the muscle of the uvula.

Muscles of the pharynx
- Three constrictors and three others: superior, middle and inferior constrictors, palatopharyngeus, stylopharyngeus and salpingopharyngeus.

Ligaments or membranes associated with the pharynx:
- Pharyngeal raphe, stylohyoid ligament, pterygomandibular raphe.

Layers of the pharynx:
- Mucous membrane, submucous layer (including the pharyngobasilar fascia at the upper end), muscular layer, and buccopharyngeal fascia.

Gaps associated with the constrictors and the structures passing through the gaps:
- Above the superior constrictor—auditory tube and ascending palatine artery (piercing pharyngobasilar fascia).
- Between superior and middle constrictors—stylopharyngeus passing down between the constrictors, and the lingual and glossopharyngeal nerves.
- Between middle and inferior constrictors—internal laryngeal nerve and superior laryngeal vessels (piercing thyrohyoid membrane).
- Below inferior constrictor: recurrent laryngeal nerve and inferior laryngeal vessels.

The hyoid bone (27) lies at the level of C3 vertebra.

The thyroid cartilage (26) lies at the level of C4 and C5 vertebrae.

The cricoid cartilage (18 and 20) lies at the level of C6 vertebra (11).

The isthmus of the thyroid gland (16) overlies tracheal rings 2-4 (17).

When enlarged the lymphoid tissue of the pharyngeal tonsil (48) is known as the adenoids.

The piriform recesses are often called the piriform fossae.

Tongue, floor of mouth and oral mucosa

Dissections of the tongue and surface features

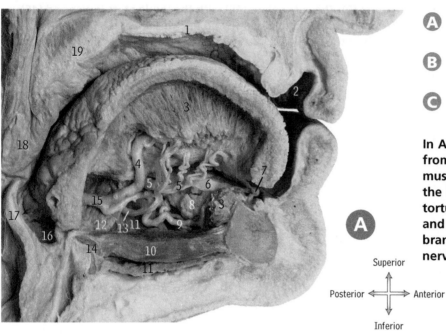

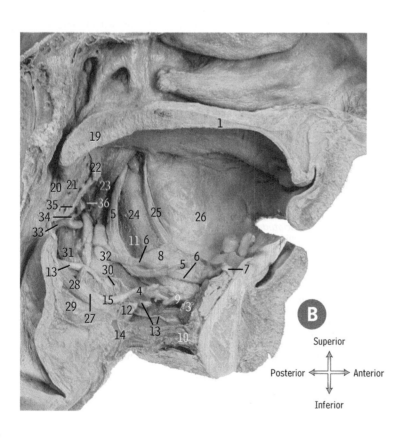

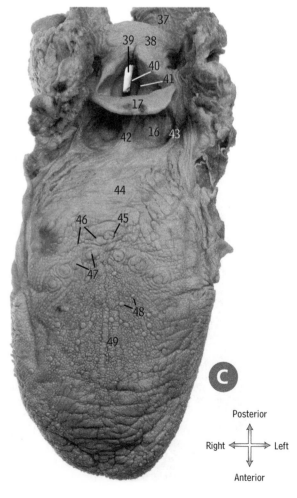

A deep dissection of the left half of the tongue, from the right

B the left half of the mouth with the tongue removed, from the right

C the tongue from above, with the inlet (aditus) of the larynx

In A and B left-sided structures are viewed from the right. In A much of the tongue musculature has been removed to show the lingual artery (15) dividing into its two tortuous main branches (the deep lingual and sublingual arteries, 4 and 9), and branches of the lingual and hypoglossal nerves (5 and 13).

Superior

Posterior ⟷ Anterior

Inferior

Superior

Posterior ⟷ Anterior

Inferior

Posterior

Right ⟷ Left

Anterior

With the whole tongue removed in B, the lingual nerve (5) is seen coming down from above to hook under the submandibular duct (6). Lower down, the lingual artery (15) and hypoglossal nerve (13) are separated by the (cut end of) hyoglossus (12); as viewed from its own side, the nerve runs superficial to the muscle and the artery deep to it (compare with page 178, A25 and 29).

Looking down on the tongue in C, the V-shaped line of vallate papillae (47) lies just in front of the sulcus terminalis (46). The valleculae (16) are in front of the epiglottis (17), and behind it is the laryngeal inlet with a view (at a lower level) of the vestibular and vocal folds (41 and 40). For details of the larynx see pages 190-193.

1 Hard palate
2 Vestibule of mouth
3 Genioglossus (anterior part)
4 Deep lingual artery
5 Lingual nerve
6 Submandibular duct
7 Orifice of submandibular duct on sublingual papilla
8 Sublingual gland
9 Sublingual artery
10 Geniohyoid
11 Mylohyoid
12 Hyoglossus
13 Hypoglossal nerve
14 Body of hyoid bone
15 Lingual artery
16 Vallecula
17 Epiglottis
18 Oral part of pharynx
19 Soft palate
20 Palatopharyngeal arch
21 Tonsil
22 Upper end of palatoglossal arch
23 Medial pterygoid
24 Upper border of body of edentulous mandible
25 Cut edge of mucous membrane
26 Mucous membrane overlying buccinator
27 Lower end of stylohyoid ligament
28 Middle constrictor of pharynx
29 Greater horn of hyoid bone
30 Vena comitans of hypoglossal nerve
31 Stylohyoid
32 Deep part of submandibular gland
33 Facial artery
34 Ascending palatine artery
35 External palatine (paratonsillar) vein
36 Styloglossus
37 Posterior wall of pharynx
38 Posterior wall of larynx
39 Rima of glottis
40 Vocal fold
41 Vestibular fold
42 Median glosso-epiglottic fold
43 Lateral glosso-epiglottic fold
44 Postsulcal part of dorsum of tongue
45 Foramen caecum
46 Sulcus terminalis
47 Vallate papillae
48 Fungiform papillae
49 Presulcal part of dorsum of tongue

All the muscles of the tongue (page 169) are supplied by the hypoglossal nerve (A and B, 13), except palatoglossus, which is supplied by the pharyngeal plexus.

The mucous membrane of the presulcal part (anterior two-thirds) of the tongue (C49) is supplied by the lingual nerve (ordinary sensation) with chorda tympani (facial nerve) fibres (which joined the lingual nerve in the infratemporal fossa) supplying taste buds.

The mucous membrane of the postsulcal part (posterior one-third) of the tongue (C44) (but including the vallate papillae, C47, which lie in front of the sulcus terminalis, C46) is supplied by the glossopharyngeal nerve (ordinary sensation and taste).

The mucous membrane of the part of the tongue that forms the front wall of the vallecula (C16) is supplied (like that of the rest of the vallecula) by the internal laryngeal branch of the vagus nerve.

The cell bodies of the taste fibres in the chorda tympani are in the genicular ganglion of the facial nerve: of those in the glossopharyngeal nerve, in the glossopharyngeal ganglia: and of those in the internal laryngeal nerve (for taste buds in the palate) in the inferior vagal ganglion. The central fibres from all these ganglia converge to synapse with the cell bodies of the nucleus of the tractus solitarius.

The *sublingual gland* (B8) lies beneath the mucous membrane of the floor of the mouth, contacting the sublingual fossa of the mandible (above the mylohyoid line, page 36, C23; page 175, D70). Important relations include:
• above—mucous membrane of the floor of the mouth (B25)
• below—mylohyoid (B11)
• in front—sublingual gland of the opposite side
• behind—deep part of the submandibular gland (B32)
• laterally—sublingual fossa of the mandible (above the mylohyoid line, page 36, C23)
• medially—genioglossus (page 174, B52) with the lingual nerve and the submandibular duct intervening (B5 and 6)

Up to 20 small sublingual ducts open separately in the floor of the mouth on the summit of the sublingual fold (page 174, B56), but some of them may open instead into the submandibular duct (page 174, B48).

The pathway for submandibular and sublingual gland secretion: from the superior salivary nucleus by the nervus intermedius part of the facial nerve, chorda tympani and lingual nerve to the submandibular ganglion (synapse) and then to the glands by lingual nerve filaments.

For notes on the parotid gland see page 134 and on the submandibular gland see page 175.

The foramen caecum (C45) marks the position of the upper end of the thyroglossal duct and the thyroid diverticulum, the embryonic outgrowth from which the thyroid gland develops.

The pyramidal lobe of the thyroid gland (page 120, C68) represents a differentiation of part of the remains of the thyroglossal duct. A fibrous or fibromuscular band may connect the lobe or isthmus to the hyoid bone: if muscular, it constitutes the levator of the thyroid gland. Parts of the duct may persist to form thyroglossal cysts or aberrant masses of thyroid tissue: for example, a lingual thyroid within the tongue.

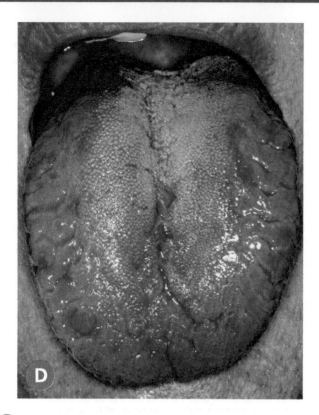

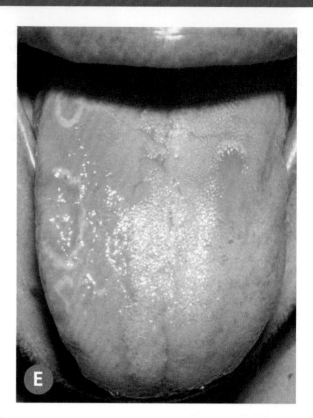

D Deeply fissured tongues (also called scrotal tongues) are normal but may be associated with Heerfordt's syndrome (parotid sarcoidosis, dry mouth and facial palsy)

E Geographic tongue (erythema migrans) is so called because of the irregular but normal turnover of the papillae of the dorsum of the tongue giving the appearance of a map of the world

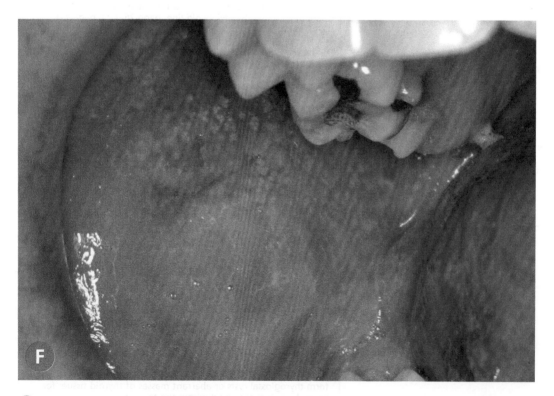

F These white spots (*Fordyce spots*) are normal but prominent sebaceous glands, often found in abundance in the buccal mucosa

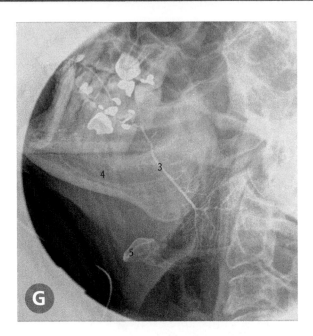

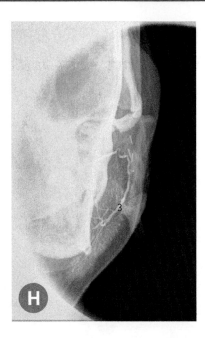

G Lateral view of a parotid sialogram. A small amount of contrast medium has been injected into the partid duct

H Frontal view of a parotid sialogram

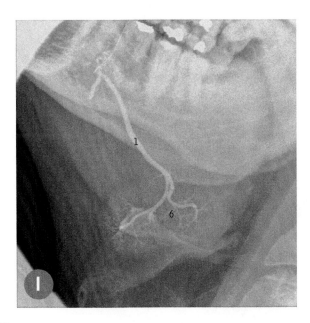

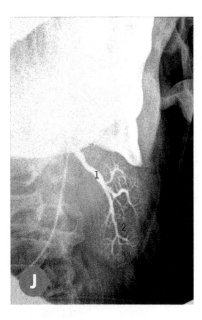

I Lateral view of a submandibular sialogram

J Frontal view of a submandibular sialogram

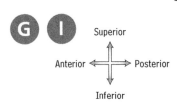

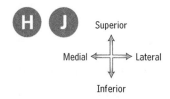

1 Submandibular duct
2 Submandibular gland
3 Parotid duct
4 Mandible
5 Body of hyoid bone
6 Secondary ductules

Mouth and salivary glands

The salivary glands, roof and floor of the mouth

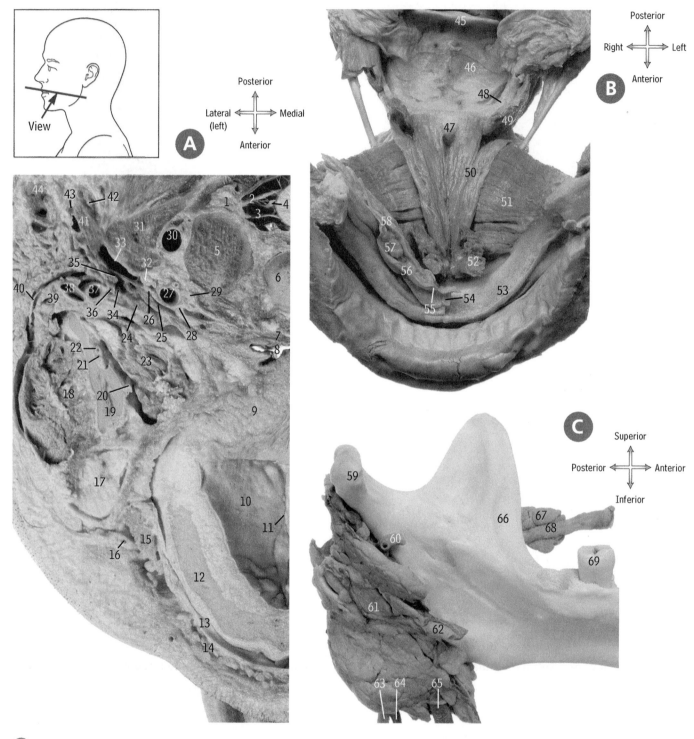

A a transverse section of the left half of the head, from below

B the floor of the mouth after removal of the tongue, from above

C the left parotid gland and the mandible, from the medial side

D the right sublingual and submandibular glands and the mandible, from the medial side

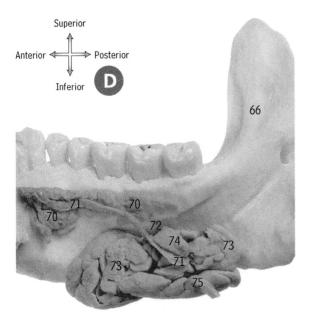

Superior

Anterior ⟷ Posterior

Inferior **D**

In A the section has passed through the alveolar process of the maxilla (12) and about halfway up the ramus of the mandible (19), at the level of the opening of the mandibular foramen containing the inferior alveolar nerve and artery (21 and 22). The lingual nerve (20) is outside the foramen and 1 cm in front of it. The parotid gland (39), C-shaped in horizontal section, clasps the ramus of the mandible (19), which has the masseter on its outer side (18), and the medial pterygoid on the inner side (23).

In B the tongue has been removed so that the floor of the mouth (mylohyoid, 51, and geniohyoid, 50) can be viewed from above.

In C and D, isolated salivary glands (61, 73 and 70) have been laid in their proper positions in relation to the mandible.

The *submandibular gland* has a large superficial and a small deep part (D73 and 74), continuous round the posterior border of mylohyoid.

The superficial part lies in the digastric triangle (page 112, 46). Important relations include:
- below—skin, platysma, investing layer of deep cervical fascia, facial vein, cervical branch of the facial nerve, submandibular lymph nodes
- laterally—submandibular fossa of the mandible (below the mylohyoid line, page 36, C22), insertion of medial pterygoid, facial artery
- medially—mylohyoid muscle, nerve and vessels, lingual nerve and submandibular ganglion, hypoglossal nerve, deep lingual vein, hyoglossus

The deep part of the gland lies on hyoglossus (page 178, A26) with the lingual nerve above, and the hypoglossal nerve and submandibular duct below (page 178, A7, 25 and 21). For secretion see page 171.

The submandibular duct is 5 cm long. It emerges from the superficial part of the gland (D71) near the posterior border of mylohyoid and passes forward between mylohyoid and hyoglossus and then between the sublingual gland and genioglossus. It opens in the floor of the mouth on the sublingual papilla (B55) at the side of the frenulum of the tongue (B54).

---

1 Dorsal root ganglion ⎤ of second
2 Dorsal root ⎥ cervical nerve
3 Ventral root ⎦
4 Spinal root of accessory nerve
5 Lateral mass of atlas
6 Dens of axis
7 Superior constrictor of pharynx
8 Nasal part of pharynx
9 Soft palate
10 Hard palate
11 Palatal raphe
12 Alveolar process of maxilla
13 Vestibule of mouth
14 Labial glands
15 Buccinator
16 Facial artery
17 Buccal fat pad
18 Masseter
19 Ramus of mandible
20 Lingual nerve
21 Inferior alveolar nerve
22 Inferior alveolar artery
23 Medial pterygoid
24 Styloglossus
25 Stylopharyngeus

26 Glossopharyngeal nerve
27 Internal carotid artery
28 Hypoglossal nerve
29 Superior cervical sympathetic ganglion
30 Vertebral artery
31 Transverse process of atlas
32 Vagus nerve
33 Internal jugular vein
34 Stylohyoid ligament
35 Stylohyoid
36 Posterior auricular artery
37 External carotid artery
38 Retromandibular vein
39 Parotid gland
40 A zygomatic branch of facial nerve
41 Posterior belly of digastric
42 Accessory nerve (spinal part)
43 Occipital artery
44 Sternocleidomastoid
45 Epiglottis
46 Vallecula
47 Body ⎤ of hyoid bone
48 Greater horn ⎦
49 Hyoglossus
50 Geniohyoid

51 Mylohyoid
52 Genioglossus
53 Edentulous body of mandible
54 Frenulum of tongue
55 Sublingual papilla
56 Sublingual fold
57 Sublingual gland
58 Submandibular duct
59 Condylar process of mandible
60 Maxillary artery
61 Parotid gland
62 External carotid artery
63 Great auricular nerve
64 Posterior division ⎤ of retromandibular
65 Anterior division ⎦ vein
66 Ramus of mandible
67 Accessory parotid gland
68 Parotid duct
69 Lower second molar tooth
70 Sublingual gland
71 Submandibular duct
72 Mylohyoid line of body of mandible
73 Superficial part ⎤ of submandibular gland
74 Deep part ⎦
75 Facial artery

Mouth and palate in sections

Oral cavity and adjacent structures

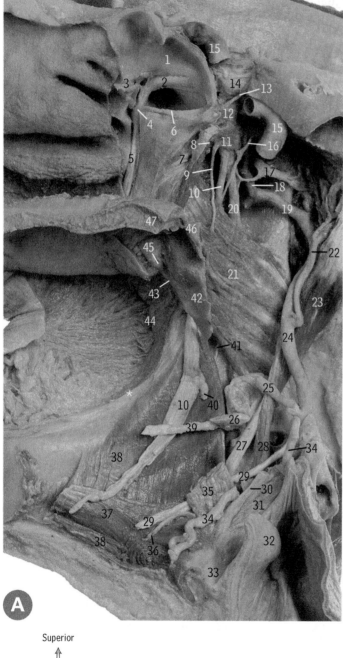

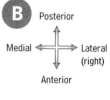

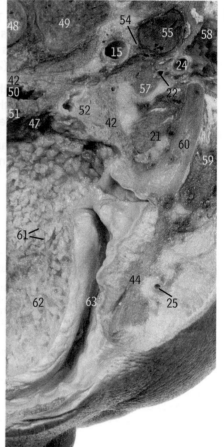

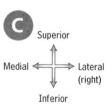

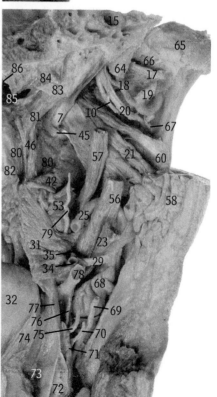

Superior

Anterior ⟷ Posterior

Inferior

A the right half of the mouth, from the left

B transverse section of the right half of the roof of the mouth, from below

C the right half of the soft palate, from behind

To understand these rather complicated but instructive specimens, they may be considered to give different views of the medial pterygoid muscle (21) and adjacent structures. In A the right muscle is seen from the medial side, with parts of the skull removed to show the trigeminal ganglion (14) with the maxillary and mandibular nerves (2 and 12) branching from it. The pterygopalatine ganglion (4) is attached to the maxillary nerve (2), the otic ganglion (11) to the mandibular nerve (12), and the submandibular ganglion (40) to the lingual nerve (10). The asterisk (*) indicates the position of the lower third molar tooth.

In B the transverse section is below the hard palate (62) and is viewed from below looking upwards. The right ramus of the mandible (60) has the medial pterygoid (21) on its medial side.

The dissection in C is viewed from behind, looking forwards. On the right of the picture the posterior border of the right ramus of the mandible (60), with the medial pterygoid (21) on its medial side, has been exposed by removing most of the parotid gland (58); on the left is seen the posterior surface of the epiglottis (32). Stylohyoid (56) passes downwards and forwards to split round the digastric (23), with styloglossus (57) more anteriorly. The glossopharyngeal nerve (79) winds round stylopharyngeus (53). Palatopharyngeus (46) runs down from the palatine aponeurosis (80), with levator veli palatini (81) approaching the aponeurosis from above, lateral to the auditory tube (83).

All the muscles of the palate (page 169) are supplied by the pharyngeal plexus, except tensor veli palatini which is supplied by the nerve to the medial pterygoid (mandibular nerve).

The mucous membrane of the palate is supplied by the nasopalatine, greater and lesser palatine and glossopharyngeal nerves.

The surface of the tonsil is pitted by downgrowths of the epithelium to form the tonsillar crypts.

A deep crypt-like structure near the upper pole of the tonsil is the intratonsillar cleft, and represents the proximal end of the embryonic second pharyngeal pouch.

The mucous membrane of the tonsil is supplied by the lesser palatine and glossopharyngeal nerves.

The lingual nerve (A10) enters the mouth by passing beneath the lower border of the superior constrictor (A42), and immediately below this the nerve lies below and behind the third molar tooth (whose position is indicated by the asterisk in A), either in contact with the periosteum of the mandible or on the upper part of mylohyoid (as here, A38).

---

1 Sphenoidal sinus
2 Maxillary nerve
3 Sphenopalatine foramen and artery
4 Pterygopalatine ganglion
5 Greater palatine nerve
6 Nerve of pterygoid canal
7 Tensor veli palatini
8 Nerve to tensor veli palatini
9 Nerve to medial pterygoid
10 Lingual nerve
11 Otic ganglion
12 Mandibular nerve
13 Greater petrosal nerve
14 Trigeminal ganglion
15 Internal carotid artery
16 Chorda tympani
17 Auriculotemporal nerve
18 Middle meningeal artery
19 Maxillary artery
20 Inferior alveolar nerve
21 Medial pterygoid
22 Occipital artery
23 Posterior belly of digastric
24 External carotid artery
25 Facial artery
26 Deep part of submandibular gland
27 Tendon of digastric
28 Stylohyoid
29 Hypoglossal nerve

30 Stylohyoid ligament
31 Middle constrictor of pharynx
32 Epiglottis
33 Vallecula
34 Lingual artery
35 Hyoglossus
36 Vena comitans of hypoglossal nerve
37 Geniohyoid
38 Mylohyoid
39 Submandibular duct
40 Submandibular ganglion
41 Nerve to mylohyoid
42 Superior constrictor of pharynx
43 Pterygomandibular raphe
44 Buccinator
45 Pterygoid hamulus
46 Palatopharyngeus
47 Soft palate
48 Dens of axis
49 Lateral mass of atlas
50 Nasal part of pharynx
51 Uvula
52 Tonsil (upper end)
53 Stylopharyngeus
54 Vagus nerve
55 Internal jugular vein
56 Stylohyoid
57 Styloglossus
58 Parotid gland

59 Masseter
60 Ramus of mandible
61 Palatal glands
62 Hard palate
63 Vestibule of mouth
64 Base of styloid process
65 Intra-articular disc of temporomandibular joint
66 Lateral pterygoid
67 Inferior alveolar artery
68 Posterior part of submandibular gland
69 Superior thyroid artery
70 Superior laryngeal artery
71 Inferior constrictor of pharynx
72 Lamina of thyroid cartilage
73 Piriform recess
74 Aryepiglottic fold
75 Internal laryngeal nerve
76 Thyrohyoid
77 Thyrohyoid membrane
78 Greater horn of hyoid bone
79 Glossopharyngeal nerve
80 Palatine aponeurosis
81 Levator veli palatini
82 Musculus uvulae
83 Cartilaginous part of auditory tube
84 Longus capitis
85 Posterior nasal aperture (choana)
86 Nasal septum (vomer)

Pharynx *External and internal surfaces of the pharynx*

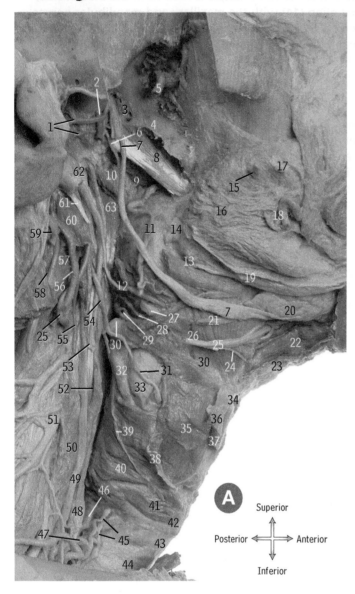

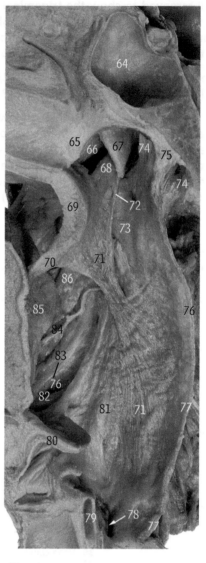

A

Superior

Posterior ⟷ Anterior

Inferior

B the right internal surface,
from the left

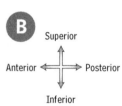

B

Superior

Anterior ⟷ Posterior

Inferior

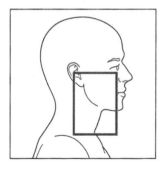

A the external surface,
from the right

Palatopharyngeus (B71) (with salpingopharyngeus joining it, B72) passes downwards internal to the constrictor muscles.

Stylopharyngeus (page 180, B11) passes downwards between the superior and middle constrictors (page 180, B32 and 30).

Fibres from palatopharyngeus and stylopharyngeus reach the posterior border of the lamina of the thyroid cartilage (page 180, B38) and, together with the inferior constrictor, they act as elevators of the larynx during swallowing.

All the muscles of the pharynx (page 169) are supplied by the pharyngeal plexus, except stylopharyngeus, which is supplied by the muscular branch of the glossopharyngeal nerve (A12). The lowest (cricopharyngeal) part of the inferior constrictor (A40) may receive an additional supply from the external laryngeal nerve (A39).

Hyoglossus (A26) is a key landmark at the side of the tongue:
• passing superficial to it—lingual nerve (7), submandibular duct (21) and hypoglossal nerve (25).
• passing deep to its posterior border—glossopharyngeal nerve (12), stylohyoid ligament (27) and lingual artery (29).

In A the mandible, mastication muscles and great vessels have been removed. The superior constrictor (11) passes back from the pterygomandibular raphe (14), with the buccinator (16) running forwards from the raphe. The narrow origin of the middle constrictor (28) passes back from the angle between the stylohyoid ligament (27, whose upper end has been cut off) and the greater horn of the hyoid bone (30). The inferior constrictor (40) runs back from a broad origin from the thyroid cartilage behind the sternothyroid attachment (38) and from the side of the cricoid cartilage (42).

In B the muscular layer of the right side of the pharynx has been exposed from the inside by removing the mucous membrane. Palatopharyngeus (71) is the innermost muscle. The glossopharyngeal nerve (84) runs down in the 'tonsillar bed' between palatoglossus (86) in front and the upper anterior part of palatopharyngeus (71) behind.

1 Roots of auriculotemporal nerve
2 Middle meningeal artery
3 Mandibular nerve
4 Lateral pterygoid plate
5 Maxillary artery entering pterygomaxillary fissure
6 Chorda tympani
7 Lingual nerve
8 Tensor veli palatini
9 Levator veli palatini
10 Pharyngobasilar fascia
11 Superior constrictor of pharynx and ascending palatine artery
12 Stylopharyngeus and glossopharyngeal nerve
13 Styloglossus
14 Pterygomandibular raphe
15 Parotid duct
16 Buccinator
17 Molar glands
18 Facial artery
19 Mucoperiosteum of mandible
20 Sublingual gland
21 Submandibular duct
22 Geniohyoid
23 Mylohyoid
24 Nerve to geniohyoid
25 Hypoglossal nerve
26 Hyoglossus
27 Stylohyoid ligament
28 Middle constrictor of pharynx

29 Lingual artery
30 Greater horn of hyoid bone
31 Internal laryngeal nerve
32 Superior horn of thyroid cartilage
33 Thyrohyoid membrane
34 Body of hyoid bone
35 Thyrohyoid
36 Superior belly of omohyoid
37 Sternohyoid
38 Sternothyroid
39 External laryngeal nerve
40 Inferior constrictor of pharynx
41 Cricothyroid
42 Arch of cricoid cartilage
43 Cricotracheal ligament
44 Trachea
45 Recurrent laryngeal nerve
46 Inferior laryngeal artery
47 Inferior thyroid artery
48 Middle cervical sympathetic ganglion
49 Vagus nerve
50 Scalenus anterior
51 Ventral ramus of fourth cervical nerve
52 Sympathetic trunk
53 Ascending pharyngeal artery
54 Superior laryngeal nerve
55 Superior root of ansa cervicalis
56 Occipital artery
57 Transverse process of atlas
58 Accessory nerve (spinal part)
59 Posterior auricular artery

60 Internal jugular vein
61 Stylohyoid
62 Styloid process
63 Longus capitis
64 Sphenoidal sinus
65 Vomer (posterior part of nasal septum)
66 Tensor veli palatini
67 Cartilaginous part of auditory tube
68 Levator veli palatini
69 Soft palate
70 Uvula
71 Palatopharyngeus
72 Salpingopharyngeus
73 Superior constrictor
74 Longus capitis
75 Attachment of pharyngeal raphe to pharyngeal tubercle
76 Middle constrictor
77 Inferior constrictor
78 Piriform recess
79 Lamina of cricoid cartilage
80 Epiglottis
81 Pharyngeal wall overlying superior horn of thyroid cartilage
82 Greater horn of hyoid bone
83 Stylohyoid ligament
84 Glossopharyngeal nerve
85 Postsulcal part of dorsum of tongue
86 Palatoglossus

C Stages of swallowing

Stages of swallowing	Bolus control	Airway protection
VOLUNTARY Bolus in mouth	1) Jaws closed *Muscles:* masseter, temporalis, medial pterygoid 2) Lips closed *Muscles:* orbicularis oris 3) Bolus accommodated on tongue, tip raised against palate *Muscles:* tongue muscles, genioglossus	Airway patent Pillars of fauces contracted over posterior surface of tongue *Muscles:* palatoglossus, palatopharyngeus
INVOLUNTARY a) Bolus passes into oropharynx	1) Posterior part of tongue moves upwards and backwards *Muscles:* mylohyoid, styloglossus 2) Pillars of fauces contract behind bolus	Nasopharynx closed Soft palate tensed and raised *Muscles:* tensor veli palatini, levator veli palatini, Passavant's ridge
INVOLUNTARY b) Bolus passes over epiglottis towards oesophagus	Pharynx raised *Muscles:* stylopharyngeus, palatopharyngeus, salpingopharyngeus	1) Larynx closed by elevation behind posterior part of tongue and epiglottis *Muscles:* stylopharyngeus, palatopharyngeus, salpingopharyngeus, thyrohyoid 2) Larynx inlet closed *Muscles:* arytenoids
INVOLUNTARY c) Bolus passes into oesophagus	Relaxation of cricopharyngeus	Airway re-opened Soft palate, pharynx and larynx return to original positions

Pharynx *Posterior surface of the pharynx*

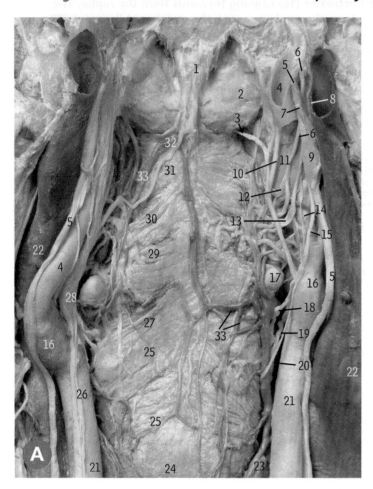

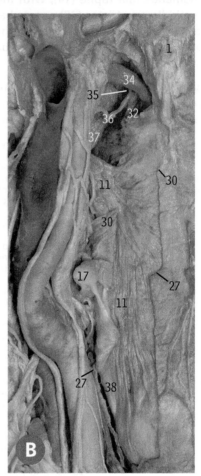

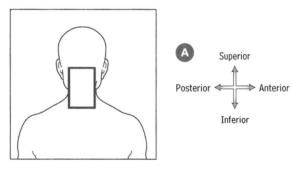

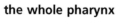

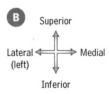

the whole pharynx

Superior

Lateral ⟷ Medial
(left)

Inferior

the left half

Posterior ⟷ Anterior

Superior

Inferior

In A the skull has been sectioned coronally at the level of the pharyngeal tubercle (1). On the right, part of the internal carotid artery (4) has been removed to show the pharyngeal branches (12 and 13) of the glossopharyngeal and vagus nerves that make up the pharyngeal plexus. The pharyngeal venous plexus (33) is particularly prominent on the right.

In B removal of the pharyngobasilar fascia seen in A (2) reveals parts of the levator and tensor veli palatini (34 and 35), and with removal of parts of the middle and inferior constrictors (30 and 27), fibres of stylopharyngeus (11) can be traced down to the posterior border of the lamina of the thyroid cartilage (38).

Fibres of all three constrictors converge in an upward direction on to the pharyngeal raphe (1); hence the importance of the inferior constrictor as an elevator of the larynx (see page 191).

The pharyngobasilar fascia (A2) is the thickened submucosa of the pharynx that extends between the upper border of the superior constrictor and the base of the skull.

The buccopharyngeal fascia (which is very much thinner than the pharyngobasilar fascia and must not be confused with it) lies on the external surface of the pharyngeal constrictors and is continuous anteriorly over the outer surface of the buccinator. It is really nothing more than the epimysium on the surface of the muscles.

Some of the uppermost fibres of the superior constrictor and of the palatopharyngeus (page 178, B73 and 71) form a muscular band which, during swallowing, raises a transverse ridge (Passavant's ridge) on the posterior pharyngeal wall. With accompanying elevation of the soft palate, it closes off the nasal part of the pharynx from the oral part. It must be noted that the ridge only becomes evident during the act of swallowing; it is not seen in the living pharynx at rest or in the cadaver.

The pharyngeal plexuses of nerves and veins are situated mainly on the posterior surface of the middle constrictor (A29).

The pharyngeal plexus of nerves is formed by the pharyngeal branches of the glossopharyngeal and vagus nerves (A12 and 13). The glossopharyngeal component is afferent only; the vagal component is motor to the pharynx and palate as well as containing afferent fibres.

Glossopharyngeal nerve paralysis:
• No detectable motor disability, as the nerve supplies only one small muscle, stylopharyngeus.
• Loss of taste from the posterior one-third of the tongue, with anaesthesia in the same area and in part of the pharyngeal mucous membrane.

Vagus and cranial accessory nerve paralysis:
• Paralysis of the soft palate on the affected side (the palate is pulled towards the unaffected side on saying 'Ah').
• Dysphagia (difficulty in swallowing) due to paralysis of pharyngeal muscles.
• Hoarseness of voice due to paralysis of laryngeal muscles.

Spinal accessory nerve paralysis:
• Paralysis of sternocleidomastoid and trapezius.

Hypoglossal nerve paralysis:
• Paralysis of the tongue on the affected side (with deviation towards the affected side on protrusion, due to the unopposed action of the intact side).

---

1 Attachment of pharyngeal raphe to pharyngeal tubercle of base of skull
2 Pharyngobasilar fascia
3 Ascending pharyngeal artery
4 Internal carotid artery
5 Vagus nerve
6 Glossopharyngeal nerve
7 Accessory nerve
8 Hypoglossal nerve
9 Inferior ganglion of vagus nerve
10 Posterior meningeal artery
11 Stylopharyngeus
12 Pharyngeal branch of glossopharyngeal nerve
13 Pharyngeal branch of vagus nerve
14 Vagal branch to carotid body
15 Superior laryngeal branch of vagus nerve
16 Carotid sinus
17 Tip of greater horn of hyoid bone
18 Internal laryngeal nerve
19 Superior thyroid artery
20 External laryngeal nerve
21 Common carotid artery
22 Internal jugular vein
23 Lateral lobe of thyroid gland
24 Cricopharyngeal part ⎫ of inferior constrictor
25 Thyropharyngeal part ⎬
26 Sympathetic trunk
27 Upper border of inferior constrictor
28 Superior cervical sympathetic ganglion
29 Middle constrictor
30 Upper border of middle constrictor
31 Superior constrictor
32 Upper border of superior constrictor
33 Pharyngeal veins
34 Levator veli palatini
35 Tensor veli palatini
36 Ascending palatine artery
37 Medial pterygoid
38 Posterior border of lamina of thyroid cartilage

Ear Components of the ear

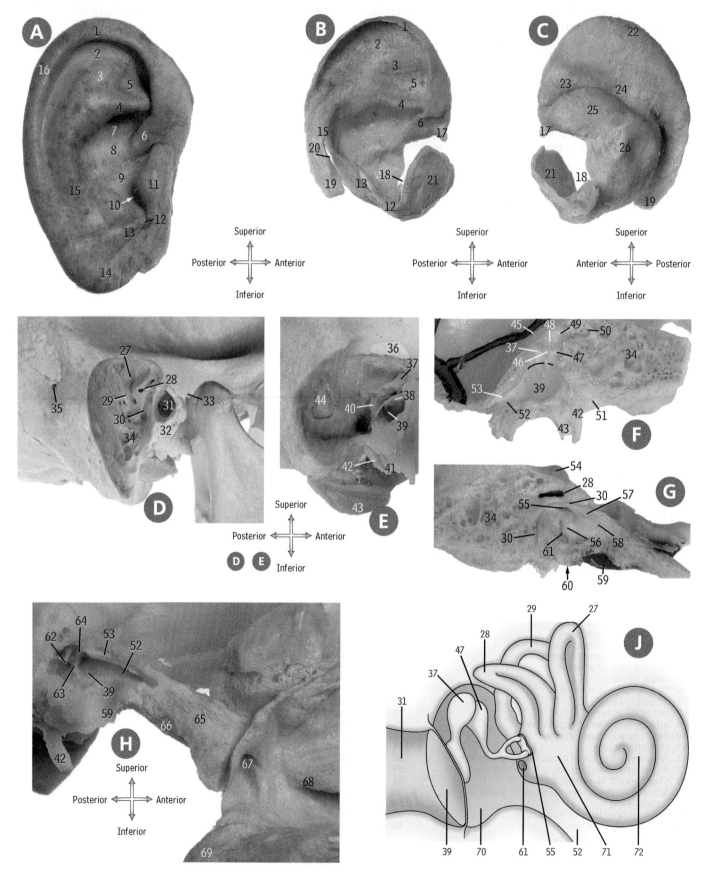

The external, middle and internal ear

A right auricle, from the right

B right auricular cartilage, from the right

C right auricular cartilage, from the left

D dissection through the right mastoid process, from the right

E similar to D but deeper, from the right and behind

F section through the right middle ear, from the left

G section through the right middle ear, from the right

H left auditory tube, from the right (enlarged)

J diagram of parts of the ear

A, B and C show the surface features and cartilaginous framework of the auricle (pinna).

In D part of the right mastoid process of a dried skull has been chipped away to open up the mastoid air cells (34) and the semicircular canals (27–29).

In E a deeper dissection of the area in D shows how near the sigmoid sinus (44) lies to the deepest mastoid air cells. The canal for the facial nerve (40) has been opened up where the chorda tympani branch (38) takes a recurrent course to pass through the mucous membrane of the tympanic membrane (39).

F and G are sections through the middle ear and adjacent parts of the temporal bone, showing the lateral (F) and medial (G) walls of the middle ear cavity. The narrow black bristle (unlabelled, below 46 and 47) indicates the course of the chorda tympani under the mucous membrane of the tympanic membrane (39).

In H the cartilaginous part of the auditory tube (65 and 66) has been dissected away from surrounding tissues but with the tubal opening (67) into the nasopharynx left intact.

The diagram (J) shows the parts of the right ear as seen from the front, with the external meatus and middle ear in coronal section.

The lobule of the ear (A14), the part most often pierced for wearing earrings, is composed of dense fibrous tissue, not cartilage.

The external ear consists of the auricle (pinna, A) and the external acoustic meatus (A10; D and J, 31), at the medial end of which lies the tympanic membrane (E, F and J, 39) separating the external ear from the middle ear.

The middle ear (tympanic cavity, J70) is an irregular space in the temporal bone, lined with mucous membrane, containing the auditory ossicles (malleus, incus and stapes) and filled with air that communicates anteriorly with the nasopharynx through the auditory tube (Eustachian tube, H52, 65 and 66). For details of the walls of the middle ear cavity, see the notes on page 185.

The epitympanic recess (F48) is the part of the tympanic cavity that projects upwards above the level of the tympanic membrane (F39) to accommodate the head of the malleus and the body of the incus (F37 and 47). It leads backwards through the aditus (F49) into the mastoid antrum (F50) which is an enlarged mastoid air cell (F34).

---

1 Helix
2 Scaphoid fossa
3 Upper crus of antihelix
4 Lower crus of antihelix
5 Triangular fossa
6 Crus of helix
7 Cymba conchae
8 Concha
9 Cavum conchae
10 External acoustic meatus
11 Tragus
12 Intertragic notch
13 Antitragus
14 Lobule
15 Antihelix
16 Position of auricular tubercle (if present)
17 Spine of helix
18 Terminal notch
19 Tail of helix
20 Antitragohelicine meatus
21 Cartilage of external acoustic meatus
22 Scaphoid eminence
23 Triangular eminence
24 Transverse antihelicine groove
25 Conchal eminence

26 Ponticulus
27 Anterior ⎫
28 Lateral ⎬ semicircular canal
29 Posterior ⎭
30 Canal for facial nerve
31 External acoustic meatus
32 Tympanic part of temporal bone
33 Postglenoid tubercle
34 Mastoid air cells
35 Mastoid foramen
36 Dura mater of middle cranial fossa
37 Head of malleus in epitympanic recess
38 Chorda tympani
39 Tympanic membrane
40 Facial nerve
41 Sheath of styloid process
42 Styloid process
43 Occipital condyle
44 Dura mater of sigmoid sinus
45 Tegmen tympani
46 Incudomallear joint
47 Body of incus
48 Epitympanic recess
49 Aditus to mastoid antrum
50 Mastoid antrum

51 Stylomastoid foramen
52 Semicanal for auditory tube
53 Semicanal for tensor tympani
54 Arcuate eminence (overlying anterior semicircular canal)
55 Oval window (fenestra vestibuli), with stapes in J
56 Promontory
57 Trochleariform (cochleariform) process
58 Position of opening of auditory tube
59 Carotid canal
60 Jugular bulb
61 Round window (fenestra cochleae)
62 Incudostapedial joint
63 Handle of malleus
64 Tendon of tensor tympani and 57
65 Medial lamina ⎫ of cartilaginous part
66 Lateral lamina ⎬ of auditory tube
67 Opening of auditory tube
68 Inferior nasal concha
69 Soft palate
70 Middle ear (tympanic cavity)
71 Vestibule
72 Cochlea

Internal structure I

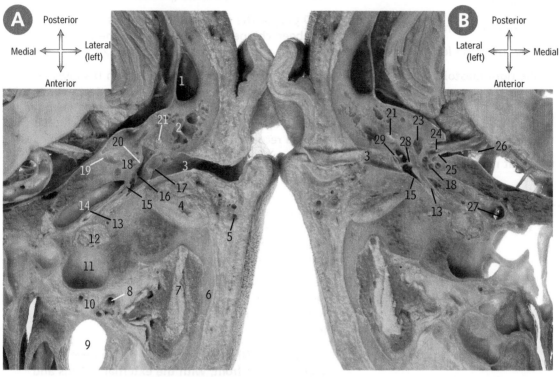

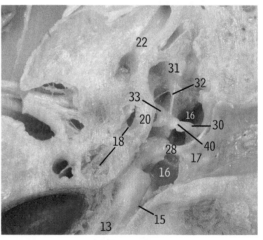

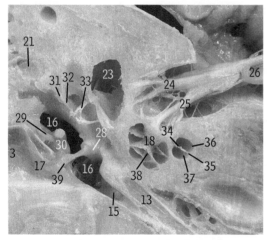

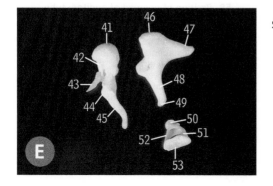

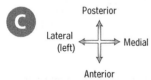

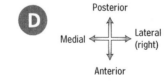

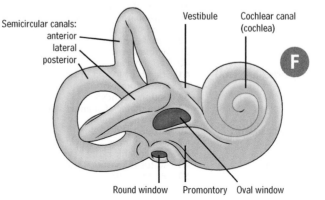

Semicircular canals:
anterior
lateral
posterior

Vestibule

Cochlear canal
(cochlea)

Round window   Promontory   Oval window

Transverse sections
through the ear,
and the auditory
ossicles

A the lower
surface of a
section
through the
left ear, from
above

B the upper
surface of the
same section,
from below

C the central
area of B,
enlarged

D the upper
surface of a
section
through the
right ear
(enlarged), at
a slightly
lower level
than the
section in B

E the right
auditory
ossicles,
disarticulated
and enlarged

F diagram of
the osseous
labyrinth

G diagram of
the
membranous
labyrinth

1 Sigmoid sinus
2 Mastoid air cells
3 External acoustic meatus
4 Intra-articular disc of temporomandibular joint
5 Superficial temporal artery
6 Zygomatic arch
7 Temporalis
8 Maxillary artery
9 Maxillary sinus
10 Pterygopalatine fossa
11 Sphenoidal sinus
12 Cavernous sinus
13 Semicanal with tensor tympani
14 Internal carotid artery in carotid canal
15 Opening of auditory tube
16 Cavity of middle ear
17 Tympanic membrane
18 Cochlea
19 Floor of internal acoustic meatus
20 Promontory
21 Facial nerve
22 Posterior semicircular canal
23 Vestibular part of osseous labyrinth
24 Vestibular part ⎱ of vestibulocochlear nerve
25 Cochlear part ⎰ in internal acoustic meatus
26 Labyrinthine artery
27 Internal carotid artery in foramen lacerum
28 Tendon of tensor tympani and trochleariform (cochleariform) process
29 Chorda tympani
30 Long limb of incus
31 Pyramid
32 Stapedius
33 Stapes
34 Osseous spiral lamina
35 Basilar membrane
36 Scala tympani
37 Scala vestibuli
38 Modiolus
39 Handle of malleus
40 Incudostapedial joint
41 Head ⎫
42 Neck ⎪
43 Anterior process ⎬ of malleus
44 Lateral process ⎪
45 Handle ⎭
46 Body ⎫
47 Short limb ⎬ of incus
48 Long limb ⎪
49 Lenticular process ⎭
50 Head ⎫
51 Posterior limb ⎬ of stapes
52 Anterior limb ⎪
53 Base (footplate) ⎭

The section in A is viewed looking down to the neck, and in B looking up to the top of the head; the sections were produced by the same saw cut and have been separated like opening a book, with the spine of the book in the centre at the auricle of the external ear. The section has passed through the external acoustic meatus (3), the middle ear cavity (16) and the horizontal part of the internal carotid artery within the carotid canal (14).

The enlargement of B in C shows the vestibular and cochlear parts of the vestibulocochlear nerve (24 and 25) in the internal acoustic meatus, coils of the cochlea (18), and the tendon of tensor tympani (28) bridging the tympanic cavity (16) to become attached to the handle of the malleus (39). The auditory tube (15) opens into the front of the cavity.

D is a similar section to C but at a slightly lower level, showing the stapedius muscle (32) emerging from the pyramid (31) to join the stapes (33). Much of the posterior semicircular canal (22) has been opened up.

E is an enlarged view of the three disarticulated auditory ossicles.

From the diagrams F and G it can be visualised that the semicircular ducts lie within the semicircular canals, the cochlear duct within the cochlear canal (cochlea), and the utricle and saccule within the vestibule.

Features of the walls of the middle ear:
• Lateral wall—tympanic membrane (page 182, F39); part of the petro-tympanic fissure (page 54, D42); anterior and posterior canaliculi for the chorda tympani (page 182, F, at either end of bristle).
• Medial wall (from above downwards)—prominence due to lateral semicircular canal (page 182, G28); prominence due to canal for facial nerve (page 182, G30); promontory (A20 and page 182, G56, due to first turn of cochlea), with oval window (fenestra vestibuli, page 182, G55) occupied by footplate of stapes above and behind promontory, and round window (fenestra cochleae, page 182, G61) below and behind promontory.
• Roof—tegmen tympani (part of petrous part of temporal bone, page 182, F45 and page 54, C32).
• Floor—above superior bulb of internal jugular vein in jugular fossa (page 54, D47) with canaliculus for tympanic branch of glossopharyngeal nerve (page 54, D45).
• Anterior wall—carotid canal (page 182, G59) with (laterally) openings of semicanals for tensor tympani and auditory tube (page 54, E49 and 50).
• Posterior wall—aditus to mastoid antrum (page 182, F49); pyramid (with stapedius emerging, C31 and 32) in front of vertical part of facial nerve (C21); fossa for incus (page 182, F47).

The internal ear consists of the osseous (bony) labyrinth and the membranous labyrinth.

The osseous labyrinth is a space within the temporal bone consisting of (from front to back) the cochlea (sometimes called the cochlear canal), the vestibule and the semicircular canals.

The membranous labyrinth is inside the bony labyrinth and consists of the cochlear duct (within the cochlea), the utricle and saccule (within the vestibule), and the semicircular ducts (within the semicircular canals).

The various parts of the membranous labyrinth are smaller than the osseous labyrinth and are separated from the walls of the osseous labyrinth by perilymph. The membranous labyrinth itself contains endolymph. These two fluids do not mix with one another, but the perilymph probably communicates with the cerebrospinal fluid in the subarachnoid space via the cochlear canaliculus.

The cochlea is spiral-shaped, like a snail shell.

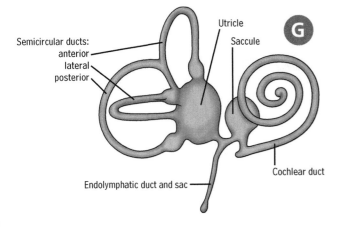

Semicircular ducts:
anterior
lateral
posterior

Utricle
Saccule

G

Cochlear duct

Endolymphatic duct and sac

Internal structure II

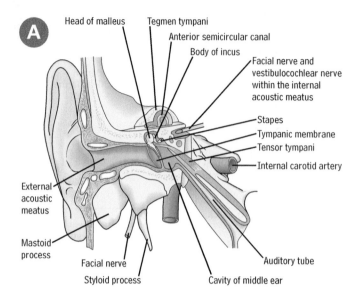

A

Head of malleus
Tegmen tympani
Anterior semicircular canal
Body of incus
Facial nerve and vestibulocochlear nerve within the internal acoustic meatus
Stapes
Tympanic membrane
Tensor tympani
Internal carotid artery
External acoustic meatus
Mastoid process
Facial nerve
Styloid process
Cavity of middle ear
Auditory tube

B

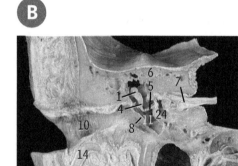

C

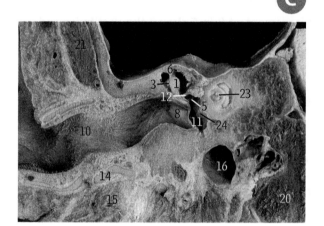

Coronal sections through the ear, and the auditory ossicles

Ⓐ diagram of a coronal section through the right ear, from the front

Ⓑ coronal section through the right ear, from the front

Ⓒ coronal section through the right ear, from the front

Ⓓ coronal section through the right ear, from behind

Ⓔ endoscopic view of adult right tympanic membrane, with descriptive diagram

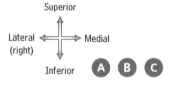

Superior

Lateral (right) ⟷ Medial

Inferior   Ⓐ Ⓑ Ⓒ

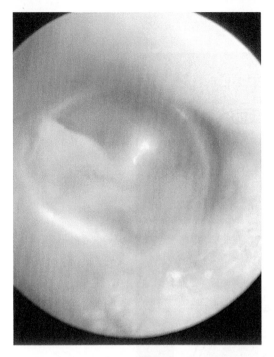

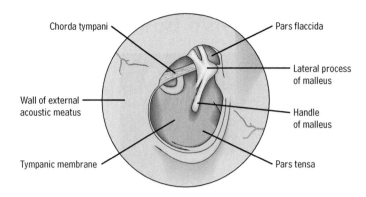

Chorda tympani

Pars flaccida

Lateral process of malleus

Wall of external acoustic meatus

Handle of malleus

Tympanic membrane

Pars tensa

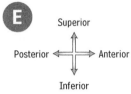

E

Superior

Posterior ⟵⟶ Anterior

Inferior

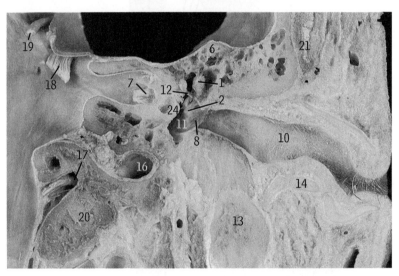

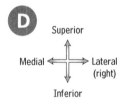

D

Superior

Medial ⟵⟶ Lateral (right)

Inferior

1 Head ⎫
2 Handle ⎬ of malleus
3 Body ⎭
4 Long limb of incus
5 Stapes
6 Tegmen tympani
7 Facial nerve and vestibulocochlear nerve within the internal acoustic meatus
8 Tympanic membrane
9 Styloid process
10 External acoustic meatus
11 Cavity of middle ear
12 Tendon of tensor tympani

13 Head of mandible
14 Auricular cartilage
15 Parotid gland
16 Internal jugular vein
17 Glossopharyngeal nerve, vagus nerve and accessory nerve entering the jugular foramen
18 Trigeminal nerve
19 Oculomotor nerve
20 Occipital condyle
21 Temporalis
22 Atlas (first cervical vertebra)
23 Cochlea
24 Promontory of middle ear

Larynx Hyoid bone and laryngeal cartilages

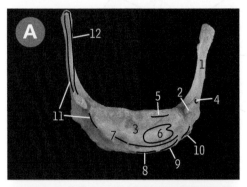

A

12
1
2
4
5
11
3
7
6
10
8
9

Posterior
Right ⬅️➡️ Left
Anterior

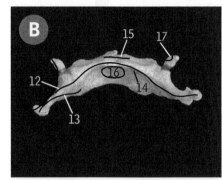

B

15
17
12
16
14
13

Superior
Left ⬅️➡️ Right
Inferior

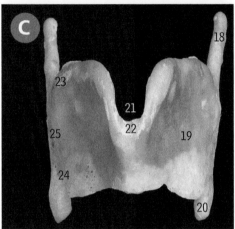

C

18
23
21
22
25
19
24
20

Superior
Right ⬅️➡️ Left
Inferior

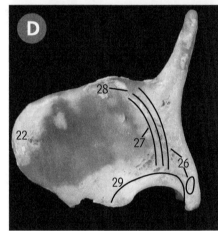

D

28
27
22
26
29

Superior
Anterior ⬅️➡️ Posterior
Inferior

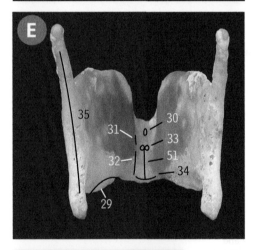

E

35
31
30
33
32
51
34
29

Superior
Left ⬅️➡️ Right
Inferior

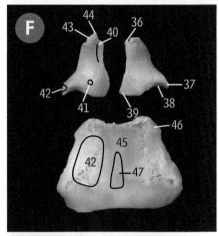

F

44
43
40
36
42
41
39
38
37
46
45
42
47

Superior
Left ⬅️➡️ Right
Inferior

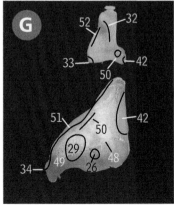

G

52
32
33
42
50
51
42
50
29
48
34
49
26

Superior
Anterior ⬅️➡️ Posterior
Inferior

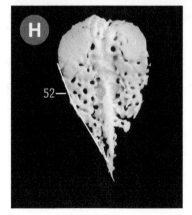

H

52

Superior
Left ⬅️➡️ Right
Inferior

The hyoid bone and the cartilages of the larynx

(A) the hyoid bone, from above and in front, with attachments

(B) the hyoid bone, from behind, with attachments

(C) the thyroid cartilage, from the front

(D) the thyroid cartilage, from the left, with attachments

(E) the thyroid cartilage, from behind, with attachments

(F) the cricoid and arytenoid cartilages, from behind, with attachments

(G) the cricoid and arytenoid cartilages, from the left, with attachments

(H) the epiglottic cartilage, from behind

On the hyoid bone and laryngeal cartilages, attachments (unless central) have been shown for simplicity on one side only, though they are of course bilateral.

The *hyoid bone*, not itself part of the larynx but attached to it by muscles and membranes, consists of a body (A3) with greater and lesser horns on each side (A1 and 2).

The *thyroid cartilage* consists of two laminae (C19) united at the front and with superior and inferior horns at the back (C18 and 20). The gap above the united thyroid laminae is the thyroid notch (C21), which is bounded below by the laryngeal prominence (Adam's apple, C22). The angle between the laminae is more acute in males than in females, in whom the prominence is less obvious.

The *cricoid cartilage* is shaped like a signet ring, with an arch at the front (G49) and a lamina at the back (F45).

The paired *arytenoid cartilages* have the shape of a three-sided pyramid, with at the base an (anterior) vocal process (F39) to which the vocal ligament is attached (G33; page 192, C32), and a (lateral) muscular process (F37) to which the posterior and lateral crico-arytenoid muscles are attached (G42 and 50; page 192, B7 and 21).

The thyroid, cricoid and almost all of the arytenoid cartilages are composed of hyaline cartilage and may undergo some degree of calcification with increasing age.

The apex of the arytenoid cartilage (F36) is composed of elastic fibrocartilage, like the epiglottic cartilage (which is leaf-shaped with numerous pits or perforations) (H) and the corniculate and cuneiform cartilages (which are like small pips or rice grains, F43 and 44). The triticeal cartilages (not shown) are very small nodules that are often found in the posterior margin of the thyrohyoid membrane (page 192, D36).

1 Greater horn ⎫
2 Lesser horn ⎬ of hyoid bone
3 Body ⎭
4 Stylohyoid ligament
5 Genioglossus
6 Geniohyoid
7 Mylohyoid
8 Sternohyoid
9 Omohyoid
10 Stylohyoid
11 Hyoglossus
12 Middle constrictor
13 Thyrohyoid
14 Thyrohyoid membrane
15 Hyoepiglottic ligament
16 Bursa
17 Chondroglossus
18 Superior horn ⎫
19 Lamina ⎬ of thyroid cartilage
20 Inferior horn ⎭
21 Thyroid notch
22 Laryngeal prominence (Adam's apple)
23 Superior ⎫
24 Inferior ⎬ tubercle of thyroid cartilage
25 Oblique line
26 Inferior constrictor

27 Sternothyroid
28 Thyrohyoid
29 Cricothyroid
30 Thyro-epiglottic ligament
31 Thyro-epiglottic muscle
32 Thyro-arytenoid
33 Vocal ligament
34 Conus elasticus
35 Stylopharyngeus and palatopharyngeus
36 Apex ⎫
37 Muscular process ⎬ of arytenoid cartilage
38 Articular surface ⎬
39 Vocal process ⎭
40 Transverse arytenoid
41 Oblique arytenoid
42 Posterior crico-arytenoid
43 Corniculate cartilage
44 Cuneiform cartilage
45 Lamina of cricoid cartilage
46 Articular surface for arytenoid cartilage
47 Tendon of oesophagus
48 Articular surface for inferior horn of thyroid cartilage
49 Arch of cricoid cartilage
50 Lateral crico-arytenoid
51 Cricothyroid ligament
52 Quadrangular membrane

Larynx and pharynx *The larynx with the pharynx, hyoid bone and trachea*

A from the right, with the cervical vertebral column removed

B as in A, after removal of the thyroid gland and part of the inferior constrictor

C from the front and the right, after removal of muscles

D in a neck dissection, from the right

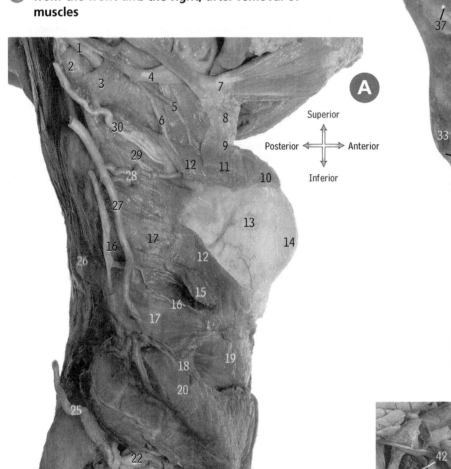

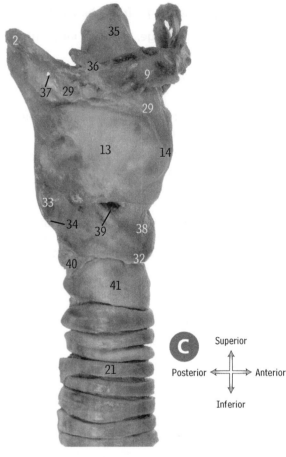

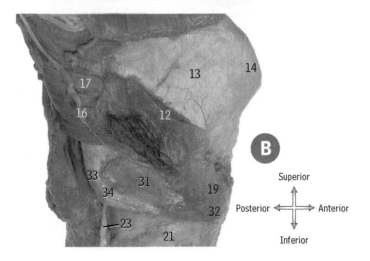

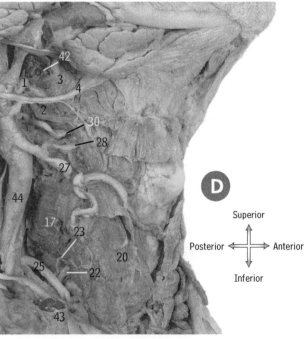

In the side view in A the lateral lobe of the thyroid gland (20) has been displaced backwards to show the part of the origin of the inferior constrictor (17) that arises from the tendinous band (18) over cricothyroid (19). The lingual artery (1) lies just above the tip of the greater horn of the hyoid bone (2) and then passes deep to the posterior border of hyoglossus (3). The internal laryngeal nerve (30) runs just below the tip of the hyoid and pierces the thyrohyoid membrane (29) with the superior laryngeal branch (28) of the superior thyroid artery (27), behind which runs the external laryngeal nerve (16). Much of thyrohyoid (12) has been removed to show part of the origin of the inferior constrictor (17) from the lamina of the thyroid cartilage (13).

In B with the thyroid gland taken away, the lowest (cricopharyngeus) part of the inferior constrictor has been removed to show the recurrent laryngeal nerve (23) passing up behind the cricothyroid joint (34).

In C all muscles, vessels and nerves have been removed to display the thyrohyoid membrane (29), the cricothyroid membrane (38 and 39), and the cricotracheal ligament (40) attached to the first tracheal ring (41, which is here unusually broad).

In D most of the internal jugular vein (43) has been removed and the common carotid artery (44) has been displaced backwards to show the inferior thyroid artery (25) and recurrent laryngeal nerve (23).

Cartilages of the larynx:
- Unpaired—thyroid, cricoid, epiglottic
- Paired—arytenoid, corniculate, cuneiform

Joints of the larynx: cricothyroid (B and C, 34), crico-arytenoid (page 192, E42), arytenocorniculate (page 192, E44).

Membranes and ligaments of the larynx:
- Extrinsic—thyrohyoid membrane (C29), hyo-epiglottic and thyro-epiglottic ligaments, cricotracheal ligament (C40).
- Intrinsic—quadrangular membrane (page 192, D37), whose upper margin forms the aryepiglottic fold (page 192, A3) and lower margin the vestibular (false vocal) fold (page 192, D28); cricothyroid ligament, whose upper margin (the vocal ligament, page 192, D32) forms the anterior part of the vocal fold (vocal cord). See notes on page 193.

The *extrinsic muscles* of the larynx (those connecting it to surrounding structures) can be divided into elevators and depressors—those directly attached to the thyroid and cricoid cartilages and which raise the larynx, e.g. during swallowing, and those that return it to the normal position:

Elevators: inferior constrictor (A17)
stylopharyngeus (page 180, B11)
palatopharyngeus (page 178, B71)   } attached to the thyroid cartilage
salpingopharyngeus (page 118, B72)
thyrohyoid (page 118, B9)

Depressors: sternothyroid (page 118, B48)—attached to thyroid cartilage
upper oesophageal attachment (page 188, F47)—to cricoid cartilage
elastic recoil of trachea

The *intrinsic muscles* of the larynx move the vocal folds and alter the shape of the laryngeal inlet, and can be classified according to their main effects on the folds or the laryngeal inlet; i.e. they alter

the shape of the rima of the glottis (the gap between the vocal folds of each side), or have a sphincteric action on the inlet:

Tensor:	cricothyroid (B19 and 31)
Relaxor:	thyro-arytenoid (page 192, B20)
Abductor:	posterior crico-arytenoid (page 192, A7)
Adductor:	lateral crico-arytenoid (page 192, B21)
	transverse arytenoid (page 192, A5)
	oblique arytenoid (page 192, A6)

The vocalis part of the thyro-arytenoid may tighten segments of the vocal fold (as when singing a high note).

The thyroepiglottic, aryepiglottic and oblique arytenoid muscles constrict the inlet; their relaxation restores the normal shape.

Cricothyroid (B19 and 31) is the only external intrinsic muscle of the larynx; it is easily seen on the outside of the larynx in dissections of the front of the neck (as on page 122, A9). The other intrinsic muscles are all inside the larynx and are only seen when the larynx itself is dissected (page 174).

The intrinsic muscles of the larynx are all supplied by the recurrent laryngeal nerve (A and B, 23) except for cricothyroid, supplied by the external laryngeal nerve (A and B, 16).

The mucous membrane of the larynx above the level of the vocal folds is supplied by the internal laryngeal nerve (A30), and below the vocal folds by the recurrent laryngeal nerve (A and B, 23).

The internal laryngeal nerve (A30) first enters the pharynx by piercing the thyrohyoid membrane (A29), and from there fibres spread into the larynx.

The recurrent laryngeal nerve (B23) lies immediately behind the cricothyroid joint (B34; page 192, B11) and enters the larynx by passing deep to the lower border of the inferior constrictor of the pharynx (A17).

---

1 Lingual artery
2 Tip of greater horn of hyoid bone
3 Hyoglossus
4 Hypoglossal nerve
5 Suprahyoid artery
6 Nerve to thyrohyoid
7 Tendon of digastric
8 Digastric sling
9 Body of hyoid bone
10 Sternohyoid
11 Superior belly of omohyoid
12 Thyrohyoid
13 Lamina of thyroid cartilage
14 Laryngeal prominence
15 Sternothyroid
16 External laryngeal nerve
17 Inferior constrictor
18 Tendinous band
19 Cricothyroid (straight part)
20 Lateral lobe of thyroid gland
21 Trachea
22 Inferior laryngeal artery
23 Recurrent laryngeal nerve
24 Oesophagus
25 Inferior thyroid artery
26 Posterior pharyngeal wall
27 Superior thyroid artery
28 Superior laryngeal artery
29 Thyrohyoid membrane
30 Internal laryngeal nerve
31 Cricothyroid (oblique part)
32 Arch of cricoid cartilage
33 Inferior horn of thyroid cartilage
34 Cricothyroid joint
35 Epiglottis
36 Lesser horn of hyoid bone
37 Aperture for internal laryngeal nerve and superior laryngeal artery
38 Conus elasticus (central part of cricothyroid ligament)
39 Cricothyroid ligament (lateral part, cricovocal membrane)
40 Cricotracheal ligament
41 First tracheal ring (unusually large)
42 Middle constrictor
43 Internal jugular vein
44 Common carotid artery

Larynx *Internal structure*

The muscles, ligaments, membranes and joints

A muscles, from behind

B muscles, from the left, after transecting the thyroid lamina and turning it forwards

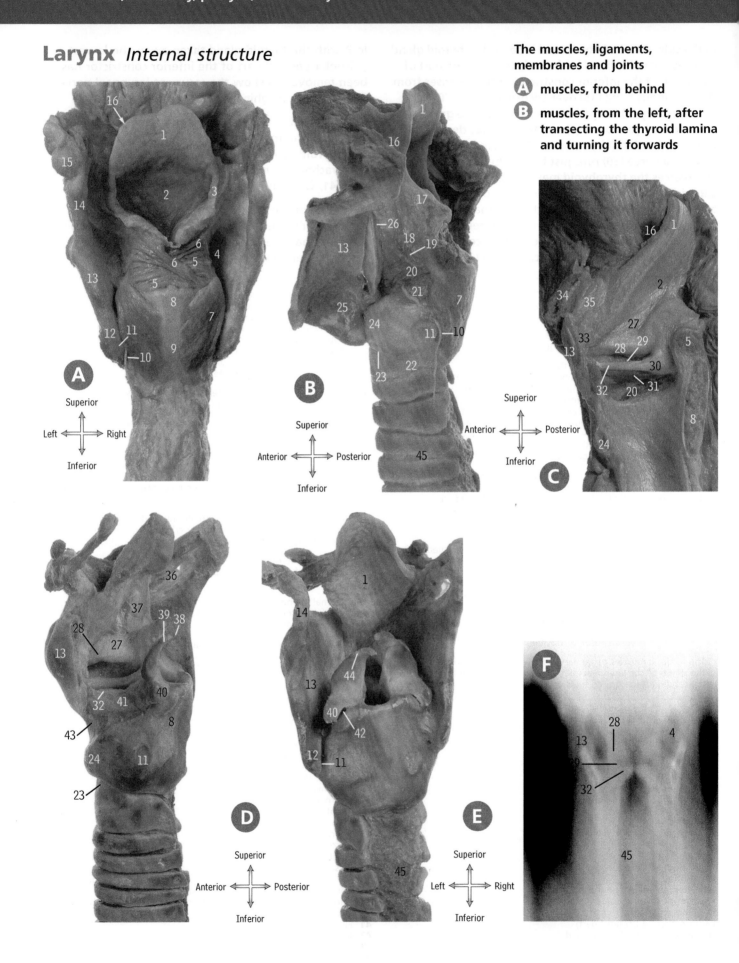

In A mucous membrane has been removed to show the most important of all laryngeal muscles, the posterior crico-arytenoid (7)—the only abductor of the vocal folds. The transverse arytenoid (5) is overlaid by the oblique arytenoids (6), whose fibres continue into the aryepiglottic fold (3) as the aryepiglottic muscles (B17).

In B most of the thyroid lamina (13) has been displaced forwards, revealing one above the other the lateral crico-arytenoid, thyro-arytenoid and thyro-epiglottic muscles (21, 20 and 18) (with some of the occasional overlying fibres that constitute the superior thyro-arytenoid, 19). The recurrent laryngeal nerve is seen passing up behind the (dislocated) cricothyroid joint (11).

In C removal of some mucous membrane below the vocal fold, formed by the vocal ligament (32) at the front and the vocal process of the arytenoid cartilage (30) at the back, shows the medial surface of the right thyro-arytenoid (20), whose upper fibres form the vocalis muscle (31). The vestibular fold (28) is at a higher level.

In D with all muscles and most of the left lamina of the thyroid cartilage removed, the left vocal ligament (32) is seen to be the upper margin of the cricovocal membrane (41). The vestibular fold (28) is the lower margin of the quadrangular membrane (37).

In E the capsules of the cricothyroid and crico-arytenoid joints (11 and 42) have been removed. This specimen is somewhat asymmetrical.

The tomogram in F, produced by a radiographic method that allows a thin 'slice' of tissue to be visualised, illustrates the vestibular and vocal folds (28 and 32) in a living subject during phonation, with the vocal folds (32) approximated.

The central (anterior) part of the cricothyroid ligament is often known as the conus elasticus (D43) (although some texts use this term for the whole ligament). The lateral part of the cricothyroid ligament is commonly known as the cricovocal membrane (D41).

The upper (free) margin of the cricovocal membrane is thickened to form the vocal ligament (D32). It is attached at the front to the lamina of the thyroid cartilage adjacent to the midline, and at the back to the vocal process of the arytenoid cartilage. Covered by mucous membrane, the vocal ligament and vocal process together form the vocal fold or vocal cord (C30 and 32).

The lower margin of the cricothyroid ligament is not free but attached to the upper border of the lamina and arch of the cricoid cartilage (D8 and 24).

The surface marking of the vocal fold is at a level midway between the laryngeal prominence and lower border of the thyroid cartilage (page 102, 16).

The quadrangular membrane, a very thin sheet of connective tissue that has been artificially thickened in D37 for emphasis, passes between the lateral side of the arytenoid cartilage (which is relatively short) to the lateral edge of the epiglottic cartilage (which is relatively long). The membrane is thus an irregular quadrilateral in shape and not rectangular.

The upper (free) margin of the quadrangular membrane is covered by mucous membrane to form the aryepiglottic fold (A3).

The lower (free) margin of the quadrangular membrane is covered by mucous membrane to form the vestibular fold (C28), also called the false vocal fold.

The slit-like space between the vestibular and vocal folds is the ventricle (or sinus) of the larynx (C29), and is continuous with the saccule, a small pouch of mucous membrane that extends upwards for a few millimetres at the anterior part of the ventricle between the vestibular fold and the inner surface of the thyroid lamina. Mucous secretion from glands in the saccule trickles down to lubricate the vocal folds.

The posterior crico-arytenoid (A7) is commonly accepted as the only muscle that can abduct the vocal folds, i.e. it opens the glottis.

The lateral crico-arytenoid (B21) and the transverse and oblique arytenoids (A5 and 6) adduct the vocal folds (close the glottis).

The cricothyroid (page 190, A19; page 120, B67) lengthens (and may increase tension in) the vocal fold.

In a *complete* recurrent laryngeal nerve lesion (e.g. complete transection during thyroidectomy), there is permanent hoarseness of the voice, and the affected vocal fold assumes a position midway between abduction and adduction.

In an *incomplete* recurrent laryngeal nerve lesion (e.g. partial transection), the affected vocal fold takes up an adducted position (for reasons which have not yet been adequately explained). Bilateral incomplete lesions are thus liable to cause respiratory embarrassment because of the very narrow airway between the folds.

In external laryngeal nerve lesions there may be no detectable abnormality. If there is any, there is some hoarseness of the voice due to loss of tension in the affected vocal fold from the paralysed cricothyroid; the fold may lie at a slightly lower level than that of the normal side. The hoarseness may disappear due to hypertrophy of the opposite cricothyroid, but with some residual loss of production of higher frequencies (as in the higher notes in singing).

C the vocal folds of the right half, in a midline sagittal section

D membranes, from the left, after resecting most of the left thyroid lamina

E joints, from behind

F Computed tomogram (CT) during phonation

1 Epiglottis	**17** Aryepiglottic muscle
2 Vestibule	**18** Thyro-epiglottic muscle
3 Aryepiglottic fold	**19** Superior thyro-arytenoid
4 Piriform recess	**20** Thyro-arytenoid
5 Transverse arytenoid	**21** Lateral crico-arytenoid
6 Oblique arytenoid	**22** First tracheal ring
7 Posterior crico-arytenoid	**23** Cricotracheal ligament
8 Lamina of cricoid cartilage	**24** Arch of cricoid cartilage
9 Site of attachment of oesophageal tendon	**25** Cricothyroid
10 Recurrent laryngeal nerve	**26** Internal laryngeal nerve
11 Cricothyroid joint	**27** Mucous membrane overlying quadrangular membrane
12 Inferior horn	**28** Vestibular fold
13 Lamina	of thyroid cartilage	**29** Ventricle of larynx
14 Superior horn	**30** Vocal process of arytenoid cartilage (posterior part of vocal fold)
15 Greater horn of hyoid bone	
16 Vallecula	

31 Vocalis part of thyro-arytenoid
32 Vocal ligament (anterior part of vocal fold)
33 Thyro-epiglottic ligament
34 Body of hyoid bone
35 Hyo-epiglottic ligament
36 Thyrohyoid membrane
37 Quadrangular membrane
38 Cuneiform cartilage
39 Corniculate cartilage
40 Muscular process of arytenoid cartilage
41 Cricovocal membrane
42 Crico-arytenoid joint
43 Conus elasticus
44 Arytenocorniculate joint
45 Trachea

Cranial cavity and brain

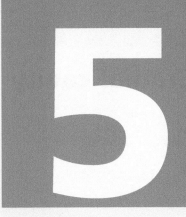

Cranial cavity

Superior

Anterior ←→ Posterior

Inferior

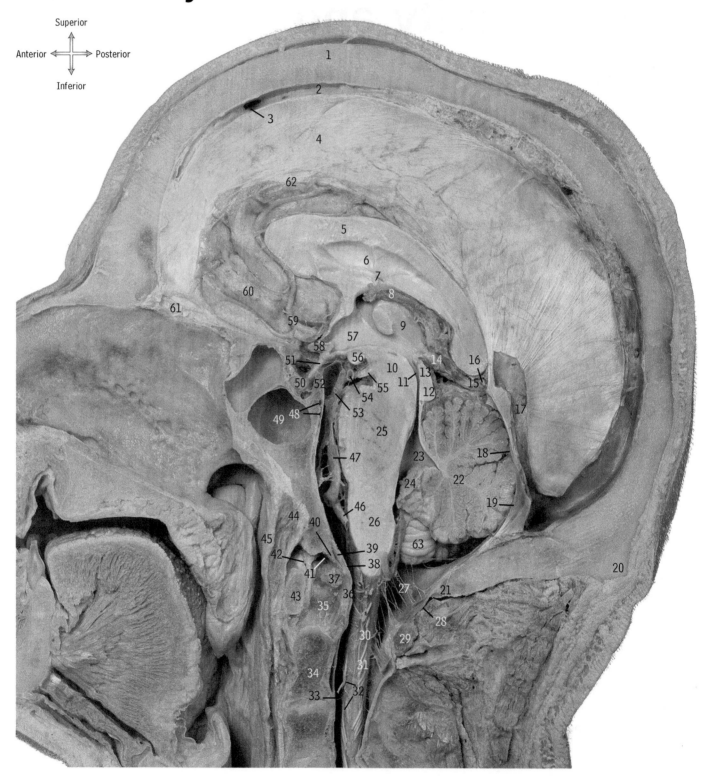

The cranial cavity, brain and meninges, in a paramedian sagittal section

The section is slightly to the left of the midline so that the dens of the axis (35) and spinal cord (30) have escaped being cut. The vault of the skull (1) is thicker than usual. The superior sagittal and straight sinuses have been opened up (2 and 17). The corpus callosum (5) lies below the falx cerebri (4), and the cerebellum (22) is below and in front of the tentorium cerebelli (18). The tonsil of the cerebellum (63) is just above the foramen magnum (21), through which the medulla oblongata (26) passes, to become the spinal cord (30)

at the level of the atlas (43 and 29). The basilar artery (47) passes up in front of the pons (25) with the posterior cerebral artery (54) arising at the upper end. The third ventricle (9) communicates with the fourth ventricle (23) via the aqueduct of the midbrain (11), and the pineal body (14) at the back of the third ventricle projects over the superior colliculus of the midbrain (13). (Details of the mouth and pharynx in this specimen are given on page 168.)

1 Vault of skull
2 Superior sagittal sinus
3 Aperture of a superior cerebral vein
4 Falx cerebri
5 Corpus callosum
6 Septum pellucidum
7 Body of fornix
8 Choroid plexus of third ventricle
9 Thalamus and third ventricle
10 Midbrain
11 Aqueduct of midbrain
12 Inferior colliculus
13 Superior colliculus
14 Pineal body
15 Great cerebral vein
16 Basal vein
17 Straight sinus
18 Tentorium cerebelli
19 Falx cerebelli
20 External occipital protuberance
21 Posterior margin of foramen magnum
22 Cerebellum
23 Fourth ventricle
24 Choroid plexus of fourth ventricle
25 Pons
26 Medulla oblongata
27 Filaments of arachnoid mater in cerebellomedullary cistern (cisterna magna)
28 Posterior atlanto-occipital membrane and overlying dura mater
29 Posterior arch of atlas
30 Spinal cord (spinal medulla)
31 Dorsal rootlets ⎱ of spinal nerves
32 Ventral rootlets ⎰

33 Spinal subarachnoid space
34 Body of axis
35 Dens of axis (left side)
36 Transverse ligament of atlas
37 Alar ligament
38 Dura mater
39 Tectorial membrane
40 Superior longitudinal band of cruciform ligament
41 Apical ligament
42 Anterior atlanto-occipital membrane
43 Anterior arch of atlas
44 Longus capitis
45 Posterior pharyngeal wall
46 Vertebral artery
47 Basilar artery
48 Basilar sinus
49 Sphenoidal sinus
50 Pituitary gland
51 Pituitary stalk
52 Dorsum sellae
53 Superior cerebellar artery
54 Posterior cerebral artery
55 Oculomotor nerve
56 Mamillary body
57 Hypothalamus
58 Optic chiasma
59 Anterior cerebral artery
60 Arachnoid mater overlying medial surface of cerebral hemisphere
61 Crista galli
62 Lower border of falx cerebri and inferior sagittal sinus
63 Tonsil of cerebellum

The cranial cavity contains:
• the brain with its vessels and membranes
• the cranial nerves
• vessels on the outermost membrane

The membranes of the brain, collectively called the meninges, consist of the dura mater, the arachnoid mater and the pia mater.

The dura mater is sometimes called the pachymeninx; the arachnoid and pia mater together constitute the leptomeninges. For further details see page 199.

Cranial vault, meninges and brain

Dissection of the scalp and cranial vault

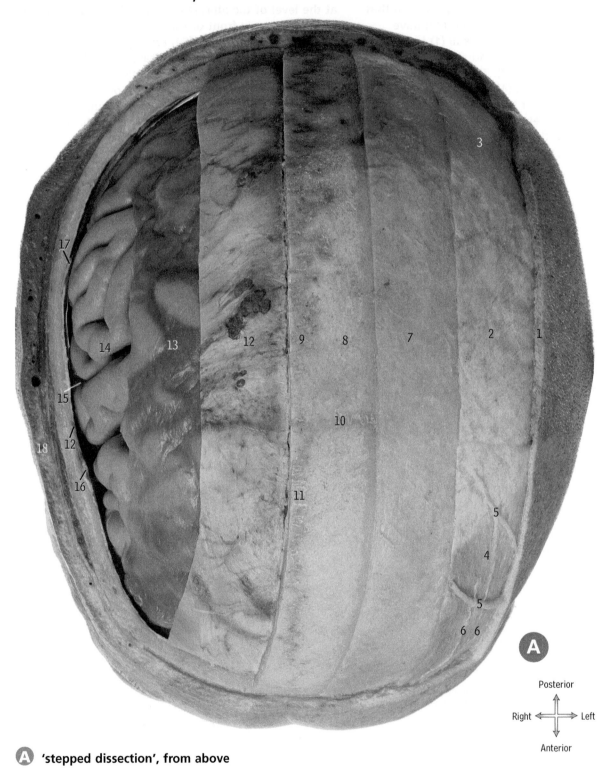

A 'stepped dissection', from above

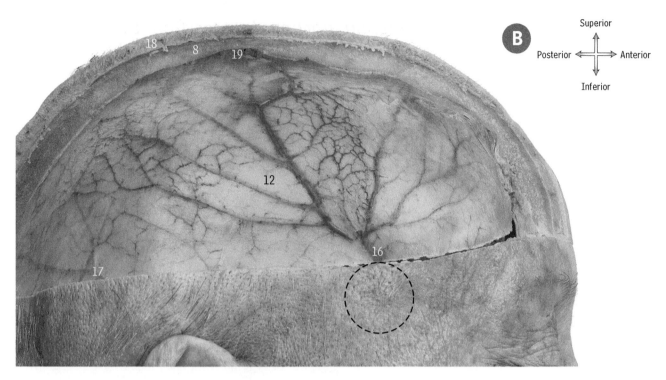

B

Superior

Posterior ←——→ Anterior

Inferior

B the dura mater and meningeal vessels on the right side

In A the bone of the cranial vault (8) has been removed on the right side of the head (left side of the picture) to show the dura mater (12), which itself has been partly removed to reveal the underlying arachnoid mater (13), in turn overlying the cerebral hemisphere (14). On the left side of the head are shown components of the scalp (1-7; see notes).

In B the scalp (18) and cranial vault (8) of the right side have been removed to display branches of the middle meningeal artery (16 and 17). The dotted circle indicates the position of pterion, the region on the surface of the skull beneath which the main trunk of the artery lies (see the note on page 9).

 1 Skin and dense subcutaneous tissue
 2 Epicranial aponeurosis (galea aponeurotica)
 3 Occipital belly ⎫
 4 Frontal belly ⎬ of occipitofrontalis
 5 Branches of superficial temporal artery
 6 Branches of supra-orbital nerve
 7 Loose connective tissue and pericranium
 8 Bone of cranial vault
 9 Sagittal suture
10 Coronal suture
11 Frontal (metopic) suture
12 Dura mater
13 Arachnoid mater
14 Cerebral hemisphere covered by pia mater
15 Subarachnoid space
16 Frontal branch ⎫
17 Parietal branch ⎬ of middle meningeal artery
18 Scalp
19 Arachnoid granulation

The scalp consists of five layers:
• skin (A1)
• dense connective tissue (A1)
• the epicranial aponeurosis and the occipitofrontalis muscle (A2, 3 and 4)
• loose connective tissue (A7)
• the pericranium (periosteum of the cranial vault, A7)

The *dura mater* (A12) is the outermost and thickest of the meninges. For further details see page 201.

The *arachnoid mater* (A13) lies inside the dura mater, separated from it by the subdural space which is merely a capillary interval: that is, the dura and arachnoid lie in contact like two pages of a closed book. Over parts of its inner surface within the cranium, the arachnoid has filamentous (spidery) projections attaching it to the pia mater (as on page 196, 27). The intervening space which is crossed by the filaments is the subarachnoid space (A15), filled with cerebrospinal fluid.

The *pia mater* (A14) adheres intimately to the surface of the brain and spinal cord. It forms the denticulate ligament at the side of the spinal cord (page 248, B31), and the subarachnoid septum at the back of the cord (page 168, 12).

The middle meningeal artery (B16 and 17) supplies the dura mater and bone but it does not supply the brain. It lies between the dura and cranial vault (B12 and 8).

Brain and meninges *The brain and arachnoid mater, from the left*

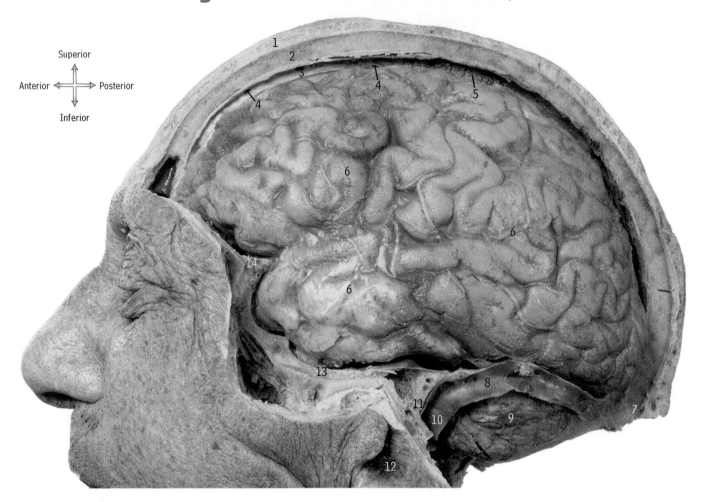

The cranial vault and part of the base of the skull and dura mater have been dissected away, leaving the arachnoid mater covering the cerebral hemisphere, and the superior sagittal sinus (3), the left transverse sinus (8) and some of the mastoid air cells (11).

 1 Scalp
 2 Cranial vault
 3 Superior sagittal sinus
 4 Openings of superior cerebral veins
 5 Arachnoid granulations
 6 Vessels and arachnoid mater overlying cerebral hemisphere
 7 External occipital protuberance
 8 Transverse sinus
 9 Cerebellar hemisphere
10 Sigmoid sinus
11 Mastoid air cells
12 External acoustic meatus
13 Floor of lateral part of middle cranial fossa
14 Floor of anterior cranial fossa

The *dura mater* has cerebral and spinal parts.

The cerebral part of the dura mater lines the inside of the cranium and consists of an outer endosteal layer (corresponding to periosteum), and an inner meningeal layer. The two layers blend with one another but in certain areas they become separated to form venous sinuses (see below).

The meningeal layer forms sheaths for the cranial nerves as they pass out through skull foramina, and also forms four processes or partitions (see page 203):
- falx cerebri (page 196, 4; page 202, 2)
- tentorium cerebelli (page 202, 25)
- falx cerebelli (page 196, 19)
- diaphragma sellae (page 206, 31)

The spinal part of the dura mater corresponds to the meningeal layer of the cerebral part and forms a sheath for the spinal cord within the vertebral canal (page 248, B35).

The venous sinuses of the dura mater lie between the endosteal and meningeal layers. Some are situated in the midline and others are paired; they can be divided into two groups:

Posterosuperior	*Antero-inferior*
Superior sagittal	Cavernous (paired)
Inferior sagittal	Intercavernous
Straight	Sphenoparietal (paired)
Transverse (paired)	Superior petrosal (paired)
Sigmoid (paired)	Inferior petrosal (paired)
Petrosquamous (paired)	Basilar
Occipital	Middle meningeal veins (paired)

Dura mater and cranial nerves

A the falx cerebri and tentorium cerebelli, from the right and above

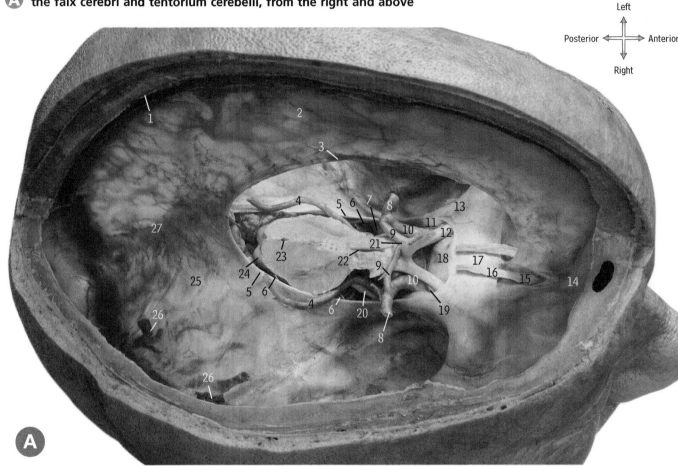

In A the brain has been removed by cutting through the brainstem at the midbrain (23) and the lowest part of the third ventricle (22), level with the free margin of the tentorium cerebelli (5), leaving intact the optic chiasma (hidden by the anterior communicating and anterior cerebral arteries, 21 and 9) with the optic nerves (12) joining it. The olfactory tracts (16) and the anterior, middle and posterior cerebral arteries (9, 8 and 4) have been severed. The straight sinus (27) lies in the dura at the junction of the falx cerebri (2) and the tentorium cerebelli (25).

In B the anterior part of the brainstem has been dissected away, leaving the cranial nerves intact.

1 Superior sagittal sinus	**17** Jugum of sphenoid bone	**34** Roots of hypoglossal nerve and
2 Falx cerebri	**18** Prechiasmatic groove	hypoglossal canal
3 Inferior sagittal sinus	**19** Ophthalmic artery	**35** Spinal root of accessory nerve
4 Posterior cerebral artery	**20** Oculomotor nerve	**36** Vertebral artery
5 Free margin of tentorium cerebelli	**21** Anterior communicating artery	**37** Dens of axis
6 Trochlear nerve	**22** Third ventricle	**38** Posterior arch of atlas
7 Attached margin of tentorium cerebelli	**23** Aqueduct of midbrain	**39** Margin of foramen magnum
and superior margin of petrous part of	**24** Inferior colliculus	**40** Medulla oblongata
temporal bone with superior petrosal	**25** Tentorium cerebelli	**41** Pons
sinus	**26** Inferior cerebral veins	**42** Midbrain
8 Middle cerebral artery	**27** Straight sinus in junction of **2** and **25**	**43** Transverse sinus
9 Anterior cerebral artery	**28** Pituitary gland	**44** Sigmoid sinus
10 Internal carotid artery	**29** Left sphenoidal sinus	**45** Nasal septum
11 Anterior clinoid process	**30** Trigeminal nerve	**46** Opening of auditory tube
12 Optic nerve	**31** Facial and vestibulocochlear nerves and	**47** Inferior margin of falx cerebri
13 Posterior margin of lesser wing of	internal acoustic meatus	**48** Internal occipital protuberance
sphenoid bone and sphenoparietal sinus	**32** Abducent nerve	
14 Crista galli	**33** Roots of glossopharyngeal, vagus and	
15 Olfactory bulb	cranial part of accessory nerves and	
16 Olfactory tract	jugular foramen	

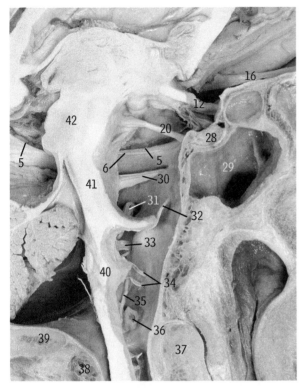

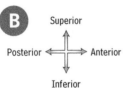

The falx cerebri (A2) is the deep midline fold of dura mater, which hangs down from the cranial vault into the longitudinal fissure between the two cerebral hemispheres (page 196, 4). The superior sagittal sinus lies in its upper border (A1; page 196, 2; page 200, 3) and the inferior sagittal sinus in its lower (free) concave margin (A3; page 196, 62 and 5). Its narrow apex at the front is attached to the crista galli (page 196, 61), and its broad base at the back to the tentorium cerebelli with the straight sinus at the junction (A27; page 196, 18 and 17; page 204, A28).

The tentorium cerebelli (A25) is the fold of dura mater forming the tent-like roof for much of the posterior cranial fossa (page 204, A27; page 206, 36). Its free margin (A5) forms the central gap over the anterior part of the fossa, which is occupied by the midbrain part of the brainstem (A23); at the front, the free margin runs forwards to form a ridge on the roof of the cavernous sinus (page 206, 33) and then becomes attached to the anterior clinoid process (A11; page 206, 32). Its attached margin adheres to the lips of the transverse and superior petrosal sinuses (page 206, 22 and 12), reaching the posterior clinoid process at the front (page 204, 8; page 206, 29). Note that the anterior end of the free margin crosses the anterior end of the attached margin before they reach their respective clinoid processes (best shown on page 206, 27 and 32, and 37 and 29).

The falx cerebelli (page 196, 19) is a very small dural fold containing the occipital sinus, in the midline below the tentorium cerebelli.

The diaphragma sellae (page 204, A17; page 206, 31) is a small circular fold of dura that forms a roof for the pituitary fossa. Part of the intercavernous sinus lies between its layers, and it is pierced by the pituitary stalk (page 204, A18; page 206, 30).

B the left half of the brainstem, with cranial nerves, in a midline sagittal section

B

Superior

Posterior ⟷ Anterior

Inferior

In C the skull has been cut para-median slightly to the right of the true median sagittal plane to reveal the falx cerebri (2) and nasal septum (45) which are mid-line structures. From this view the position of the anterior (A), middle (M) and posterior (P) cranial fossa in relationship to the falx cerebri (2) and tentorium cerebelli (25) may be appreciated.

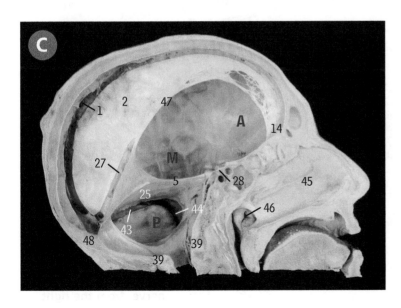

C the falx cerebri and tentorium cerebelli, from the right

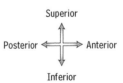

Superior

Posterior ⟷ Anterior

Inferior

Dura mater

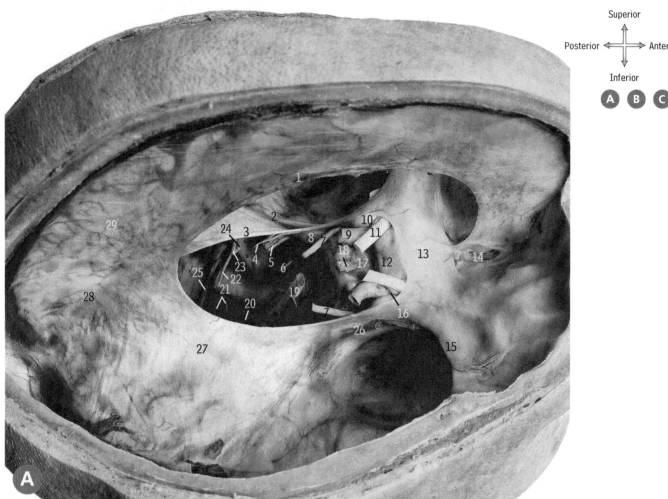

Superior
Posterior ← → Anterior
Inferior

Ⓐ Ⓑ Ⓒ

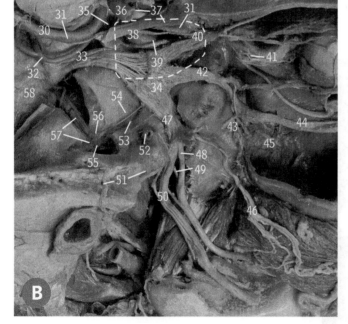

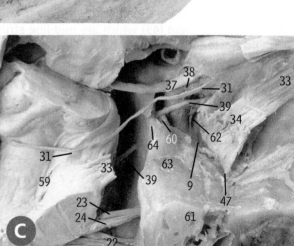

Ⓑ Ⓒ

Ⓐ the falx and tentorium, from the right, above and behind

Ⓑ the right cavernous sinus and trigeminal nerve, from the right

Ⓒ the right cavernous sinus, from the right

The falx cerebri, tentorium cerebelli, cavernous sinus and the trigeminal nerve

In A the brainstem has been removed from the specimen shown on page 202 so that cranial nerves can be seen piercing the dura. The oculomotor nerve (7) enters the roof of the cavernous sinus (26); other nerves enter it from behind. The trochlear nerve (4) pierces the dura at the junction of the free and attached margins of the tentorium cerebelli (3 and 2), with the abducent nerve (6) lower down. The trigeminal nerve (5) runs forwards over the tip of the petrous part of the temporal bone, the facial and vestibulocochlear nerves (24 and 23) enter the internal acoustic meatus, and the roots of the glossopharyngeal, vagus and cranial part of the accessory nerves (22), with the spinal root of the accessory nerve (25), enter the jugular foramen. Compare with page 203, B, C.

In B much of the skull base of the right side has been dissected away and the superior orbital fissure (40), foramen rotundum (42) and foramen ovale (47) have been opened up, with removal of most of the dura but leaving part of the free margin of the tentorium (35) as a landmark. The dashed line indicates the extent of the cavernous sinus, whose contents (see notes) are seen from the lateral side. Bone of the petrous temporal has been removed to show the facial nerve (57) with its genicular ganglion (56) giving off the greater petrosal nerve (54) which runs forwards to the (hidden) foramen lacerum. The lesser petrosal nerve (53) emerges from the middle ear (55) to join the otic ganglion, hidden on the medial side of the mandibular nerve (47).

In C the lateral wall of the cavernous sinus has been opened up. The trigeminal nerve (33) has been transected and turned forwards, lifting the trigeminal ganglion (34) away from the trigeminal impression on the petrous bone (63) and giving a view of the oculomotor, trochlear and abducent nerves (37, 31 and 39) in the sinus.

The cavernous sinus (A26; page 206, 33) contains the internal carotid artery with its sympathetic plexus (C38 and 62); the abducent nerve on the lateral side of the artery (B39); and the oculomotor, trochlear, ophthalmic and maxillary nerves in the lateral wall (B37, 31, 40 and 42).

The trigeminal ganglion (B34) lies in the trigeminal cave of dura mater, in the trigeminal impression (C63; page 54, C37) at the apex of the petrous part of the temporal bone, below and behind the cavernous sinus.

The facial nerve (B57) enters the internal acoustic meatus and runs laterally in the facial canal above the vestibule of the inner ear to the genicular ganglion (B56) in the medial wall of the epitympanic recess. The nerve then takes a right-angled turn backwards in the medial wall of the middle ear (B55) above the promontory, passes downwards in the medial wall of the aditus to the mastoid antrum, and finally emerges through the stylomastoid foramen.

The greater petrosal nerve (B54, from the facial) is joined by the deep petrosal nerve (from the sympathetic plexus of the internal carotid artery, C62) within the foramen lacerum to form the nerve of the pterygoid canal (page 176, A6).

After emerging from the brainstem between the pons and pyramid (page 236, A11), the abducent nerve runs forwards and slightly upwards and laterally through the cisterna pontis to pierce the dura mater on the clivus (C, lower 39). The nerve continues upwards beneath the dura to bend forwards over the tip of the petrous part of the temporal bone and beneath the petrosphenoidal ligament (C64) to enter the cavernous sinus. The nerve can be damaged in fractures of the skull that involve the petrous temporal or clivus, or by stretching if the brainstem is forced downwards. Displacement of the midbrain may also damage the oculomotor and trochlear nerves.

---

1 Inferior margin of falx cerebri and inferior sagittal sinus
2 Attached margin of tentorium cerebelli and superior petrosal sinus
3 Free margin of tentorium cerebelli
4 Trochlear nerve
5 Trigeminal nerve
6 Abducent nerve
7 Oculomotor nerve
8 Posterior clinoid process
9 Internal carotid artery
10 Anterior clinoid process
11 Optic nerve
12 Prechiasmatic groove
13 Jugum of sphenoid bone
14 Cribriform plate of ethmoid bone
15 Posterior margin of lesser wing of sphenoid bone and sphenoparietal sinus
16 Ophthalmic artery
17 Diaphragma sellae
18 Pituitary stalk
19 Basilar artery
20 Left vertebral artery
21 Hypoglossal nerve

22 Roots of glossopharyngeal, vagus and cranial part of accessory nerves
23 Facial nerve
24 Vestibulocochlear nerve
25 Spinal root of accessory nerve
26 Cavernous sinus
27 Tentorium cerebelli
28 Straight sinus in junction between 27 and 29
29 Falx cerebri
30 Posterior cerebral artery
31 Trochlear nerve
32 Superior cerebellar artery
33 Trigeminal nerve
34 Trigeminal ganglion
35 Free margin of tentorium cerebelli
36 Middle cerebral artery
37 Oculomotor nerve
38 Internal carotid artery
39 Abducent nerve
40 Ophthalmic nerve entering superior orbital fissure
41 Ciliary ganglion
42 Maxillary nerve in foramen rotundum

43 Posterior superior alveolar nerve
44 Infra-orbital nerve
45 Maxillary sinus
46 Buccal nerve
47 Mandibular nerve in foramen ovale
48 Lingual nerve
49 Chorda tympani
50 Inferior alveolar nerve
51 Auriculotemporal nerve
52 Middle meningeal artery in foramen spinosum
53 Lesser petrosal nerve
54 Greater petrosal nerve
55 Middle ear (tympanic cavity)
56 Genicular ganglion of facial nerve
57 Facial nerve
58 Cerebellum
59 Pons
60 Apex of petrous part of temporal bone
61 Upper margin of foramen lacerum
62 Sympathetic plexus (internal carotid nerve)
63 Trigeminal impression
64 Petrosphenoidal ligament

The cranial fossae, from above

Anterior

Left ⟵⟶ Right

Posterior

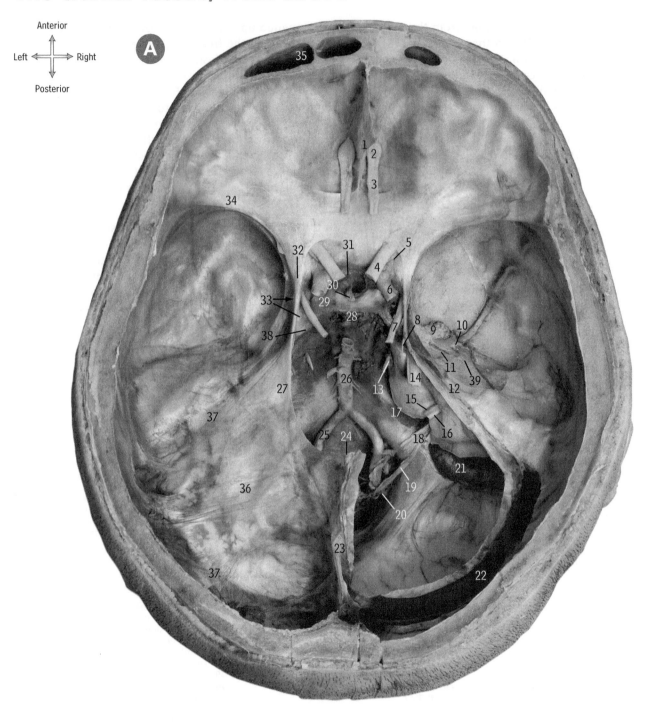

A The right half of the tentorium cerebelli (36) has been removed. The right transverse, sigmoid and superior petrosal sinuses (22, 21 and 12) and the straight sinus (23) have been opened up, and part of the dura has been stripped off from the right lateral part of the middle cranial fossa to reveal the middle meningeal artery (10), the mandibular nerve (9) and the groove for the greater petrosal nerve (11). Compare this view of the various cranial nerves piercing the dura with that on page 204, A

1 Falx cerebri attached to crista galli
2 Olfactory bulb
3 Olfactory tract
4 Optic nerve emerging from optic canal
5 Ophthalmic artery
6 Internal carotid artery
7 Oculomotor nerve
8 Trochlear nerve
9 Mandibular nerve and foramen ovale
10 Middle meningeal artery and foramen spinosum
11 Groove for greater petrosal nerve
12 Superior petrosal sinus and cut edges of attached margin of tentorium cerebelli
13 Abducent nerve
14 Trigeminal nerve
15 Facial nerve
16 Vestibulocochlear nerve
17 Inferior petrosal sinus
18 Roots of glossopharyngeal, vagus and cranial part of accessory nerves
19 Spinal root of accessory nerve
20 Hypoglossal nerve
21 Sigmoid sinus
22 Transverse sinus
23 Straight sinus at junction of falx cerebri and tentorium cerebelli
24 Great cerebral vein
25 Vertebral artery
26 Basilar artery
27 Free margin of tentorium cerebelli
28 Upper part of basilar plexus
29 Posterior clinoid process
30 Pituitary stalk
31 Diaphragma sellae
32 Anterior clinoid process
33 Cavernous sinus
34 Posterior margin of lesser wing of sphenoid bone and sphenoparietal sinus
35 Frontal sinus
36 Tentorium cerebelli
37 Attached margin of tentorium
38 Attached margin of tentorium passing to **29**
39 Groove for lesser petrosal nerve
40 Adenohypophysis (anterior lobe of pituitary gland)
41 Neurohypophysis (posterior lobe of pituitary gland)

The tentorium cerebelli (36) forms the roof of the posterior cranial fossa; the anterior and middle cranial fossae have no defined upper boundary.

The *anterior cranial fossa* contains:
• the front parts of the frontal lobes of the cerebral hemispheres (page 200, 14)
• the olfactory nerves, olfactory bulbs and olfactory tracts (2 and 3)
• the anterior ethmoidal nerves and vessels (page 148, C32 and 35).

The *middle cranial fossa* contains in its median part:
• the pituitary stalk and gland and the diaphragma sellae (30 and 31)
• the optic nerves (4) and optic chiasma (page 236, A3 and 4)
• the intercavernous sinus (below the pituitary gland) and in its lateral parts
• the cavernous sinus (33) containing the internal carotid artery and sympathetic plexus, the oculomotor, trochlear and abducent nerves, and the ophthalmic and maxillary branches of the trigeminal nerve (see pages 204 and 205)
• the trigeminal ganglion and the mandibular branch of the trigeminal nerve (see pages 204 and 205)
• the greater and lesser petrosal nerves (11 and 39)
• the middle meningeal (10) and accessory meningeal vessels, and meningeal branches of the ascending pharyngeal, ophthalmic and lacrimal arteries
• the temporal lobes of the cerebral hemispheres (page 206, 13).

The *posterior cranial fossa* contains:
• the lowest part of the midbrain, and the pons, medulla oblongata and cerebellum (page 196, 10, 25, 26 and 22)
• the vertebral and basilar arteries and their branches (25 and 26), and meningeal branches of the ascending pharyngeal and occipital arteries
• the sigmoid (21), inferior petrosal (17), basilar and occipital sinuses, with the straight, transverse and superior petrosal sinuses in the tentorium cerebelli that forms the roof (23, 22 and 12)
• the trigeminal (14), abducent (13), facial (15), vestibulocochlear (16), glossopharyngeal, vagus and accessory (18 and 19) and hypoglossal nerves (i.e. the fifth to twelfth cranial nerves), and meningeal branches of upper cervical nerves
• the falx cerebelli (page 196, 19).

The posterior (lower) end of the superior sagittal sinus is known as the confluence of the sinuses, where there is communication with the straight and occipital sinuses and the transverse sinuses of both sides.

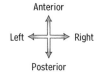

Anterior

Left ⟷ Right

Posterior

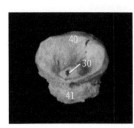

B an isolated pituitary gland (shown enlarged to approx. 167% of actual size as presented at dissection, from above)

(See pages 30-32, 212-217 for pituitary fossa and pituitary gland in situ.)

Cranial nerves and their connections

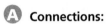

Connections:
Red– Sympathetic
Yellow– Parasympathetic
Orange– Sensory

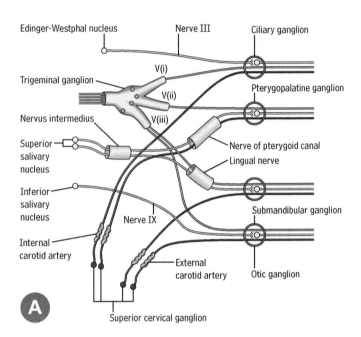

Edinger-Westphal nucleus

Nerve III

Ciliary ganglion

V(i)

Trigeminal ganglion

V(ii)

Pterygopalatine ganglion

Nervus intermedius

V(iii)

Superior salivary nucleus

Nerve of pterygoid canal

Lingual nerve

Inferior salivary nucleus

Nerve IX

Submandibular ganglion

Internal carotid artery

External carotid artery

Otic ganglion

Superior cervical ganglion

A

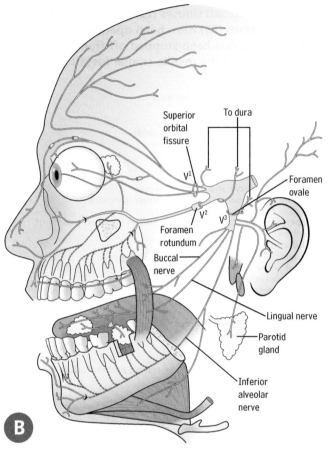

Superior orbital fissure

To dura

V¹

Foramen ovale

Foramen rotundum

V²

V³

Buccal nerve

Lingual nerve

Parotid gland

Inferior alveolar nerve

B

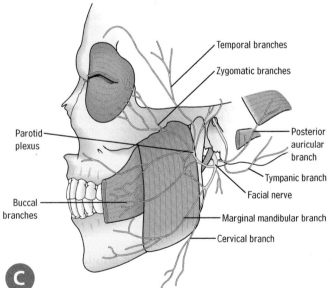

Temporal branches

Zygomatic branches

Parotid plexus

Posterior auricular branch

Tympanic branch

Facial nerve

Buccal branches

Marginal mandibular branch

Cervical branch

C

A diagram of the connections of the cranial ganglia

B diagram of the branches of the trigeminal nerve V

C diagram of the branches of the facial nerve VII

D diagram of the branches of the hypoglossal nerve XII

E diagram of the branches of the glossopharyngeal nerve IX

F diagram of the branches of the vagus nerve X

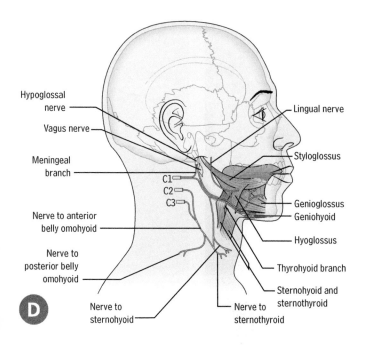

D

Hypoglossal nerve

Vagus nerve

Meningeal branch

Nerve to anterior belly omohyoid

Nerve to posterior belly omohyoid

Nerve to sternohyoid

C1
C2
C3

Lingual nerve

Styloglossus

Genioglossus
Geniohyoid

Hyoglossus

Thyrohyoid branch

Sternohyoid and sternothyroid

Nerve to sternothyroid

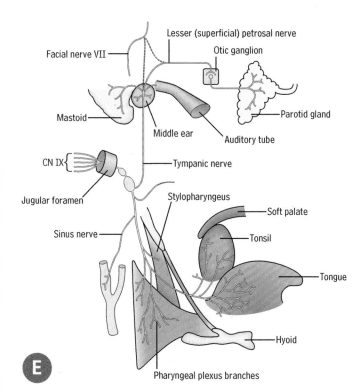

E

Facial nerve VII

Mastoid

CN IX

Jugular foramen

Sinus nerve

Lesser (superficial) petrosal nerve

Otic ganglion

Middle ear

Auditory tube

Parotid gland

Tympanic nerve

Stylopharyngeus

Soft palate

Tonsil

Tongue

Hyoid

Pharyngeal plexus branches

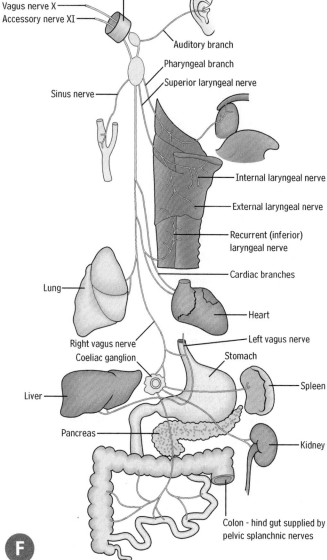

F

Vagus nerve X
Accessory nerve XI

Sinus nerve

Jugular foramen

Auditory branch

Pharyngeal branch
Superior laryngeal nerve

Internal laryngeal nerve

External laryngeal nerve

Recurrent (inferior) laryngeal nerve

Cardiac branches

Lung

Right vagus nerve
Coeliac ganglion

Liver

Pancreas

Heart

Left vagus nerve

Stomach

Spleen

Kidney

Colon - hind gut supplied by pelvic splanchnic nerves

Cranial fossae, cavernous sinus and trigeminal nerve

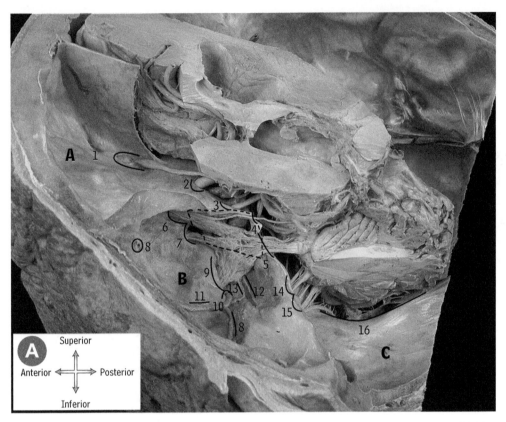

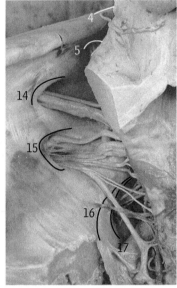

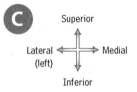

Anterior cranial fossa – A

1 *Foramina in the cribriform plate of the ethmoid bone*
 • Olfactory nerve filaments I
 • Anterior ethmoidal nerve and vessels

Middle cranial fossa – B

2 *Optic canal:* in the sphenoid bone between the body and the two roots of the lesser wing
 • Optic nerve II
 • Ophthalmic artery
3 *Roof of cavernous sinus*
 • Dura pierced by oculomotor nerve III
4 *Junction of free and attached margins of tentorium cerebelli*
 • Dura pierced by trochlear nerve IV
5 *Cavernous sinus*
 • Dura pierced by trigeminal nerve V entering from behind and running forwards over the tip of the petrous part of the temporal bone
6 *Superior orbital fissure:* in the sphenoid bone between the body and the greater and lesser wings, with a fragment of the frontal bone at the lateral extremity
 • Oculomotor nerve III
 • Trochlear nerve IV
 • Abducent nerve VI
 • Lacrimal nerve
 • Fontal nerve
 • Nasociliary nerve
 • Filaments from the internal carotid (sympathetic) plexus
 • Orbital branch of the middle meningeal artery
 • Recurrent branch of the lacrimal artery
 • Superior ophthalmic vein
7 *Foramen rotundum:* in the greater wing of the sphenoid bone
 • Maxillary nerve V2

8 *Groove for the middle meningeal artery* – parietal branch
9 *Foramen ovale:* in the greater wing of the sphenoid bone
 • Mandibular nerve V3
 • Lesser petrosal nerve (usually)
 • Accessory meningeal artery
 • Emissary veins (from cavernous sinus to pterygoid plexus)
10 *Foramen spinosum:* in the greater wing of the sphenoid bone
 • Middle meningeal vessels
 • Meningeal branch of the mandibular nerve
11 *Groove for middle meningeal artery* – frontal branch
12 *Hiatus and groove for greater petrosal nerve:* in the tegmen tympani of the petrous temporal bone, in front of the arcuate eminence
 • Greater petrosal nerve
 • Petrosal branch of the middle meningeal artery
13 *Hiatus and groove for lesser petrosal nerve:* in tegmen tympani of the petrous temporal bone, about 3 mm in front of the hiatus for the greater petrosal nerve
 • Lesser petrosal nerve

Posterior cranial fossa – C

14 *Internal acoustic meatus:* in the posterior surface of the petrous temporal bone
 • Facial nerve VII
 • Vestibulocochlear nerve VIII
 • Labyrinthine artery
15 *Jugular foramen:* between the jugular fossa of the petrous temporal bone and the occipital bone
 • Glossopharyngeal nerve IX
 • Vagus nerve X
 • Accessory nerves XI

Note: in A, lines to denote 14 and 15 have been marked on the superior margin of the petrous part of the temporal bone, however, it must be appreciated that the actual opening of the internal acoustic meatus (14) is in fact positioned inferiorly on the posterior surface of the petrous part of the temporal bone. Similarly, the jugular foramen (15) is positioned more inferiorly and is formed by the gap between the jugular notch of the occipital bone and the petrous part of the temporal bone. Picture C clarifies the actual positions of 14 and 15.

 • Meningeal branches of the vagus nerve
 • Inferior jugular vein
 • A meningeal branch of the occipital artery
16 *Foramen magnum:* in the occipital bone
 • Apical ligament of the odontoid process of the axis
 • Tectorial membrane
 • Medulla oblongata and meninges (including first digitations of denticulate ligament)
 • Spinal parts of the accessory nerves
 • Meningeal branches of the upper cervical nerves
 • Vertebral arteries
 • Anterior spinal artery
 • Posterior spinal artery

Posterior cranial fossa – C

17 *Hypoglossal canal:* in the occipital bone above the anterior part of the condyle
 • Hypoglossal nerve XII and its (recurrent) meningeal branch
 • A meningeal branch of the ascending pharyngeal artery
 • Emissary vein (from the basilar plexus to the internal jugular vein)

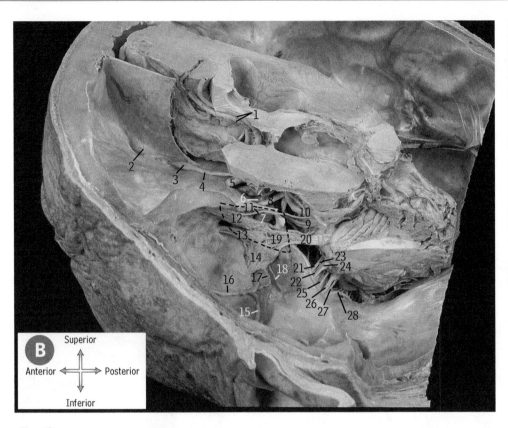

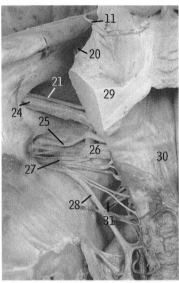

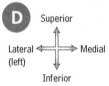

B Superior ↑ / Anterior ←→ Posterior / Inferior

D Superior ↑ / Lateral (left) ←→ Medial / Inferior

A **B**   the left cavernous sinus and trigeminal nerve from the left, above and behind

C **D**   the left half of the lower brainstem and upper part of the cervical spinal cord from behind

1	Cortical branches of middle cerebral artery
2	Falx cerebri attached to crista galli
3	Olfactory bulb
4	Olfactory tract
5	Optic nerve II
6	Pituitary gland
7	Internal carotid artery
8	Oculomotor nerve III
9	Superior cerebellar artery
10	Posterior cerebellar artery
11	Trochlear nerve IV
12	Ophthalmic nerve V¹
13	Maxillary nerve V²
14	Mandibular nerve V³
15	Middle meningeal artery parietal branch
16	Middle meningeal artery frontal branch
17	Lesser petrosal nerve
18	Greater petrosal nerve
19	Trigeminal ganglion
20	Trigeminal nerve V
21	Facial nerve VII
22	Nervous intermedius
23	Labyrinthine artery
24	Vestibulocochlear nerve VIII
25	Glossopharyngeal nerve IX
26	Vagus nerve X
27	Cranial part of accessory nerve
28	Spinal root of accessory nerve
29	Middle cerebellar peduncle
30	Floor of the fourth ventricle
31	Hypoglossal nerve XII

In **A, B**, the left half of the brain and portions of the cerebellum have been removed, and dura has been stripped off the lateral part of the middle cranial fossa to reveal structures within the cavernous sinus and branches of the trigeminal nerve, middle meningeal vessels and petrosal nerves.

In **A**, the approximate margins of skull foramina and grooves within the anterior, middle and posterior cranial fossae at the base of the skull have been highlighted with lines. The accompanying annotated list gives their position and the key structures which pass through them.

In **A, B**, the dashed line indicates the extent of the cavernous sinus.

In **C, D**, the posterior part of the skull and upper vertebrae have been removed to show continuity of the brainstem with the spinal cord.

Cranial cavity, brain, cranial nerves

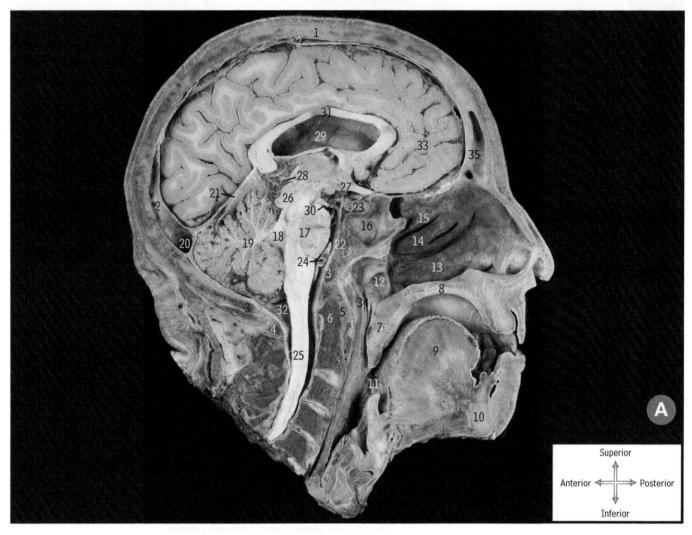

Superior

Anterior ← → Posterior

Inferior

A The cranial cavity and brain in a median sagittal section, from the right

In A the section has passed through the median sagittal plane and the action of the 1 mm saw cut has removed both the falx cerebri (page 196) and the nasal septum (page 166A; page 196).

1 Vault of skull	**18** Fourth ventricle	**33** Medial surface of left cerebral
2 Superior sagittal sinus	**19** Cerebellum	hemisphere
3 Margin of foramen magnum	**20** Transverse sinus	**34** Nasal part of pharynx (nasopharynx)
4 Posterior arch of atlas ⎱ first cervical	**21** Tentorium cerebelli	**35** Frontal sinus
5 Anterior arch of atlas ⎰ vertebra	**22** Clivus	**36** Optic nerve II
6 Dens of axis—second cervical vertebra	**23** Pituitary gland	**37** Olfactory tract
7 Soft palate	**24** Basilar artery	**38** Olfactory bulb
8 Hard palate	**25** Spinal cord (spinal medulla)	**39** Ophthalmic artery
9 Tongue	**26** Midbrain	**40** Trochlear nerve IV
10 Mandible	**27** Optic chiasma	**41** Trigeminal nerve V
11 Oral part of pharynx (oropharynx)	**28** Pineal body	**42** Facial nerve VII, vestibulocochlear
12 Opening of auditory tube	**29** Lateral ventricle	nerve VIII
13 Inferior nasal concha	**30** Oculomotor nerve III	**43** Roots of glossopharyngeal nerve
14 Middle nasal concha	**31** Corpus callosum	IX, vagus nerve X, cranial part of
15 Superior nasal concha	**32** Cerebellomedullary cistern (cisterna	accessory nerve XI
16 Sphenoidal sinus	magna)	**44** Abducent nerve VI
17 Pons		

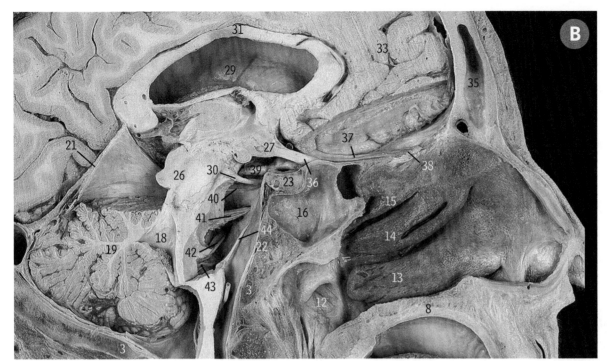

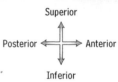

B As A (enlargement of the central area)

In B the inferior aspect of the frontal lobe of the brain,
pons, medulla oblongata and the anterior lobe of the
cerebellum have been dissected to expose cranial nerves.

Superior
Posterior ⟷ Anterior
Inferior

Cranial nerves and their principal function—see also p. 290, p. 291 and p. 237		
I Olfactory	Smell	Not a single nerve but about 20 small filaments passing through the roof of the nose to the olfactory bulb on the under-surface of the brain
II Optic	Vision	Passing back from the retina of the eye to the optic chiasma on the under-surface of the brain
III Oculomotor	Motor/ parasympathetic	To four of the muscles which move the eye, and also containing parasympathetic fibres which constrict the pupil and alter the curvature of the lens
IV Trochlear	Motor	To one of the eye muscles (superior oblique)
V Trigeminal	Sensory/motor	Main sensory nerve of the head including the face and the surface of the eye, and the motor nerve to muscles of mastication (chewing), moving the lower jaw
VI Abducent	Motor	To one of the eye muscles (lateral rectus)
VII Facial	Motor/sensory/ parasympathetic	To the muscles of the face, and containing some taste fibres and parasympathetic lacrimal, salivary and nasal glands
VIII Vestibulocochlear	Motor/sensory	Combined nerve for balance (vestibular part) and hearing (cochlear part)
IX Glossopharyngeal	Sensory/ parasympathetic	Some taste fibres, and other sensory fibres for the lining of the throat, and small but parasympathetic fibres for reflex control of blood pressure
X Vagus	Motor/sensory/ parasympathetic	To larynx, pharynx and soft palate (for speech and swallowing), and gastric secretion and movement, and slowing heart rate. Afferent from many thoracic and abdominal viscera
XI Accessory	Motor	The spinal part goes to the sternocleidomastoid and the trapezius, with other fibres (the cranial part) joining the vagus to supply the larynx, pharynx and soft palate
XII Hypoglossal	Motor	To tongue muscles

Cranial cavity, cranial nerves

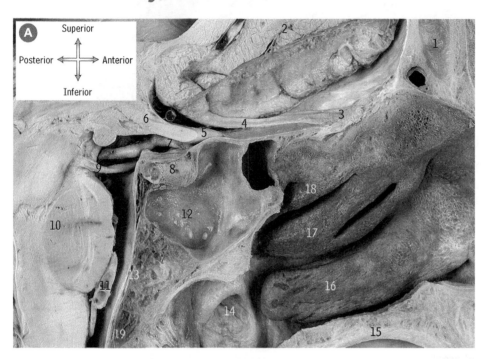

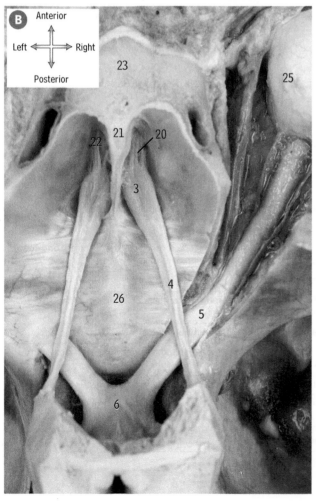

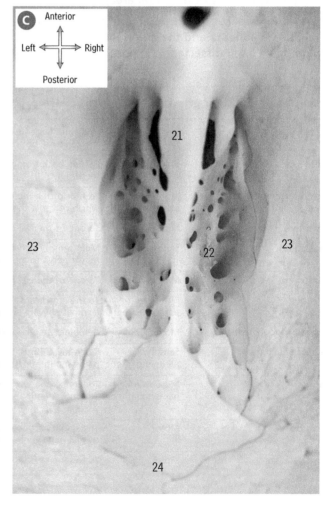

A   as B (page 213), enlargement of the lateral wall of the nasal cavity

B   central floor of the anterior cranial fossa, from above

C   cribriform plate of ethmoid bone in a skull, from above

D   as B (page 213), enlargement of pons, clivus and sphenoidal sinus area

E   as B (page 213), enlargement of the dorsal surface of the brainstem, from the right, above and behind

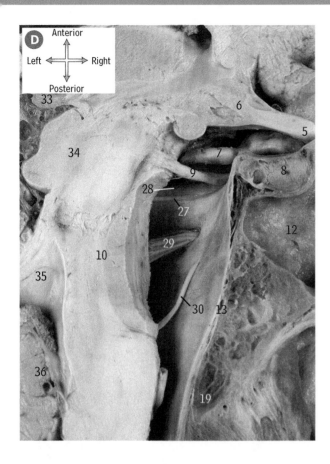

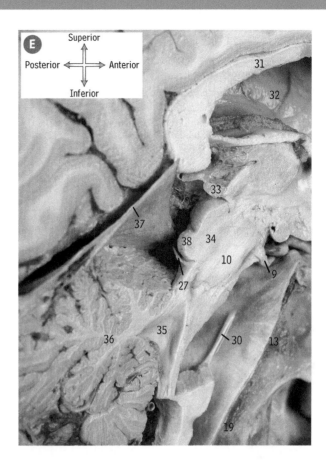

In A, a portion of tissue has been removed from the inferior aspect of the frontal lobe of the brain along with arachnoid mater and associated blood vessels to expose the olfactory tract (4), olfactory bulb (3) and optic nerve (5).

In B the cerebral hemispheres of the brain have been removed at the level of the third ventricle and a wedge of bone from the roof of the right orbit to expose: olfactory tracts (4), olfactory bulbs (3), filaments of olfactory nerves (20), optic chiasma (6) and extent of the right optic nerve (5). Olfactory nerve filaments (20), twenty or so in number, pass from the olfactory mucous membrane through the perforations of the cribriform plate of the ethmoid bone (22) ensheathed in dura mater (26), and pia arachnoid.

C complements B by illustrating the multiple perforations (foramina) in the cribriform plate of the ethmoid bone (22) through which pass filaments of olfactory nerve (20).

In D a portion of the pons, arachnoid mater and associated blood vessels have been removed to expose the oculomotor nerve (9), trochlear nerve (27), trigeminal nerve (29) and abducent nerve (30).

In E the anterior lobe of the cerebellum has been removed with arachnoid mater and associated blood vessels to expose the trochlear nerve (27) emerging from the dorsal surface of the brainstem.

1	Frontal sinus	**21**	Crista galli
2	Medial surface of the left cerebral hemisphere	**22**	Cribriform plate of ethmoid bone
3	Olfactory bulb	**23**	Frontal bone
4	Olfactory tract	**24**	Jugum of sphenoid bone
5	Optic nerve II	**25**	Eyeball
6	Optic chiasma	**26**	Dura overlying floor of the anterior cranial fossa
7	Ophthalmic artery	**27**	Trochlear nerve IV
8	Pituitary gland	**28**	Free margin of tentorium cerebelli
9	Oculomotor nerve III	**29**	Trigeminal nerve V
10	Pons	**30**	Abducent nerve VI
11	Basilar artery	**31**	Corpus callosum
12	Sphenoidal sinus	**32**	Lateral ventricle
13	Clivus	**33**	Pineal body
14	Opening of auditory tube	**34**	Midbrain
15	Hard palate	**35**	Fourth ventricle
16	Inferior nasal concha	**36**	Cerebellum
17	Middle nasal concha	**37**	Tentorium cerebelli
18	Superior nasal concha	**38**	Inferior colliculus
19	Margin of foramen magnum		
20	Filaments of olfactory nerve I		

Cranial nerves

Notes on: The Olfactory nerve I

Traditionally, the *olfactory bulb* and the *olfactory tract* have been rather erroneously referred to as the **olfactory nerve I**.

Probably, because these two interconnected structures are easily located and observed at the base of the brain, (3 and 4 p. 232) and in the floor of the anterior cranial fossa, (B 3 and 4 p. 211), using basic dissection technique.

Whereas, the true **olfactory nerves I**, (B 20 p. 214) are rarely seen in the dissecting room, requiring skilled dissection under magnification, in order to reveal them.

The **olfactory nerve I** is in fact, not a single nerve, but about 20 small filaments which have their origins in the olfactory nasal

mucosa in the nasal cavity. They collect in bundles and together form a criss-cross plexiform network in the mucosa, each nerve filament ensheathed in dura mater and pia arachnoid. The nerves, in their sheaths, arise through, the multiple bony perforations in the cribriform plate of the ethmoid bone (C 22 p. 214), in lateral and medial groups, to end in the glomeruli of the olfactory bulbs, via the bulbs undersurface.

Therefore, in strict terminology, it can be considered that the *olfactory bulb* and the *olfactory tract*, although integral parts, are not the true **olfactory nerve I**.

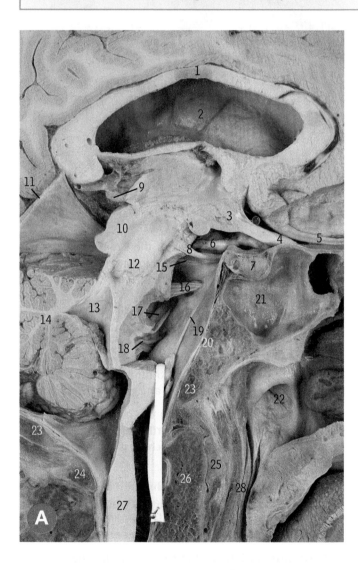

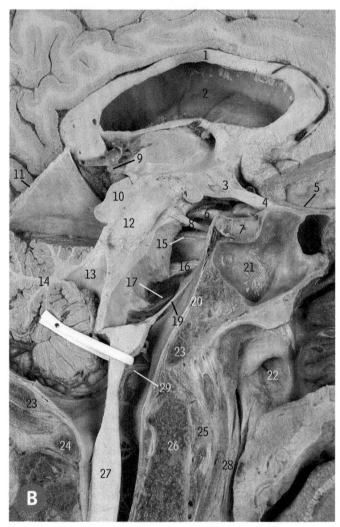

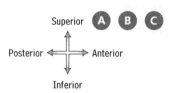

A **B** **C**   as B (page 213), enlargement of the pons, clivus and sphenoidal sinus area

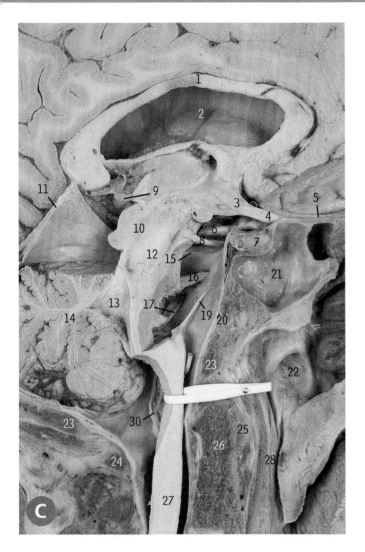

In A further dissection has been carried out with removal of more tissue from the pons, and a white plastic band has been used to displace the spinal cord. Exposed superiorly to inferiorly are: olfactory tract (5), optic chiasma (3), optic nerve (4), oculomotor nerve (8), trochlear nerve (15), trigeminal nerve (16), facial nerve (17), vestibulocochlear nerve (17), roots of the glossopharyngeal nerve (18), vagus nerve (18) and cranial root of the accessory nerve (18).

In B a small portion of tissue has been removed from the anterior aspect of the medulla oblongata which has been displaced by a white plastic band to display roots of the hypoglossal nerve (29).

In C a portion of tissue from the posterior aspect of the medulla oblongata has been removed and the medulla displaced by a white plastic band to display the spinal root of the accessory nerve (30).

1	Corpus callosum	**17**	Facial nerve VII, vestibulocochlear nerve VIII
2	Lateral ventricle	**18**	Roots of glossopharyngeal nerve IX, vagus nerve X, cranial part of accessory nerve XI
3	Optic chiasma		
4	Optic nerve II	**19**	Abducent nerve VI
5	Olfactory tract	**20**	Clivus
6	Ophthalmic artery	**21**	Sphenoid sinus
7	Pituitary gland	**22**	Opening of auditory tube
8	Oculomotor nerve III	**23**	Margin of foramen magnum
9	Pineal body	**24**	Posterior arch of atlas
10	Midbrain	**25**	Anterior arch of atlas—first cervical vertebra
11	Tentorium cerebelli	**26**	Dens of axis—second cervical vertebra
12	Pons	**27**	Spinal cord (spinal medulla)
13	Fourth ventricle	**28**	Nasal part of pharynx (nasopharynx)
14	Cerebellum	**29**	Roots of hypoglossal nerve XII
15	Trochlear nerve IV	**30**	Spinal root of accessory nerve XI
16	Trigeminal nerve V		

Brain Brain and meninges

The brain within the meninges, from above

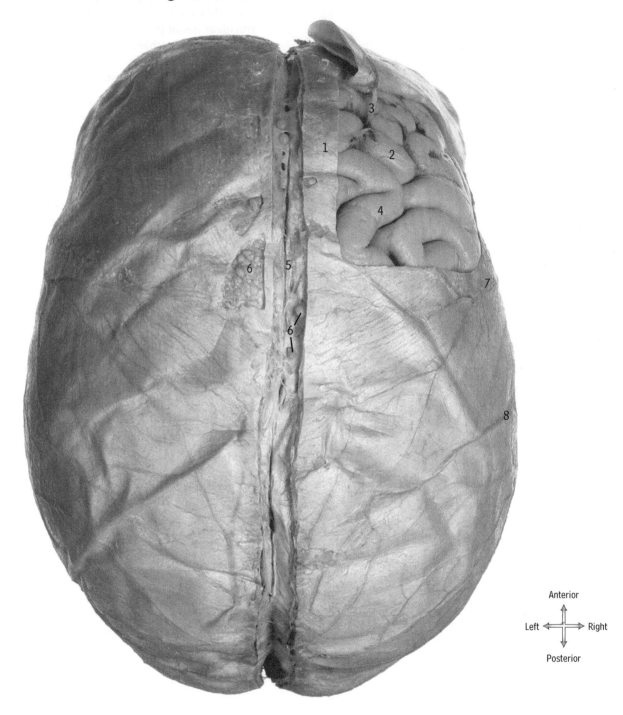

Anterior

Left ⟷ Right

Posterior

Here the whole of the dura mater has been stripped off from the inside of the cranial vault and removed intact with the brain; this is an unusual dissection—the dura is normally left within the cranium (as on page 199, B) and the brain removed with the arachnoid surrounding it (as on pages 220 and 222). A window has been cut in the dura over the front of the right cerebral hemisphere, and the flap of dura turned forwards to show the underlying filmy and transparent arachnoid mater; some arachnoid has been removed, and it is labelled (2) at the cut edge. The dura forming the roof of the superior sagittal sinus (5) has also been removed, to show the arachnoid granulations (6) projecting into the sinus (cerebrospinal fluid drains into the venous blood through the walls of these projections).

1 Dura mater
2 Arachnoid mater (cut edge)
3 A superior cerebral vein
4 Cerebral hemisphere (and pia mater)
5 Superior sagittal sinus
6 Arachnoid granulations
7 Frontal branch ⎤
8 Parietal branch ⎦ of middle meningeal artery

For notes on the meninges see page 197.

The central nervous system consists of the brain and spinal cord (properly known as the spinal medulla).

The brain consists of:
• the hindbrain (rhombencephalon), comprising the medulla oblongata (myelencephalon), pons (metencephalon) and the cerebellum
• the midbrain (mesencephalon)
• the forebrain (prosencephalon), comprising the diencephalon (structures surrounding the third ventricle) and the cerebral hemispheres (telencephalon)

The cavity of the hindbrain is the fourth ventricle.

The cavity of the midbrain is the aqueduct.

The cavities of the forebrain are the third ventricle (centrally) and the lateral ventricles (one in each cerebral hemisphere).

For notes on the ventricles see page 239.

The brainstem (see page 229) consists of:
• the midbrain
• the pons
• the medulla oblongata

The peripheral nervous system consists of:
• the cranial nerves (12 pairs)
• the spinal nerves (31 pairs)
• the autonomic system of nerves and their associated ganglia

Cerebral hemispheres and cerebellum

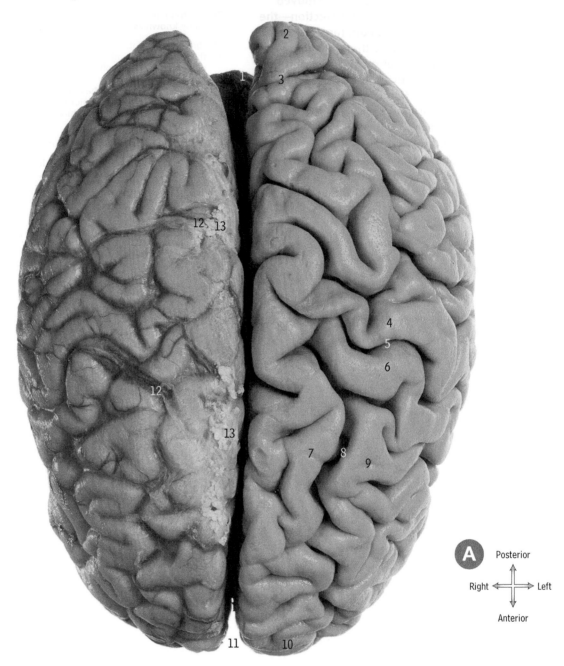

The cerebral and cerebellar hemispheres

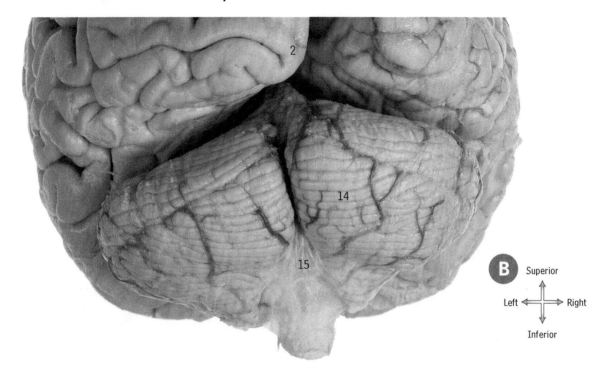

B   Superior

Left ⟷ Right

Inferior

Ⓐ the cerebral hemispheres, from above

Ⓑ the lower part of the brain, from behind, showing the cerebellum

The arachnoid, with the underlying blood vessels, remains intact over the right cerebral hemisphere in A and B, and over the cerebellum in B, but it has been removed from the left hemisphere. In life, cerebrospinal fluid would raise the arachnoid from the brain surface. The larger gaps beneath the arachnoid form various cisterns (cisternae), such as the cerebellomedullary cistern (cisterna magna, 15).

The cerebral cortex is thrown into broad convoluted folds known as gyri (singular—gyrus). The spaces between the gyri are the sulci (singular—sulcus).

No two brains have identical gyri and sulci, but the general pattern is sufficiently constant to allow the gyri and sulci to be named. Only those of major clinical importance are identified here and on pages 224 and 230.

The cerebellar cortex is thrown into narrow closely packed folds known as folia. Unlike the gyri of the cerebral cortex, the cerebellar folia are not individually identified, but names are given to particular areas.

1 Cerebellum
2 Occipital pole
3 Parieto-occipital sulcus
4 Postcentral gyrus
5 Central sulcus
6 Precentral gyrus
7 Superior frontal gyrus
8 Superior frontal sulcus
9 Middle frontal gyrus
10 Frontal pole
11 Longitudinal fissure
12 Superior cerebral veins
13 Arachnoid granulations
14 Cerebellar hemisphere
15 Arachnoid mater of cerebellomedullary cistern (cisterna magna)

Cerebral veins *The external cerebral veins, from the right*

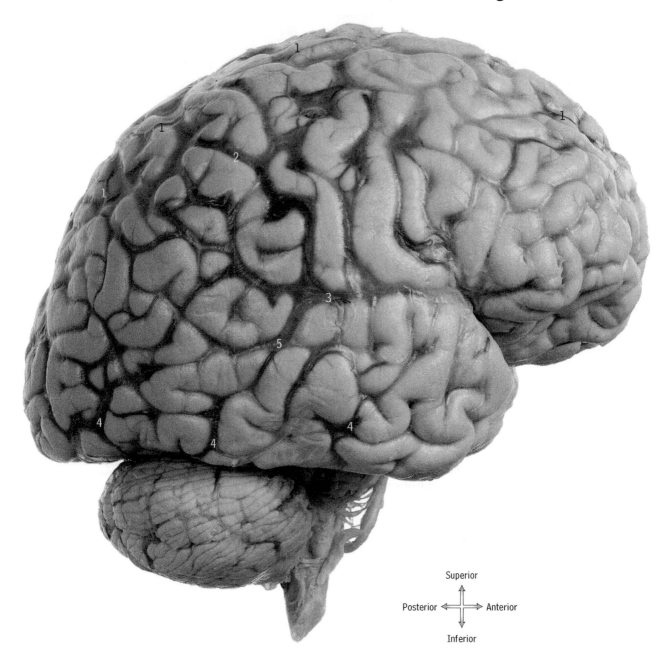

Superior

Posterior ⟷ Anterior

Inferior

The arachnoid mater has been left intact over the cerebral hemispheres, leaving vessels visible underneath the arachnoid. The larger ones are veins and the more important are identified. (For arteries see page 235.)

1 Superior cerebral veins
2 Superior anastomotic vein
3 Superficial middle cerebral vein overlying posterior ramus of lateral sulcus
4 Inferior cerebral veins
5 Inferior anastomotic vein

Most cerebral veins do not accompany arteries and are named differently. The main exceptions are the anterior cerebral veins.

Veins of the brain can be divided into internal and external groups.

The two internal cerebral veins (right and left) receive blood from the inner parts of the brain, and unite to form the great cerebral vein (page 228, 14; page 196, 15).

Various external veins drain the surfaces: superior and inferior cerebral veins, superficial and deep middle cerebral veins, superior and inferior anastomotic veins, and the basal vein. Most of them enter the nearest convenient venous sinus.
- The superior cerebral veins (as at 1), 8-12 in number, drain into the superior sagittal sinus (page 218, 5; page 196, 2 and 3), the more posterior veins entering obliquely in a forward direction (against the normal current in the sinus, which is from front to back).
- The superficial middle cerebral vein (3) runs forwards along the surface of the main part of the lateral sulcus and drains into the cavernous sinus (page 206, 33).
- The inferior cerebral veins (4) are small. Those under the frontal lobe join superior cerebral veins and drain into the superior sagittal sinus. From the temporal lobe they drain into the cavernous, superior petrosal and transverse sinuses (page 206, 33, 12 and 22).
- The superior anastomotic vein (2) runs upwards and backwards from the superficial middle cerebral vein (3) to the superior sagittal sinus, and the inferior anastomotic vein (5) passes downwards and backwards to the transverse sinus (page 206, 22).

The internal cerebral vein (page 239, B31) is formed by the union of the thalamostriate and choroidal veins (with some smaller adjacent veins from the choroid plexus, page 239, B8) and runs backwards in the tela choroidea of the roof of the third ventricle (see the note on page 239), to unite with its fellow of the opposite side beneath the splenium of the corpus callosum to form the great cerebral vein (page 239, B32; page 228, 14; page 196, 15).

The basal vein (page 196, 16) is formed by the union of the anterior cerebral vein (which accompanies the artery of the same name, page 196, 59), the deep middle cerebral vein (from the insula, page 224, B), and the striate veins (from the anterior perforated substance, page 236, B32). It passes backwards round the lateral side of the cerebral peduncle to join the great cerebral vein (page 196, 15).

Cerebral hemispheres *The right cerebral hemisphere*

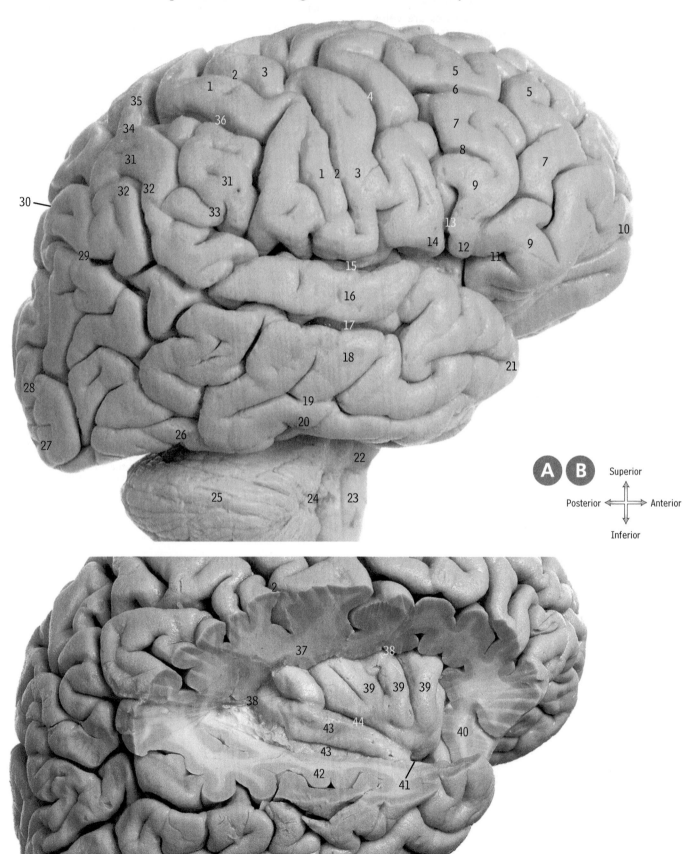

A the superolateral surface, from the right

B the insula, from the right

C diagram of principal cortical areas, superolateral surface

D diagram of principal cortical areas, medial surface

In A the major sulci and gyri are identified.

In B the cortex bounding the lateral sulcus (A15) has been removed to show the insula—the cortex buried in the depths of the lateral sulcus and only seen when the overlapping margins of the sulcus (the opercula or lids) are displaced or removed. On the diagrams in C and D the principal functional areas of the cortex are indicated.

The cerebral hemisphere has frontal, parietal, occipital and temporal lobes.
- The frontal lobe is the part lying in front of the central sulcus (2).
- The parietal lobe is bounded in front by the central sulcus (2) and behind by the upper part of a line drawn from the parieto-occipital sulcus (30) to the pre-occipital notch (26). The lower limit is the posterior ramus of the lateral sulcus (15) (and an arbitrary line continued backwards in the main line of this ramus to the posterior boundary).
- The occipital lobe lies behind the line joining the parieto-occipital sulcus (30) to the pre-occipital notch (26).
- The temporal lobe lies below the lateral sulcus (15), and is bounded behind by the lower part of the line drawn from the parieto-occipital sulcus (30) to the pre-occipital notch (26).

The lateral sulcus consists of short anterior and ascending rami (A11 and 13) and a longer posterior ramus (15), which itself is commonly known as the lateral sulcus.

The areas around the anterior and ascending rami of the lateral sulcus (A11 and 13) of the *left* cerebral hemisphere constitute the motor speech area (of Broca).

1 Postcentral gyrus
2 Central sulcus
3 Precentral gyrus
4 Precentral sulcus
5 Superior frontal gyrus
6 Superior frontal sulcus
7 Middle frontal gyrus
8 Inferior frontal sulcus
9 Inferior frontal gyrus
10 Frontal pole
11 Anterior ramus of lateral sulcus
12 Pars triangularis of inferior frontal gyrus
13 Ascending ramus of lateral sulcus
14 Pars opercularis of inferior frontal gyrus
15 Lateral sulcus (posterior ramus)
16 Superior temporal gyrus
17 Superior temporal sulcus
18 Middle temporal sulcus
19 Inferior temporal sulcus
20 Inferior temporal gyrus
21 Temporal pole
22 Pons
23 Medulla oblongata
24 Flocculus
25 Cerebellar hemisphere
26 Pre-occipital notch
27 Occipital pole
28 Lunate sulcus
29 Transverse occipital sulcus
30 Parieto-occipital sulcus
31 Inferior parietal lobule
32 Angular gyrus
33 Supramarginal gyrus
34 Intraparietal sulcus
35 Superior parietal lobule
36 Postcentral sulcus
37 Frontoparietal operculum
38 Circular sulcus of insula
39 Short gyri of insula
40 Frontal operculum
41 Limen of insula
42 Temporal operculum
43 Long gyri of insula
44 Central sulcus of insula

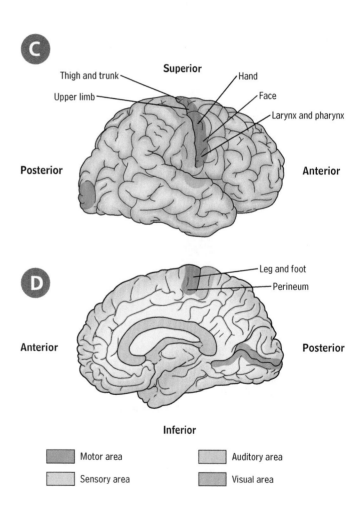

C

Thigh and trunk — Superior — Hand
Upper limb — Face
Larynx and pharynx
Posterior — Anterior

D

Leg and foot
Perineum
Anterior — Posterior
Inferior

Motor area   Auditory area
Sensory area   Visual area

Cerebral hemispheres *Blood supply of the cerebral cortex*

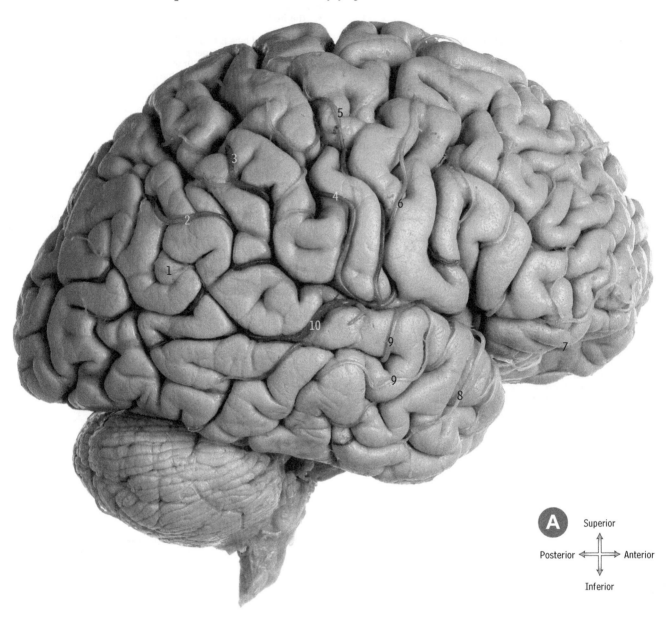

A

Superior

Posterior ⟷ Anterior

Inferior

1 Artery of angular gyrus
2 Posterior parietal artery
3 Anterior parietal artery
4 Artery of postcentral sulcus   branches of terminal (cortical) part
5 Artery of central sulcus
6 Artery of precentral sulcus
7 Lateral frontobasal artery
8 Anterior temporal artery   branches of insular part
9 Intermediate temporal artery
10 Posterior temporal artery

A the right middle cerebral artery, from the right

B diagram of cortical blood supplies, superolateral surface

C diagram of cortical blood supplies, medial surface

In A the arachnoid mater and all veins have been removed. Branches of the middle cerebral artery emerge from the lateral sulcus to spread out over much of the superolateral surface of the cortex.

The diagrams in B and C indicate the areas of cortex supplied by the three cerebral arteries.

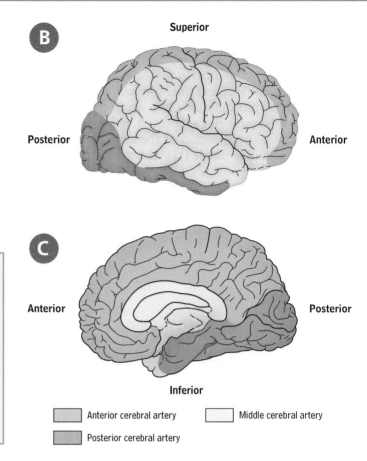

The middle cerebral artery supplies a large part of the superolateral aspect of the cerebral cortex, except for a strip about 1 cm wide along the upper border (B, anterior cerebral, extending over from the medial surface, C, and page 231), and the lower border (B and C, posterior cerebral, and page 231).

The cortex supplied by the middle cerebral artery includes much of the motor area of the precentral gyrus (but excluding the perineal and leg areas, page 225, D), and the insula in the depths of the lateral sulcus (page 224, B).

Some small middle cerebral branches extend as far back as the most lateral part of the visual area (page 231).

For branches of the anterior and posterior cerebral arteries see page 232, B.

Brain and brainstem *The right half of the brain and brainstem*

In A the brain has been cut in half longitudinally, exactly in the midline, and the right half is seen from the left. The corpus callosum (3-6), which connects the two cerebral hemispheres together, forms an obvious central feature. The aqueduct of the midbrain (22) connects the third ventricle (11) with the fourth

ventricle (19). The optic chiasma (31) is at the front lower corner of the third ventricle, with the stalk of the pituitary gland (30) just behind the chiasma. Compare this section with the MR image in B and with the similar section within the cranial cavity (page 196).

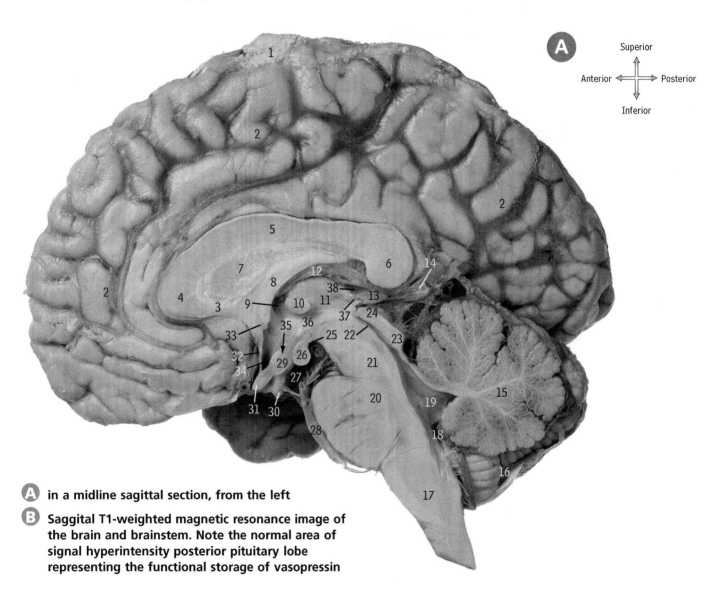

A in a midline sagittal section, from the left

B Saggital T1-weighted magnetic resonance image of the brain and brainstem. Note the normal area of signal hyperintensity posterior pituitary lobe representing the functional storage of vasopressin

1 Arachnoid granulations	**14** Great cerebral vein	**27** Interpeduncular cistern
2 Arachnoid mater and vessels overlying medial surface of cerebral hemisphere	**15** Cerebellum	**28** Basilar artery
	16 Cerebellomedullary cistern (cisterna magna)	**29** Tuber cinereum
3 Rostrum		**30** Pituitary stalk (infundibulum)
4 Genu } of corpus callosum	**17** Medulla oblongata	**31** Optic chiasma
5 Body	**18** Choroid plexus of fourth ventricle	**32** Lamina terminalis
6 Splenium	**19** Fourth ventricle	**33** Anterior commissure
7 Septum pellucidum	**20** Pons	**34** Optic recess
8 Body of fornix	**21** Midbrain	**35** Infundibular recess
9 Interventricular foramen	**22** Aqueduct of midbrain	**36** Hypothalamus
10 Interthalamic adhesion	**23** Inferior colliculus	**37** Pineal recess
11 Third ventricle	**24** Superior colliculus	**38** Suprapineal recess
12 Choroid plexus of third ventricle	**25** Posterior perforated substance	**39** Anterior pituitary gland
13 Pineal body	**26** Mamillary body	**40** Posterior pituitary gland

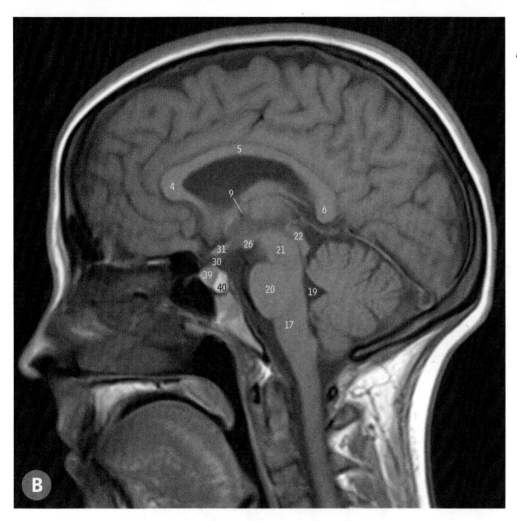

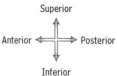

The brainstem consists of the midbrain (21), pons (20) and medulla oblongata (17).

The midbrain consists of the two cerebral peduncles (page 236, A26; page 236, B39).

Each cerebral peduncle consists of a ventral part, the crus of the peduncle (basis pedunculi), and a dorsal part, the tegmentum. Between the crus and tegmentum is a layer of pigmented grey matter, the substantia nigra.
- The tegmentum contains the aqueduct of the midbrain (22), and the part of the tegmentum dorsal to the aqueduct is the tectum, which includes the superior and inferior colliculi (24 and 23).

When removing the brain from the cranial cavity, the pituitary stalk (30) is torn, leaving the gland in the pituitary fossa (page 196, 50).

The pituitary gland (hypophysis cerebri) consists of two developmentally and functionally different parts, the adenohypophysis and neurohypophysis.
- The adenohypophysis (the more anterior part of the gland) is developed from an outgrowth of ectoderm (Rathke's pouch) from the primitive mouth, and consists histologically of the pars distalis (pars anterior), pars tuberalis and pars intermedia.
- The neurohypophysis (the more posterior part of the gland) is developed from an outgrowth of neuro-ectoderm from the primitive forebrain, and consists of the pars nervosa, the infundibulum and the median eminence.

The term 'anterior pituitary' or 'anterior lobe of the pituitary' is commonly understood to mean the pars distalis of the adenohypophysis, and 'posterior pituitary' or 'posterior lobe of the pituitary' to mean the pars nervosa.

The infundibulum is the upper hollow part of the pituitary stalk (30) and contains the infundibular recess of the third ventricle (35).

The tuber cinereum, the part of the floor of the third ventricle between the mamillary bodies (26) and the optic chiasma (31), includes an area at the base of the infundibulum known as the median eminence. This is the site of the neurosecretory cells whose products (regulatory factors) enter the hypophysial portal system of blood vessels to control the release of hormones from the cells of the anterior pituitary.

The main hormones of the anterior pituitary (39) are growth hormone, prolactin, TSH, ACTH, LH and FSH.

The hormones of the posterior pituitary (40) are produced in neurosecretory cells of the paraventricular and supra-optic nuclei in the lateral wall of the third ventricle. The axons of these cells run down in the pituitary stalk to the posterior pituitary, and the secretory products are stored within the nerve fibres.

The main hormones of the posterior pituitary are oxytocin and vasopressin (ADH).

Cerebral hemispheres and brainstem

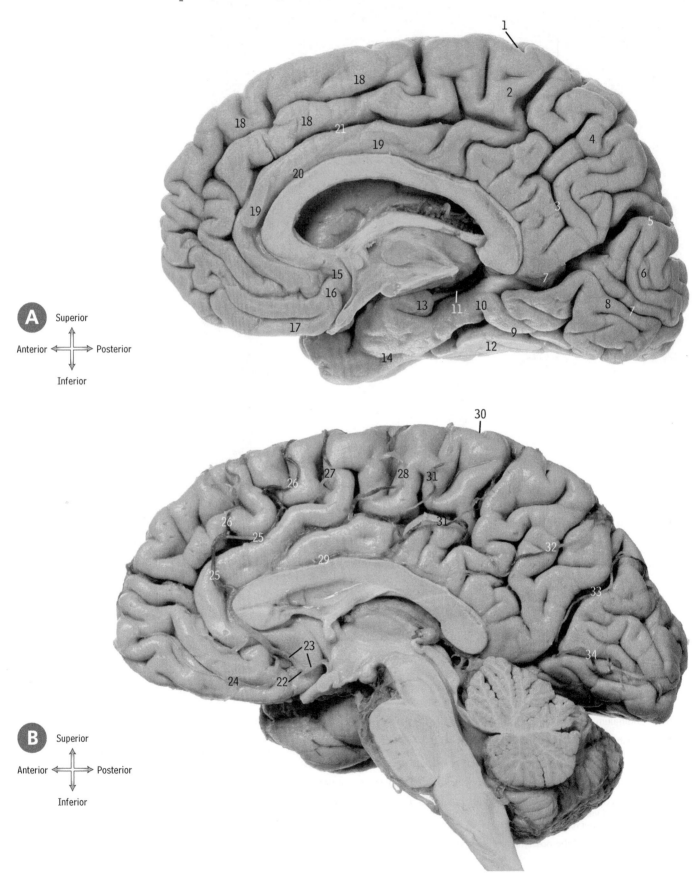

The medial surface of the hemispheres and cerebral arteries

1 Central sulcus
2 Paracentral lobule
3 Subparietal sulcus
4 Precuneus
5 Parieto-occipital sulcus
6 Cuneus
7 Calcarine sulcus
8 Lingual gyrus
9 Collateral sulcus
10 Parahippocampal gyrus
11 Dentate gyrus
12 Medial occipitotemporal gyrus
13 Uncus
14 Rhinal sulcus
15 Paraterminal gyrus
16 Subcallosal area
17 Gyrus rectus
18 Medial frontal gyrus
19 Cingulate gyrus
20 Corpus callosal sulcus
21 Cingulate sulcus
22 Anterior communicating artery
23 Anterior cerebral artery
24 Medial frontobasal artery ⎫
25 Callosomarginal artery   ⎪
26 Anteromedial frontal artery ⎪
27 Intermediomedial frontal artery ⎬ from the anterior
28 Posteromedial frontal artery ⎪ cerebral artery
29 Pericallosal artery   ⎪
30 Central sulcus   ⎪
31 Paracentral artery   ⎪
32 Precuneal artery   ⎭
33 Parieto-occipital branch ⎫ of posterior cerebral artery
34 Calcarine branch   ⎭

A the medial surface of the right cerebral hemisphere, in a midline sagittal section with the brainstem removed, from the left

B the right half of a midline sagittal section of the brain and brainstem, with branches of the anterior and posterior cerebral arteries, from the left

In A removal of the brainstem allows more of the medial surface of the temporal lobe to be seen, e.g. the parahippocampal gyrus (10), the collateral sulcus (9) and the anterior part of the calcarine sulcus (7).

In B various cortical branches of the anterior and posterior cerebral arteries are shown; the most important are the posterior cerebral branches to the visual cortex. (For branches of the middle cerebral artery, see page 226.)

On the surface of the cerebral hemisphere the anterior cerebral artery (B23) supplies the cortex on the medial aspect as far back as the parieto-occipital sulcus (A5), and a strip on the upper part of the superolateral surface adjacent to the midline (page 227, B). The cortex supplied includes the perineal and leg areas on the medial surface (page 225, D).

The posterior cerebral artery (page 234, A and B, 9) supplies the cortex of the occipital lobe and an area continuing forwards on the medial and inferior surfaces of the temporal lobe as far as and including the uncus (A13), but not including the temporal pole which has a middle cerebral supply. The cortex supplied includes the visual area (striate cortex, page 225, D; page 240, B39).

Base of the brain *The brain with the brainstem, from below*

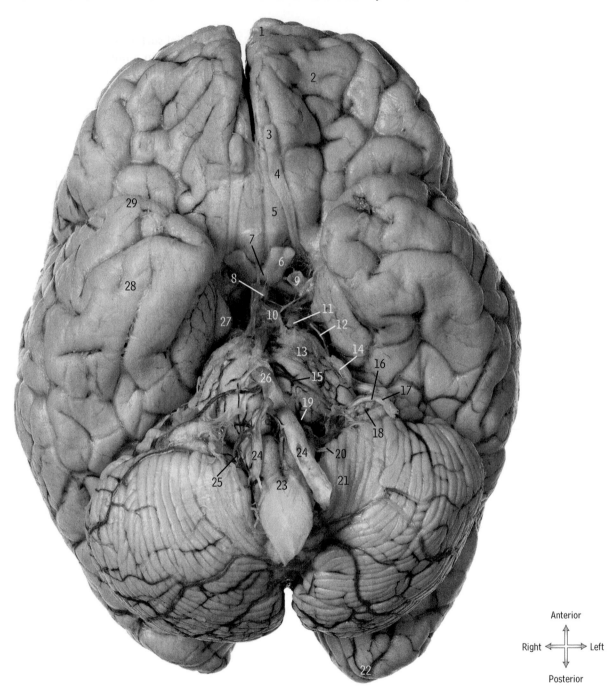

Anterior

Right ⟷ Left

Posterior

This is the view of the base of the brain as typically seen after removal from the cranial cavity; some arachnoid mater is still adherent. The medulla oblongata (23), and the two vertebral arteries (24), internal carotid arteries (9) and optic nerves (6) are the largest structures which have to be cut through in order to remove the brain. The remaining cranial nerves must also be cut, although the filaments of the olfactory nerve are invariably avulsed from the olfactory bulb (3) if the bulb itself is removed with the brain. The pituitary stalk (8) is severed, leaving the gland in its fossa in the base of the skull (page 196, 50). Details of the blood vessels and nerves are given on pages 234–239.

1 Frontal pole
2 Inferior surface of frontal lobe
3 Olfactory bulb
4 Olfactory tract
5 Gyrus rectus
6 Optic nerve
7 Optic chiasma
8 Pituitary stalk
9 Internal carotid artery
10 Arachnoid mater overlying mamillary bodies
11 Oculomotor nerve
12 Trochlear nerve
13 Pons
14 Trigeminal nerve
15 Labyrinthine artery
16 Facial nerve
17 Vestibulocochlear nerve
18 Flocculus
19 Abducent nerve
20 Rootlets of glossopharyngeal, vagus and cranial part of accessory nerves
21 Tonsil of cerebellum
22 Occipital pole
23 Medulla oblongata
24 Vertebral artery
25 Posterior inferior cerebellar artery
26 Basilar artery
27 Uncus
28 Inferior surface of temporal lobe
29 Temporal pole

The inferior surface of the frontal lobe (2) shows a slight concavity due to the convexity of the orbital part of the frontal bone in the anterior cranial fossa (page 30, A10).

The inferior surface of the temporal lobe (28) lies in the lateral part of the middle cranial fossa (page 30, A21).

The pons (13) and the overlying basilar artery (26) lie behind the clivus (page 30, A42).

The medulla oblongata (23) has been transected at the level where it passes through the foramen magnum (page 30, A40) to become continuous with the spinal cord (page 196, 30).

The tonsils of the cerebellum (21) lie just above the lateral margins of the foramen magnum (page 196, 63); increased intracranial pressure may force them into the top of the foramen and so impede the circulation of cerebrospinal fluid into the spinal subarachnoid space.

Base of the brain *The arteries of the base of the brain and brainstem*

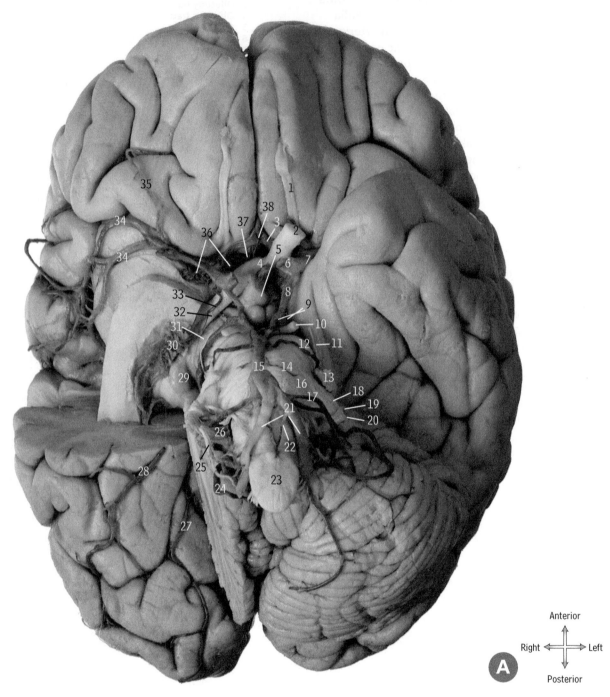

Anterior

Right ←→ Left

Posterior

A the brain, from below, with arteries in place

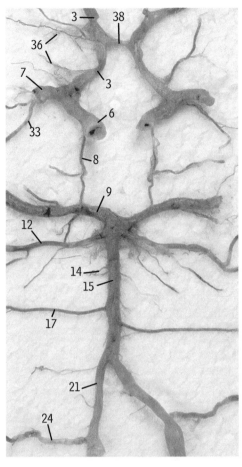

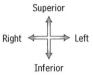

Superior

Right ⟵ ⟶ Left

Inferior

1 Olfactory tract
2 Optic nerve
3 Anterior cerebral artery
4 Optic chiasma
5 Pituitary stalk
6 Internal carotid artery
7 Middle cerebral artery
8 Posterior communicating artery
9 Posterior cerebral artery
10 Oculomotor nerve
11 Trochlear nerve
12 Superior cerebellar artery
13 Trigeminal nerve
14 Labyrinthine artery
15 Basilar artery
16 Pons
17 Anterior inferior cerebellar artery
18 Middle cerebellar peduncle
19 Facial nerve
20 Vestibulocochlear nerve
21 Vertebral artery
22 Anterior spinal artery
23 Medulla oblongata
24 Posterior inferior cerebellar artery
25 Spinal root of accessory nerve
26 Rootlets of glossopharyngeal, vagus and cranial part of accessory
    nerves
27 Posterior temporal ⎫ branch of posterior
28 Middle temporal   ⎭ cerebral artery
29 Lateral geniculate body
30 Choroid plexus of inferior horn of lateral ventricle
31 Cerebral peduncle
32 Optic tract
33 Anterior choroidal artery
34 Cortical branches of middle cerebral artery
35 Lateral frontobasal artery
36 Striate branches of middle and anterior cerebral arteries
37 Long central (recurrent) branch of anterior cerebral artery
38 Anterior communicating artery

B the arterial circle and associated vessels

The arteries taking part in the arterial circle (see note) are displayed: anterior communicating (38, in the midline), and on each side the anterior cerebral (3), internal carotid (6), posterior communicating (8) and posterior cerebral (9, from the basilar, 15).

In A removal of the front part of the right temporal lobe has opened up the lateral sulcus to show how the middle cerebral artery courses laterally through it, giving off the cortical branches (as at 34 and 35), which emerge on to the lateral surface of the cerebral hemisphere (page 226). Also revealed is the optic tract (32), passing back from the optic chiasma (4) round the side of the cerebral peduncle (31) to the lateral geniculate body (29). Superficial to the optic tract lies the anterior choroidal artery (33), running into the choroid plexus of the inferior horn of the lateral ventricle (30) and so forming the main supply of the choroid plexus of the lateral and third ventricles.

In B the various arteries have been removed en bloc and spread out to indicate their anastomotic connections.

The arterial circle (of Willis) is an anastomosis between the internal carotid and vertebral systems of vessels. It is hexagonal rather than circular in shape. The anterior cerebral branches (3) of each internal carotid artery (6) are joined by the (single) anterior communicating artery (38). On each side a posterior communicating artery (8) joins the internal carotid (6) to the posterior cerebral artery (9), the two posterior cerebrals being the terminal branches of the (single midline) basilar artery (15) which itself has been formed by the union of the two vertebral arteries (21). At the point where the anterior and posterior communicating vessels come off the internal carotid (passing forwards and backwards, respectively), the middle cerebral artery (7) runs laterally.

The various striate branches of the middle and anterior cerebral arteries (36) which enter the anterior perforated substance (page 236, B32) supply (among other structures) the internal capsule (page 241). One such branch of the middle cerebral artery has become known as the 'artery of cerebral haemorrhage', since it is particularly liable to rupture and damage the corticonuclear and corticospinal fibres that course through the capsule. This type of cerebral damage causes varying degrees of paralysis, especially of the limbs, and is commonly called a 'stroke'.

The third (oculomotor) and fourth (trochlear) nerves (10 and 11) pass between the posterior cerebral and superior cerebellar arteries (9 and 12).

Base of the brain *The brainstem, cranial nerves and geniculate bodies*

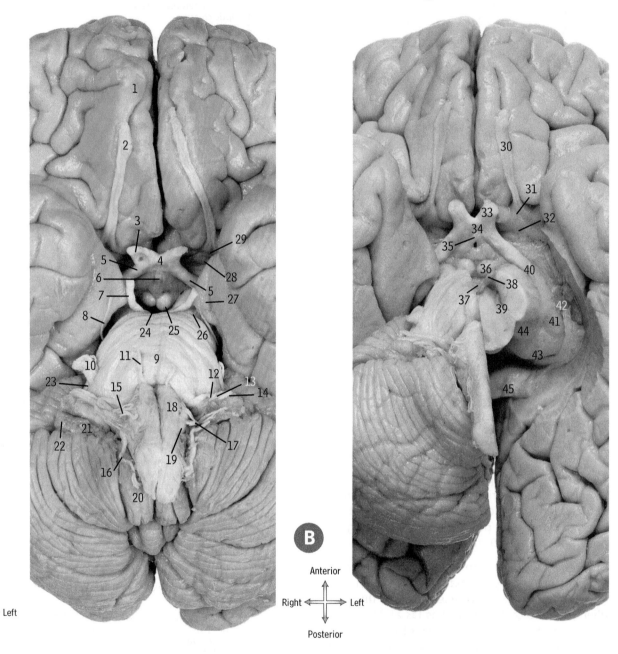

A

Anterior

Right ←→ Left

Posterior

B

Anterior

Right ←→ Left

Posterior

1 Olfactory bulb	**16** Spinal part of accessory nerve	**31** Olfactory trigone
2 Olfactory tract	**17** Rootlets of hypoglossal nerve	**32** Anterior perforated substance
3 Optic nerve	**18** Pyramid of medulla oblongata	**33** Optic nerve
4 Optic chiasma	**19** Olive	**34** Optic chiasma
5 Optic tract	**20** Tonsil of cerebellum	**35** Pituitary stalk
6 Pituitary stalk	**21** Choroid plexus of fourth ventricle	**36** Mamillary body
7 Oculomotor nerve	**22** Flocculus	**37** Posterior perforated substance
8 Trochlear nerve	**23** Middle cerebellar peduncle	**38** Oculomotor nerve
9 Pons	**24** Posterior perforated substance	**39** Cerebral peduncle
10 Trigeminal nerve	**25** Mamillary body	**40** Optic tract
11 Abducent nerve	**26** Cerebral peduncle	**41** Lateral geniculate body
12 Motor root ⎫ of facial nerve	**27** Uncus	**42** Choroid plexus of inferior horn of lateral
13 Sensory root ⎭	**28** Anterior perforated substance	ventricle
14 Vestibulocochlear nerve	**29** Olfactory trigone	**43** Pulvinar
15 Roots of glossopharyngeal, vagus and	**30** Olfactory tract	**44** Medial geniculate body
cranial part of accessory nerves		**45** Splenium of corpus callosum

A brain with the brainstem, from below

B with most of the left half of the brainstem removed

C optic pathway and patterns of visual field loss

In **A** all vessels have been removed to give a clear view of the cranial nerves and their relationship to the brainstem (see notes).

In **B** the left half of the brainstem has been removed at midbrain level to show the optic tract (40) winding backwards round the side of the cerebral peduncle (39) and leading to the lateral geniculate body (41), with the medial geniculate body adjacent (44).

C shows a schematic of the optic pathway and how pathology in different locations along the path will result in different patterns of visual field loss.

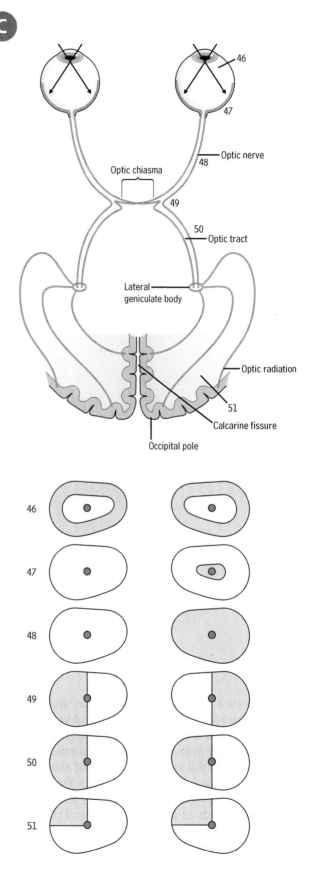

Optic chiasma

Optic nerve — 48

49

50 — Optic tract

Lateral geniculate body

Optic radiation

Calcarine fissure

51

Occipital pole

The cranial nerves are numbered (by long tradition with Roman numerals) as well as named:

I	First	Olfactory
II	Second	Optic
III	Third	Oculomotor
IV	Fourth	Trochlear
V	Fifth	Trigeminal
VI	Sixth	Abducent
VII	Seventh	Facial
VIII	Eighth	Vestibulocochlear
IX	Ninth	Glossopharyngeal
X	Tenth	Vagus
XI	Eleventh	Accessory
XII	Twelfth	Hypoglossal

The *olfactory nerve* (I) consists of about 20 filaments that pass through the cribriform plate of the ethmoid bone to enter the olfactory bulb (A1) at the front end of the olfactory tract (A2), on the undersurface of the frontal lobe.

The *optic nerve* (II) (A3) passes backwards from the eye through the optic canal (page 206, 4) to the optic chiasma (A4).

The *oculomotor nerve* (III) (A7; B38) emerges on the medial side of the cerebral peduncle (A26).

The *trochlear nerve* (IV) (A8) is the only cranial nerve to emerge from the dorsal surface of the brainstem (from the midbrain, behind the inferior colliculus, page 246, C and D, 38). It winds round the lateral side of the cerebral peduncle.

The *trigeminal nerve* (V) (A10) emerges from the lateral side of the pons (A9), where the pons continues into the middle cerebellar peduncle (A23).

The *abducent nerve* (VI) (A11) emerges near the midline at the junction of the pons (A9) and the pyramid of the medulla (A18).

The *facial nerve* (VII) (A12 and 13) and the *vestibulocochlear nerve* (VIII) (A14) emerge from the lateral pontomedullary angle.

The *glossopharyngeal* (IX) and *vagus* (X) nerves and the cranial part of the *accessory nerve* (XI) (A15) emerge from the medulla lateral to the olive (A19).

The spinal part of the accessory nerve (A16) emerges as a series of roots from the lateral side of the upper five or six cervical segments of the spinal cord, dorsal to the denticulate ligament (page 246, F47), and runs up at the side of the medulla to join the cranial part.

The *hypoglossal nerve* (XII) (A17) emerges from the medulla between the pyramid and the olive (A18 and 19).

46 Concentric diminution (tunnel vision)
47 Central scotoma
48 Complete field loss
49 Bitemporal hemianopia
50 Homonymous hemianopia
51 Quadrantic hemianopia

Interior of the cerebral hemispheres *Ventricles of the brain*

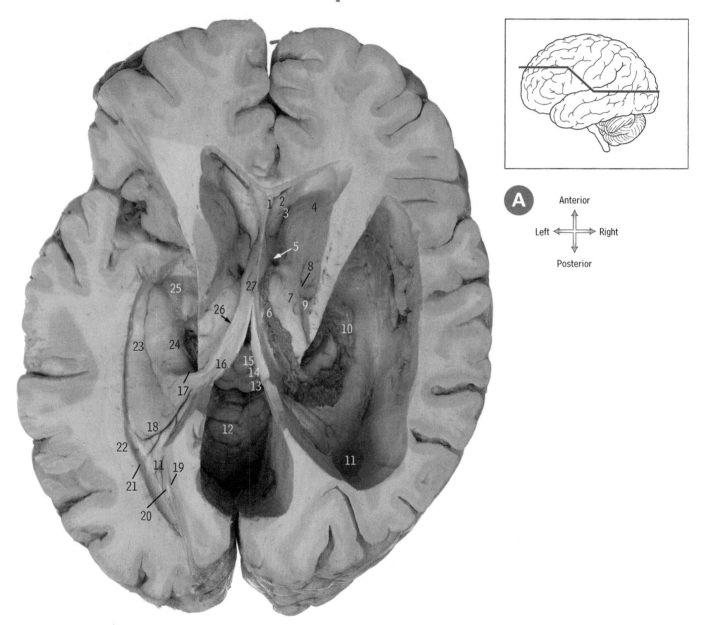

A

Anterior

Left ⟷ Right

Posterior

In A the cerebral hemispheres have been dissected away from above, to open up the lateral ventricles. On the right side, the body of the lateral ventricle (the region containing in its floor the key numbers 6–9) becomes the anterior horn (3) in front of the interventricular foramen (5). At the back the ventricle curves downwards and forwards as the inferior horn (10) and backwards as the posterior horn (11). On the left side, there has been further dissection of the inferior and posterior horns. In the floor of the inferior horn are seen the hippocampus (24 and 25) and the collateral eminence (23, the bulge produced by the collateral sulcus seen on page 230, A9). The collateral trigone (18) is at the junction of the inferior and posterior horns. The bulb (19, caused by fibres of the corpus callosum) and the calcar (20, caused by the bulge of the calcarine sulcus seen on page 230, A7) are in the medial wall of the posterior horn. The optic radiation (22) is immediately lateral to the posterior horn.

In B the front part of the bluish diamond-shaped area with the key numbers 30 and 31 is the roof of the third ventricle (B30).

A the lateral ventricles and their horns, from above

B the lateral ventricles and the roof of the third ventricle, from above

1 Septum pellucidum
2 Rostrum of corpus callosum (posterior surface)
3 Anterior horn of lateral ventricle
4 Head of caudate nucleus
5 Interventricular foramen
6 Choroid plexus of body of lateral ventricle
7 Thalamus
8 Thalamostriate vein
9 Body of caudate nucleus
10 Choroid plexus of inferior horn of lateral ventricle
11 Posterior horn of lateral ventricle
12 Vermis of cerebellum
13 Inferior colliculus
14 Superior colliculus
15 Pineal body
16 Crus of fornix
17 Fimbria
18 Collateral trigone
19 Bulb
20 Calcar
21 Tapetum of corpus callosum
22 Optic radiation
23 Collateral eminence
24 Hippocampus
25 Pes hippocampi
26 Choroid fissure
27 Body of fornix
28 Anterior column of fornix
29 Tela choroidea of third ventricle
30 Choroid plexus in third ventricle (visible below **29**)
31 Internal cerebral vein
32 Great cerebral vein

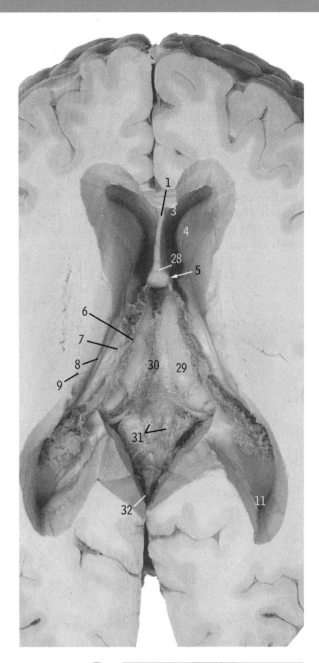

The ventricles of the brain:
• the third ventricle (page 228, 11), with on each side an interventricular foramen (5; page 228, 9) leading into
• the lateral ventricle, consisting of a body (6) with anterior, inferior and posterior horns (3, 10 and 11)
• the aqueduct of the midbrain (page 228, 22) connecting the third ventricle (page 228, 11) with
• the fourth ventricle, behind the lower part of the pons and upper part of the medulla oblongata (page 228, 17), with a median aperture in the roof (page 246, E40) and a lateral aperture in each lateral recess (page 246, C31) through which cerebrospinal fluid escapes into the subarachnoid space.

Tela choroidea is the name given to a double layer of pia mater (as at B29). When it contains a mass of capillary blood vessels and is covered by ependyma (the epithelium lining the ventricles) it becomes the choroid plexus (as at A and B, 6).

Cerebrospinal fluid is produced by the choroid plexuses. One mass of choroid plexus is in the roof of the third ventricle (B30) and extends on each side through the interventricular foramen (A and B, 5) into the body of the lateral ventricle (A and B, 6) and then into its inferior horn (A10) (but not into its anterior or posterior horns, 3 and 11).

A separate choroid plexus, not connected with the above, lies in the roof of the fourth ventricle (page 228, 18; page 246, D, 39) and extends out through the lateral recesses to become visible on the undersurface of the brain near the pontomedullary angle (page 236, A21).

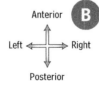

Anterior

B

Left ⟷ Right

Posterior

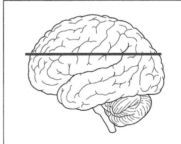

Interior of the cerebral hemispheres

The internal capsule and basal nuclei

In A the left hemisphere has been sectioned at the level of the interventricular foramen (6), and the right hemisphere about 1 cm higher. On the left side the internal capsule (27-29) is seen between the caudate nucleus (7) and thalamus (26) medially and the lentiform nucleus (30 and 31) laterally. In the higher section on the right, the nerve fibres that form the internal capsule occupy the corona radiata (13). The view on the right looks down into the body of the lateral ventricle with the choroid plexus (11) and the

upper surface of the thalamus (10) in the floor of the ventricle. At the lower level on the left the thalamus is seen in section (26). The anterior horn of the lateral ventricle (4) extends forwards into the frontal lobe, and the posterior horn (18) backwards into the occipital lobe. The optic radiation (20) runs lateral to the posterior horn, separated from it by the tapetum (19), which is a thin sheet of fibres derived from the corpus callosum (14) whose main bulk lies medial to the horn as the forceps major (15).

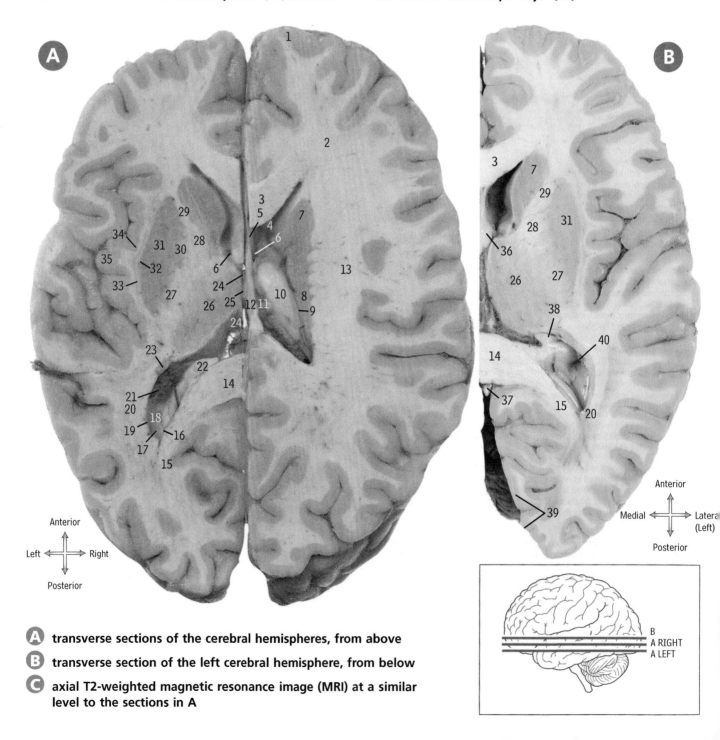

A transverse sections of the cerebral hemispheres, from above

B transverse section of the left cerebral hemisphere, from below

C axial T2-weighted magnetic resonance image (MRI) at a similar level to the sections in A

In B, looking upwards at a similar level to that on the left side of A, the third ventricle (24) is in the midline, communicating at the front with the anterior horn of the lateral ventricle (4) through the interventricular foramen (6), which is bounded medially by the anterior column of the fornix (36) and laterally by the thalamus (26). Compare with major features in the Magnetic Resonance Image (MRI) (C).

1 Frontal pole
2 Forceps minor
3 Genu of corpus callosum
4 Anterior horn of lateral ventricle
5 Septum pellucidum
6 Interventricular foramen
7 Head ⎫
8 Body ⎬ of caudate nucleus
9 Thalamostriate vein
10 Thalamus
11 Choroid plexus of body of lateral ventricle
12 Body of fornix
13 Corona radiata
14 Splenium of corpus callosum
15 Forceps major
16 Bulb
17 Calcar
18 Posterior horn of lateral ventricle
19 Tapetum of corpus callosum
20 Optic radiation
21 Choroid plexus passing forwards into inferior horn of lateral ventricle
22 Crus of fornix
23 Tail of caudate nucleus
24 Third ventricle
25 Interthalamic adhesion
26 Thalamus
27 Posterior limb ⎫
28 Genu ⎬ of internal capsule
29 Anterior limb ⎭
30 Globus pallidus ⎫
31 Putamen ⎬ lentiform nucleus
32 External capsule
33 Claustrum
34 Extreme capsule
35 Insula
36 Anterior column of fornix
37 Pineal body
38 Fimbria
39 Visual (striate) area of cerebral cortex
40 Junction of posterior and inferior horns of lateral ventricle

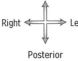

Anterior
Right ⟷ Left
Posterior

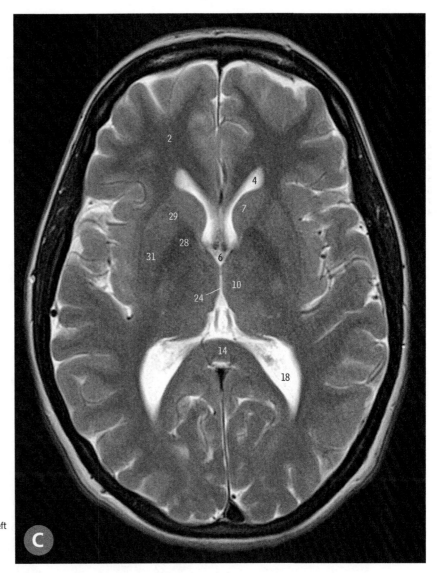

The *internal capsule* consists of:
• the anterior limb
• the genu
• the posterior limb
• the sublentiform part
• the retrolentiform part

The anterior limb (29) lies between the head of the caudate nucleus (7) and the lentiform nucleus (30 and 31). Its main fibre constituents are those passing between the various parts of the frontal cortex and thalamus (in both directions) and to pontine nuclei.

The genu (28) is between the anterior and posterior limbs (29 and 27). Its most important fibres are the corticonuclear fibres (formerly called corticobulbar), passing from the head and neck area of the motor cortex (precentral gyrus) to the motor nuclei of cranial nerves.

The posterior limb (27) lies between the thalamus (26) and the lentiform nucleus (30 and 31). Apart from fibres to pontine nuclei, it also contains those fibres of the sensory pathway that run from the thalamus to the postcentral gyrus (thalamocortical fibres), and the corticospinal fibres from the motor cortex to the anterior horn cells of the spinal cord. These motor fibres mainly occupy the anterior two-thirds of the posterior limb.

The sublentiform part consists of fibres passing below the posterior end of the lentiform nucleus. Among its most important fibres are those of the auditory radiation, running from the medial geniculate body to the auditory area of the cortex.

The retrolentiform part consists of fibres at the posterior end of the posterior limb, passing from the lateral geniculate body to the visual area of the cortex and constituting the optic radiation (20).

Clinically the most important parts of the internal capsule are the genu and anterior two-thirds of the posterior limb, because this is where the motor fibres from the cortex to cranial nerve nuclei and anterior horn cells are situated. It is damage to these 'upper motor neurons' by haemorrhage or thrombosis that causes the characteristic paralysis of a stroke (page 235).

Interior of the cerebral hemispheres

The hemispheres and brainstem in coronal section

1 Corpus callosum
2 Septum pellucidum
3 Body of fornix
4 Choroid plexus
5 Body of lateral ventricle
6 Thalamus
7 Thalamostriate vein
8 Body of caudate nucleus
9 Corona radiata
10 Internal capsule
11 External capsule
12 Extreme capsule
13 Insula
14 Tail of caudate nucleus
15 Inferior horn of lateral ventricle
16 Collateral sulcus
17 Parahippocampal gyrus
18 Hippocampus

19 Choroid plexus of inferior horn of lateral ventricle
20 Choroid fissure
21 Optic tract
22 Corticospinal and corticonuclear fibres in cerebral peduncle
23 Corticospinal and corticonuclear fibres in pons
24 Corticospinal fibres in pyramid of medulla oblongata
25 Substantia nigra
26 Red nucleus
27 Subthalamic nucleus
28 Third ventricle
29 Globus pallidus ⎫
30 Putamen ⎭ lentiform nucleus
31 Claustrum
32 Basilar artery
33 Sphenoidal sinus
34 Mandible
35 Odontoid process
36 mandible

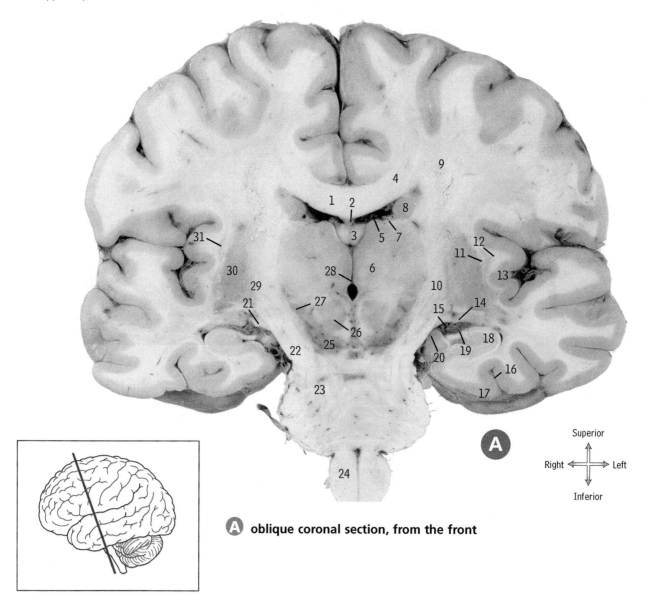

Superior
Right ⟷ Left
Inferior

A oblique coronal section, from the front

The section in A, looking from front to back, has been cut slightly obliquely in order to show how the motor fibres of the internal capsule (10) pass from the hemispheres and down through the midbrain (cerebral peduncle, 22), pons (23) and medulla (24). The sloping floor of the body of the lateral ventricle (5) is formed by the thalamus (6) and caudate nucleus (8) with the thalamostriate vein (7) in between. The roof is the corpus callosum (1), with the septum pellucidum (2) separating the two ventricles in the midline. The hippocampus (18) is in the floor of the inferior horn (15), with the tail of the caudate nucleus (14) in its roof.

The coronal magnetic resonance image (MRI) in B is at a more anterior and vertical level than A, and shows the sphenoidal sinus (33), the mandible (34) and the pteygoid muscles (35).

The **basal nuclei** (still often known clinically by their old name, basal ganglia) include certain subcortical cell groups in the white matter of the cerebral hemispheres, in particular the caudate and lentiform nuclei (A8, 29 and 30). On functional grounds it is now usual to include the substantia nigra (A25) and the subthalamic nucleus (A27) (both in the midbrain, not in the cerebrum), and to exclude the amygdaloid nucleus (at the front end of the tail of the caudate nucleus) because it is functionally associated with the limbic system.

The basal nuclei are functionally part of the extrapyramidal system. Extrapyramidal diseases do not cause paralysis but lead to abnormal involuntary movements and disturbances of reflexes and muscle tone: for example, Parkinsonism, where there is loss of the neurotransmitter dopamine in the substantia nigra.

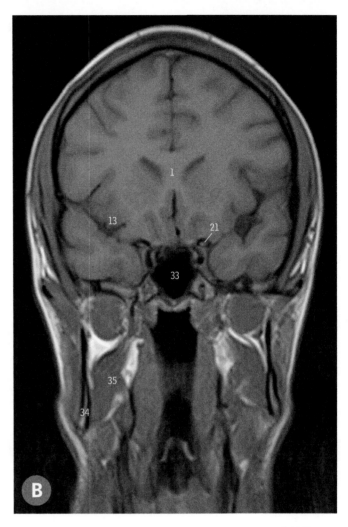

B coronal T1-weighted magnetic resonance image (MRI)

Superior

Right ⬄ Left

Inferior

Cerebellum *The cerebellum and the brainstem*

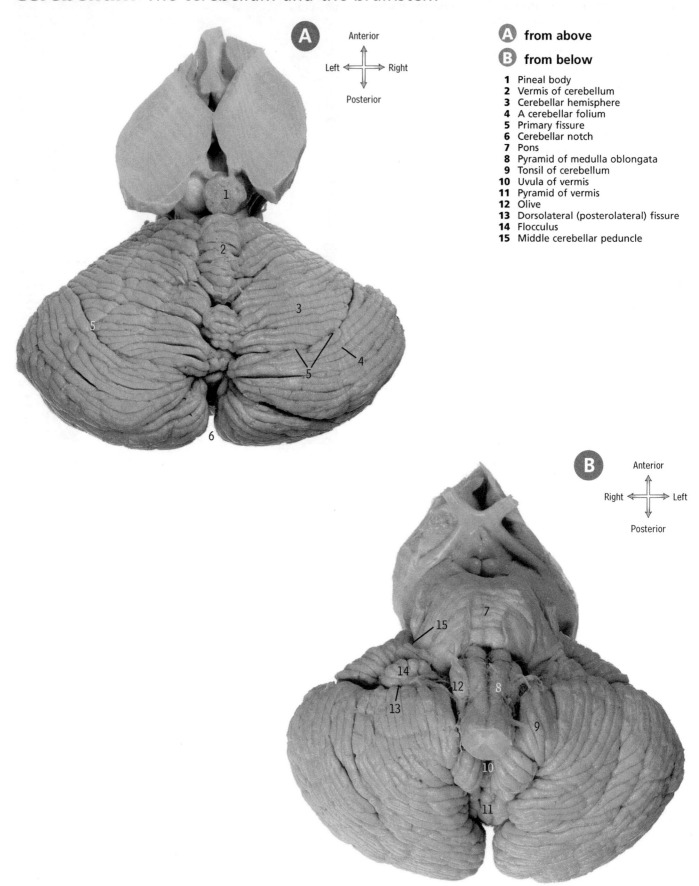

A from above

B from below

1 Pineal body
2 Vermis of cerebellum
3 Cerebellar hemisphere
4 A cerebellar folium
5 Primary fissure
6 Cerebellar notch
7 Pons
8 Pyramid of medulla oblongata
9 Tonsil of cerebellum
10 Uvula of vermis
11 Pyramid of vermis
12 Olive
13 Dorsolateral (posterolateral) fissure
14 Flocculus
15 Middle cerebellar peduncle

The view in A, looking down from above, shows the central vermis of the cerebellum (2) with the hemispheres on each side (3). The pineal body (1) projects backwards from the (unlabelled) third ventricle to overlie the midbrain (compare with the side view on page 228, 13).

In B the anterior or ventral view shows the pons (7) passing laterally to become the middle cerebellar peduncle, which disappears into the cerebellar hemisphere (as on page 236, A23). The flocculus (14) lies behind the peduncle, and the tonsil (9) is the part of the hemisphere that overlies the margin of the foramen magnum (as on page 196, 63).

The cerebellum occupies much of the posterior cranial fossa (page 196, 22) and is covered by the tentorium cerebelli (page 206, 36).

The cerebellum consists of a central longitudinal region, the vermis (A2), with a cerebellar hemisphere on each side (A3).

Like the cerebrum, the cerebellum has a cortex of grey matter on the surface, with underlying white matter.

In each hemisphere the white matter contains four subcortical cell groups—the dentate, globose, emboliform and fastigial nuclei. The nuclei give rise to most of the fibres that leave the cerebellum; the most important is the dentate nucleus (page 246, B23).

The cerebellum is connected to the brainstem by three pairs of peduncles, one pair to each part of the brainstem:
- by the superior cerebellar peduncles to the midbrain (page 246, C24)
- by the middle cerebellar peduncles to the pons (B15; page 246, C25)
- by the inferior cerebellar peduncles to the medulla oblongata (page 246, C26)

The following notes, correlating cerebellar form and function, are a simplified synopsis of a complicated organ, but are sufficient to give a general understanding of its significance.

Functionally, the cerebellum is concerned with the co-ordination of muscular movement; it has nothing to do with conscious sensation. Each cerebellar hemisphere affects its own side of the body (the ipsilateral side): for example, the left cerebellar hemisphere helps to control the left arm and leg, in contrast to the left cerebral hemisphere, which exerts its influence on the right arm and leg (the contralateral side), due to the decussation of corticospinal fibres in the medulla oblongata.

The various named parts are best appreciated in a midline sagittal section (as on page 246, A), and can conveniently be grouped according to their phylogenetic (evolutionary) significance.

The lingula at the front (page 246, A21), and the nodule at the back (page 246, A10), which is continuous at each side with the flocculus (A14, forming the flocculonodular lobe), constitute the oldest or vestibular part of the cerebellum (archaeocerebellum) and are mainly concerned with vestibular functions (balance).

The central lobule and culmen of the front part of the vermis (page 246, A20 and 19), the uvula and pyramid of the back part of the vermis (page 246, A11 and 13) and the hemisphere in front of the primary fissure (A5; page 246, A18) forming the anterior lobe, constituting the palaeocerebellum or spinal part, receiving fibres from the spinal cord and being largely concerned with posture and muscle tone.

The remainder of the vermis (page 246, A15-17) and the hemisphere behind the primary fissure (page 246, A11-18) constitute the middle lobe (sometimes also known confusingly as the posterior lobe). This is the largest and most recently evolved part of the cerebellum, the neocerebellum, and receives input from the cerebral cortex via the pontine nuclei. It is mainly concerned with the control of muscle tone and fine movements.

It follows from the above that disturbances of cerebellar function, e.g. by the pressure of tumours, result in disorders of balance and incoordinated movements of the arms and legs (ataxia), with loss of muscle tone (hypotonia) and nystagmus (oscillating eye movements) but no paralysis.

Cerebellum, brainstem and spinal cord

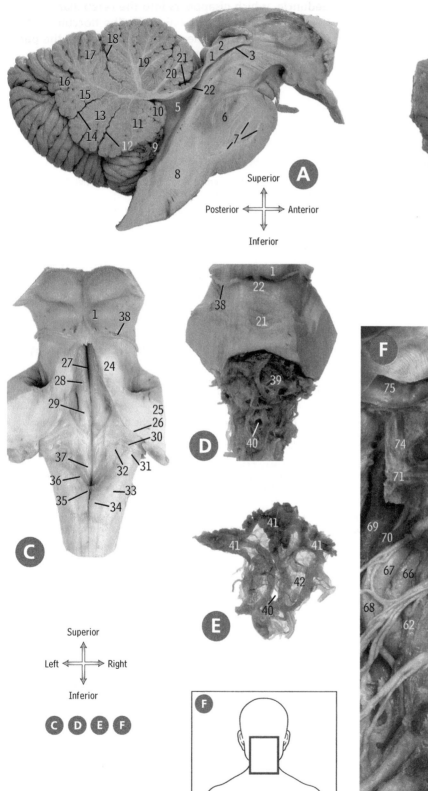

A

Superior

Posterior ⟷ Anterior

Inferior

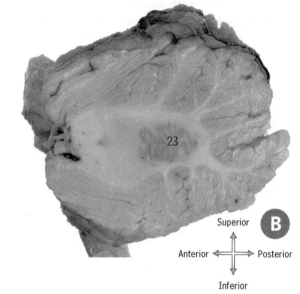

B

Superior

Anterior ⟷ Posterior

Inferior

C

D

E

Superior

Left ⟷ Right

Inferior

C D E F

F

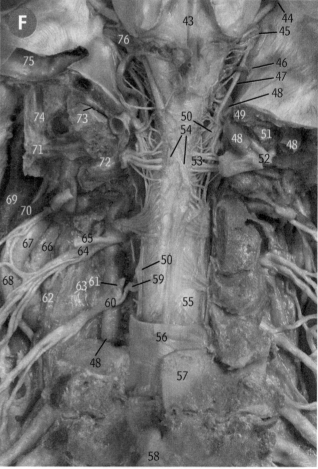

Sections of the cerebellum and brainstem, and the cervical cord

Ⓐ the left half of the brainstem and cerebellum, in a midline sagittal section, from the right

Ⓑ the right cerebellar hemisphere in an oblique sagittal section, from the left

Ⓒ the floor of the fourth ventricle, from behind

Ⓓ the roof of the fourth ventricle, from behind

Ⓔ the isolated choroid plexus of the fourth ventricle, from behind

Ⓕ the lower brainstem and cervical part of the spinal cord, from behind

In the sagittal section in A, various parts of the cerebellum are labelled (9-21). In the pons (6) corticospinal and corticonuclear fibres (7) are seen coursing down through the ventral part to reach the medulla (8).

The section of a hemisphere in B shows the dentate nucleus (23), the largest of the subcortical cerebellar nuclei.

At the side of the floor of the fourth ventricle in C are seen the cut edges of the three cerebellar peduncles (24-26) which connect the cerebellum to the midbrain, pons and medulla.

In D the tela choroidea and choroid plexus (39) of the posterior part of the roof of the fourth ventricle are shown in situ.

In E they have been dissected free to emphasise the T-shaped plexus (41) and the median aperture (40) in the tela (42).

In F the posterior parts of the skull and upper vertebrae have been removed to show the continuity of the brainstem with the spinal cord, from which dorsal nerve rootlets are seen to emerge (as at 53). The spinal root of the accessory nerve (47) runs up through the foramen magnum (49) to join the cranial part in the jugular foramen (45). Ventral nerve rootlets (as at 59), ventral to the denticulate ligament (50), unite to form a ventral nerve root which joins with a dorsal nerve root (61, whose formative rootlets dorsal to the ligamentum have been cut off from the cord in order to make the ventral rootlets visible) to form a spinal nerve immediately beyond the dorsal root ganglion (60). The nerve immediately divides into ventral and dorsal rami (as at 64 and 65).

1 Inferior colliculus
2 Tectum ⎫
3 Aqueduct ⎬ of midbrain
4 Tegmentum ⎭
5 Fourth ventricle
6 Pons
7 Corticonuclear and corticospinal fibres
8 Medulla oblongata
9 Choroid plexus of fourth ventricle
10 Nodule
11 Uvula of vermis
12 Secondary (postpyramidal) fissure
13 Pyramid of vermis
14 Prepyramidal fissure
15 Tuber of vermis
16 Folium of vermis
17 Declive
18 Primary fissure
19 Culmen
20 Central lobule
21 Lingula
22 Superior medullary velum
23 Dentate nucleus
24 Superior ⎫
25 Middle ⎬ cerebellar peduncle
26 Inferior ⎭
27 Median groove
28 Medial eminence
29 Facial colliculus
30 Medullary striae
31 Lateral recess
32 Vestibular area
33 Cuneate tubercle
34 Gracile tubercle
35 Obex
36 Vagal triangle
37 Hypoglossal triangle
38 Trochlear nerve
39 Tela choroidea and choroid plexus
40 Median aperture
41 Choroid plexus
42 Tela choroidea
43 Floor of the fourth ventricle
44 Internal acoustic meatus with facial and vestibulocochlear nerves and labyrinthine artery
45 Roots of glossopharyngeal, vagus and cranial part of accessory nerves and jugular foramen
46 Posterior inferior cerebellar artery
47 Spinal root of accessory nerve
48 Vertebral artery
49 Margin of foramen magnum
50 Denticulate ligament
51 Lateral mass of atlas
52 First cervical nerve and posterior arch of atlas
53 Dorsal rootlets of second cervical nerve
54 Posterior spinal arteries
55 Arachnoid mater
56 Dura mater
57 Lamina of sixth cervical vertebra
58 Spinous process of seventh cervical vertebra
59 Ventral rootlets ⎫
60 Dorsal root ganglion ⎬ of fourth cervical nerve
61 Dorsal root ⎭
62 Scalenus anterior
63 Longus capitis
64 Ventral ramus ⎫ of third cervical nerve
65 Dorsal ramus ⎭
66 External carotid artery
67 Internal carotid artery
68 Vagus nerve
69 Internal jugular vein
70 A vein from vertebral venous plexuses
71 Transverse process of atlas
72 Capsule of lateral atlanto-axial joint
73 Atlanto-occipital joint
74 Rectus capitis lateralis
75 Sigmoid sinus
76 Choroid plexus emerging from lateral recess of fourth ventricle

Cervical vertebral column and suboccipital region

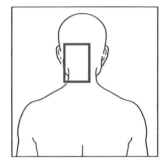

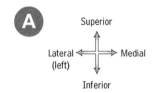

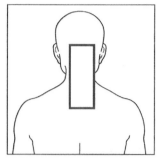

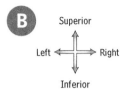

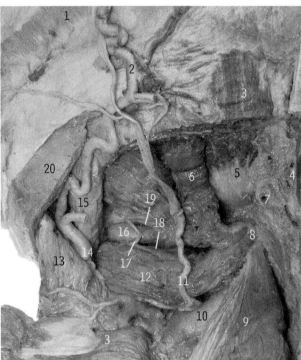

A the left suboccipital triangle

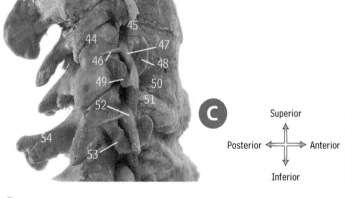

C intervertebral foramina and spinal nerves, from the right

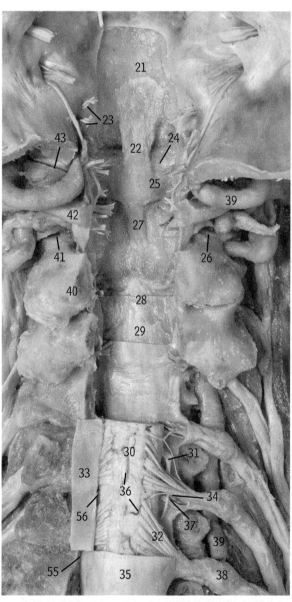

B the vertebral column and spinal cord, from behind

Cervical vertebral column *Posterior neck and vertebral joints*

The suboccipital region, vertebral column and spinal nerves

In A the suboccipital region has been exposed by removing trapezius and parts of splenius (20) and semispinalis (3). The principal structure in the suboccipital triangle (see the note below) is the vertebral artery (16).

In B the vertebral arches and much of the skull have been removed, together with parts of the meninges and spinal cord. The tectorial membrane (28) is the upward continuation of the posterior longitudinal

ligament (29). The transverse ligament of the atlas (25) forms the transverse part of the cruciform ligament (22 and 27); all are displayed by removing the tectorial membrane.

The side view of the cervical vertebral column in C shows a typical dorsal root ganglion (as at 52) in an intervertebral foramen (see page 231), and spinal nerves dividing into a small dorsal ramus (as at 46) and a large ventral ramus (47).

The suboccipital triangle:
- Boundaries—rectus capitis posterior major (A6), obliquus capitis superior (15) and obliquus capitis inferior (12).
- Floor—posterior atlanto-occipital membrane (19) and posterior arch of atlas (18).
- Contents—vertebral artery (16); dorsal ramus of C1 nerve (17).

Do not confuse the three spaces associated with the meninges: the *extradural space* (sometimes called the epidural space), outside the dura in the vertebral canal; the *subdural space*, inside the dura (between the dura and arachnoid); and the *subarachnoid space*, inside the arachnoid (between the arachnoid and the pia mater on the surface of the brain and spinal cord) and filled with cerebrospinal fluid.

---

1 Occipital belly of occipitofrontalis
2 Occipital artery
3 Semispinalis capitis
4 Ligamentum nuchae
5 Rectus capitis posterior minor
6 Rectus capitis posterior major
7 Posterior tubercle of atlas
8 Spinous process of axis
9 Semispinalis cervicis
10 Lamina of axis
11 Greater occipital nerve
12 Obliquus capitis inferior
13 Longissimus capitis
14 Transverse process of atlas
15 Obliquus capitis superior
16 Vertebral artery
17 Dorsal ramus of first cervical nerve
18 Posterior arch of atlas
19 Posterior atlanto-occipital membrane
20 Splenius capitis
21 Basilar part of occipital bone and position of attachment of tectorial membrane
22 Superior longitudinal band of cruciform ligament
23 Hypoglossal nerve and canal
24 Alar ligament
25 Transverse ligament of atlas
26 Superior articular surface of axis
27 Inferior longitudinal band of cruciform ligament
28 Tectorial membrane

29 Posterior longitudinal ligament
30 Spinal cord
31 Denticulate ligament
32 Dorsal rootlets of spinal nerve
33 Arachnoid and dura mater (reflected)
34 Radicular artery
35 Dura mater
36 Posterior spinal arteries
37 Ventral rootlets of spinal nerve
38 Dural sheath over dorsal root ganglion
39 Vertebral artery
40 Lamina of axis
41 Lateral atlanto-axial joint
42 Posterior arch of atlas
43 Atlanto-occipital joint
44 Zygapophysial joint
45 Vertebral artery
46 Dorsal ramus ⎱
47 Ventral ramus ⎰ of fourth cervical nerve
48 Anterior tubercle ⎱
49 Posterior tubercle ⎰ of transverse process
50 Body of fourth cervical vertebra
51 Intervertebral disc
52 Dorsal root ganglion of fifth cervical nerve in intervertebral foramen
53 Groove for (ventral ramus of) spinal nerve
54 Spinous process of fifth cervical vertebra
55 Extradural space
56 Subarachnoid space

Clinical imaging

6

Skull *and paranasal sinuses*

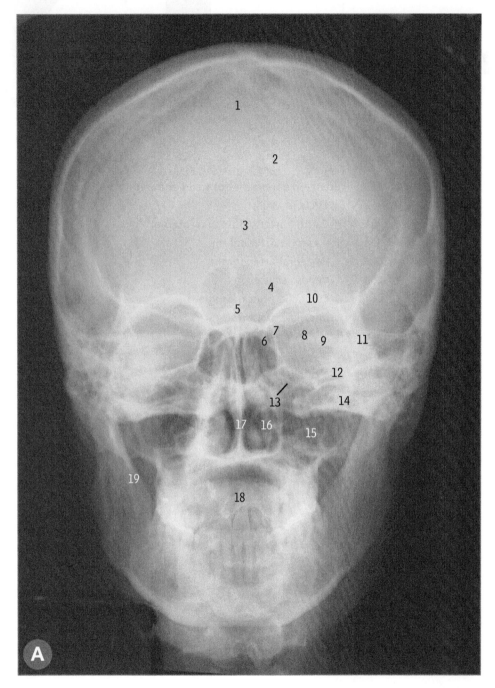

1   Sagittal suture
2   Lambdoid suture
3   Calcification within the falx cerebri
4   Frontal sinus
5   Crista galli of ethmoid
6   Ethmoidal air cells
7   Lesser wing of sphenoid
8   Superior orbital fissure
9   Greater wing of sphenoid
10 Supra-orbital margin
11 Frontozygomatic suture
12 Infra-orbital margin
13 Foramen rotundum
14 Petrous part of temporal bone
15 Maxillary sinus
16 Inferior nasal concha
17 Nasal septum
18 Dens (odontoid peg) of axis (CII) vertebra
19 Coronoid process of mandible

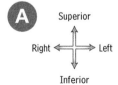

A posteroanterior view

Superior

Right ←→ Left

Inferior

When imaging a complicated structure such as the skull there is considerable overlapping of bony structures.

The more obvious features in **A**, a standard Posteroanterior view, are the orbits (upper (10) and lower (12) margins) and the nasal septum (17), with the crista galli (5) of the ethmoid bone at a higher level. The frontal sinuses (4) are small and there is some calcification (3) in the falx cerebri which would otherwise not be visualised. The ethmoidal air cells (6) lie medial to the orbits, through which are seen the lesser wing of the sphenoid (7) and the superior orbital fissure (8). At a lower level the foramen rotundum (13) is visible, with, below it the translucency of the maxillary sinus (15).

Skull *Lateral view*

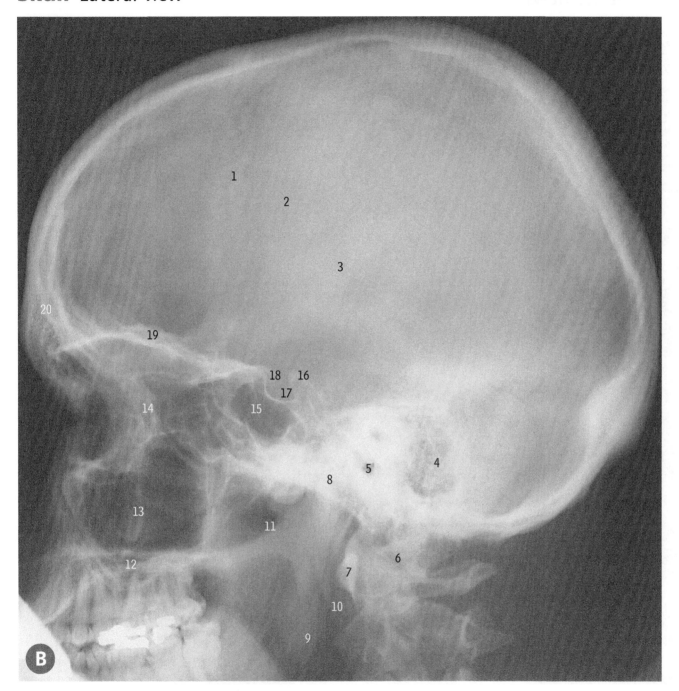

The central feature of the lateral view **B** are the pituitary fossa (17), with the anterior (18) and posterior (16) clinoid processes. In the vault of the skull, suture lines (as at 1) must not be confused with vascular markings (as at 2 and 3). The position of the external acoustic meatus (5) is indicated, and so is the head of the mandible (8); the density of overlapping bones, especially the petrous temporal, obscures details in this region, but towards the back the honeycomb of mastoid air cells (4) is clear. The opacities in the teeth are dental restorations.

1 Coronal suture
2 Frontal branch ⎫ of middle meningeal artery
3 Parietal branch ⎭
4 Mastoid air cells
5 External acoustic meatus
6 Mastoid process
7 Anterior arch of atlas (CI) vertebra
8 Head ⎫ of mandible
9 Angle ⎭
10 Oral part ⎫ of pharynx
11 Nasal part ⎭
12 Hard palate
13 Maxillary sinus
14 Ethmoidal air cells
15 Sphenoidal sinus
16 Posterior clinoid process
17 Pituitary fossa
18 Anterior clinoid process
19 Floor of anterior cranial fossa
20 Frontal sinus

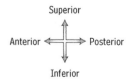

Superior

Anterior ⟵⟶ Posterior

Inferior

Skull *Facial views*

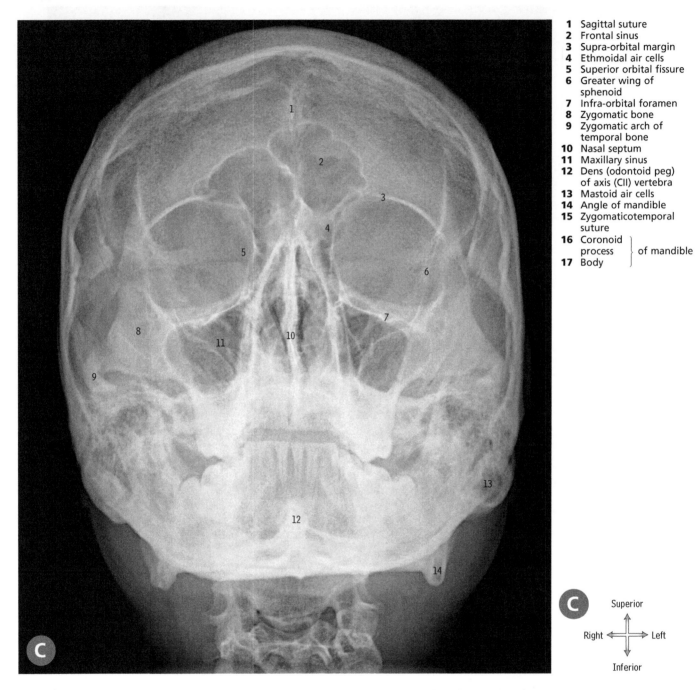

1 Sagittal suture
2 Frontal sinus
3 Supra-orbital margin
4 Ethmoidal air cells
5 Superior orbital fissure
6 Greater wing of sphenoid
7 Infra-orbital foramen
8 Zygomatic bone
9 Zygomatic arch of temporal bone
10 Nasal septum
11 Maxillary sinus
12 Dens (odontoid peg) of axis (CII) vertebra
13 Mastoid air cells
14 Angle of mandible
15 Zygomaticotemporal suture
16 Coronoid process ⎫ of mandible
17 Body ⎭

C Superior

Right ←→ Left

Inferior

C occipitomental radiograph showing the paranasal sinuses.

The mastoid air cells (13) and petrous apex should be projected below the maxila in order to fully visualise the sinuses.

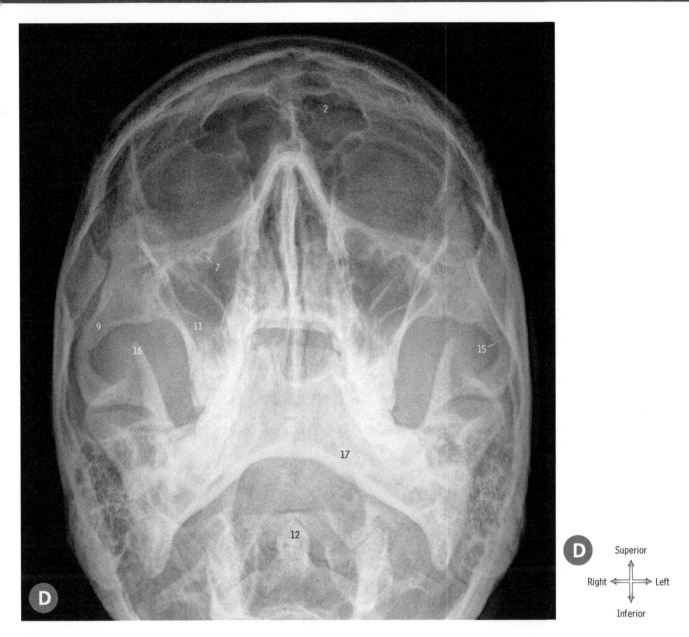

D

Superior

Right ⬌ Left

Inferior

D occipitomental 30° (OM30) view

In C, the patient's chin is tilted upwards at 45° with the x-ray beam horizontal. This avoids superimposition of the dense bones of the base of the skull. Therefore the frontal sinuses (2), above and medial to the orbits, and the maxillary sinuses (11), below the orbits, are emphasised.

A second radiograph (D) is taken with the patient in the same position but the beam at 30° of caudal angulation. The orbits are demonstrated less well but the zygomatic arches (9) and the walls of the maxillary sinuses (11) are seen clearly.

Skull *Paranasal sinuses*

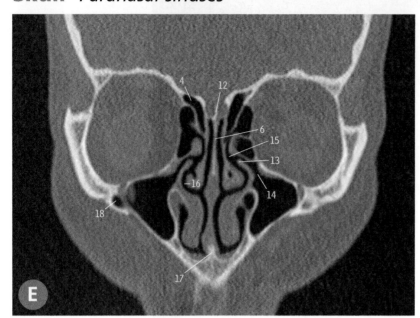

1 Cribriform plate of ethmoid
2 Roof of nasal cavity
3 Ethmoidal air cells
4 Infundibulum draining frontal sinus
5 Middle nasal concha
6 Nasal septum
7 Inferior nasal concha
8 Maxillary sinus
9 Inferior meatus
10 Hard palate
11 Alveolar process of maxilla
12 Crista galli   ⎫
13 Uncinate process   ⎬ of ethmoid
                          ⎭
14 Ostium and duct of maxillary sinus
15 Ostiomeatal complex
16 Middle meatus
17 Anterior nasal spine
18 Infra-orbital foramen

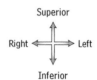

Superior

Right ⟷ Left

Inferior

E coronal CT of the paranasal sinuses and nasal cavity

The ostiomeatal complex (15) is seen, a unit that links the infundibulum (4) draining the frontal sinus, anterior and middle ethmoid air cells and maxillary sinus (8) into the middle meatus.

F coronal CT of the paranasal sinuses

Vertebral column *cervical part*

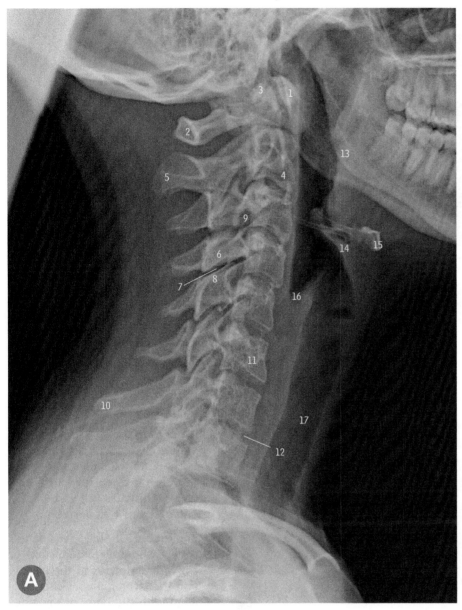

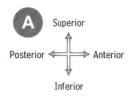

A

Superior

Posterior ⟵ ✚ ⟶ Anterior

Inferior

A **lateral radiograph of the cervical spine**

There are three standard views for radiological evaluation of the cervical spine: lateral view (A); anteroposterior view (AP) (B)—and the odontoid peg (*or opened mouth*) view (C). The odontoid peg (dens of the axis) view (C) is commonly omitted when assessing degenerative change.

The lateral view in A shows the vertebral bodies (as 11) and the obliquely angled zygapophyseal joints (as 7). The anterior (1) and posterior (2) arches of the atlas (first cervical (CI) vertebra) are clearly seen, but the dens (3) (odontoid peg) of the axis (second cervical (CII) vertebra), is largely obscured. Note the large size of the spine (5) of the axis (second cervical (CII) vertebra) and also that the spine (10) of the seventh cervical (CVII) vertebra projects farthest back than the others hence its *latin* name (*vertebra prominens*). In front of the vertebral column there is translucency due to the air-filled pharynx, larynx and trachea (17).

1 Anterior arch ⎫
2 Posterior arch ⎬ of atlas (CI) vertebra
3 Dens (odontoid peg) ⎫
4 Body ⎬ of axis (CII) vertebra
5 Spinous process ⎭
6 Inferior articular process of fourth (CIV) vertebra

7 Zygapophyseal joint
8 Superior articular process of fifth (CV) vertebra
9 Intervertebral foramen
10 Spinous process of seventh (CVII) vertebra (vertebra prominens)
11 Body of sixth (CVI) vertebra

12 Intervertebral disc space between seventh (CVII) and first (TI) vertebra
13 Angle of mandible
14 Epiglottis
15 Tip of greater horn of hyoid bone
16 Vallecula
17 Trachea

Cervical vertebrae

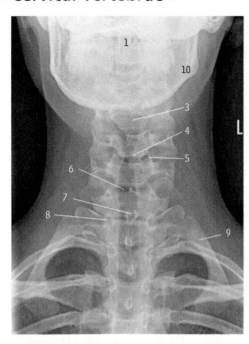

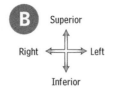

1 Dens (odontoid peg) ⎫
2 Body   ⎬ of axis (CII) vertebra
3 Body of fourth (CIV) vertebra
4 Region of vocal cords
5 Superior articular process of sixth (CVI) vertebra
6 Intervertebral disc space
7 Spinous process of seventh (CVII) vertebra (vertebra prominens)
8 Pedicle
9 First (TI) rib
10 Angle of mandible
11 Bifid spinous process of axis (CII) vertebra
12 Inferior articular surface of lateral mass of atlas (CI) vertebra
13 Superior articular surface of lateral mass of atlas (CII) vertebra
14 Lateral atlanto-axial joint

B **anteroposterior radiograph of the cervical spine**

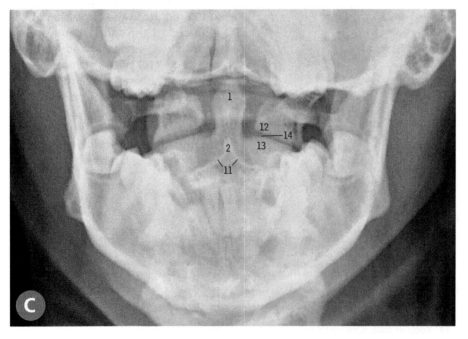

C An odontoid peg *(open mouth)* **view showing the alignment of the atlanto-axial joint (14) between the articular surfaces (12) of the atlas (CI) vertebra and (13) axis (CII) vertebra.**

The (odontoid peg), dens of the axis (1) should lie equidistant to the lateral masses of the atlas and the lateral masses should align with the body of the axis inferiorly.

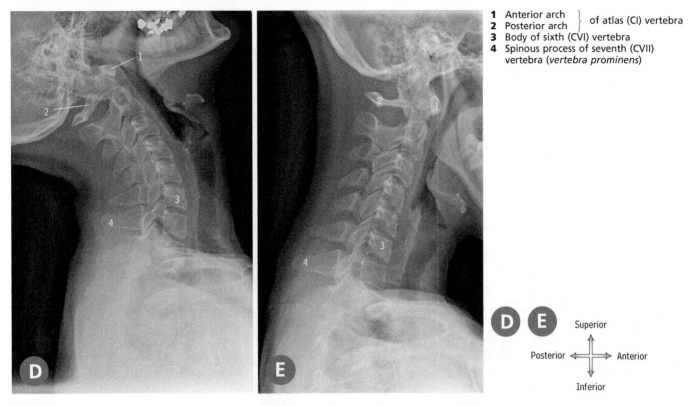

1 Anterior arch ⎫ of atlas (CI) vertebra
2 Posterior arch ⎭
3 Body of sixth (CVI) vertebra
4 Spinous process of seventh (CVII)
vertebra (*vertebra prominens*)

Superior
Posterior ⟷ Anterior
Inferior

D **E** cervical spine radiographs with the patient in extension (D) and flexion
(E) to assess intervertebral body motion and ligamentous damage

Vertebral column *cervical and upper thoracic part*

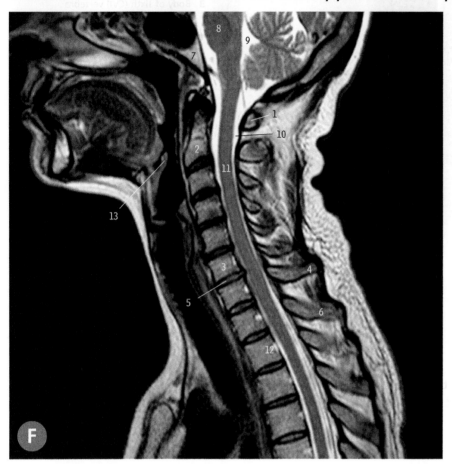

1 Posterior arch ⎫ of atlas (CI) vertebra
2 Body ⎭
3 Body of sixth (CVI) vertebra
4 Spinous process of seventh (CVII) vertebra
    (vertebra prominens)
5 Intervertebral disc between sixth (CVI) and
    seventh (CVII) vertebra
6 Spinous process of first thoracic (TI) vertebra
7 Clivus
8 Pons
9 Fourth ventricle
10 Cerebrospinal fluid (CSF)
11 Spinal medulla (spinal cord)
12 Basivertebral veins
13 Epiglottis

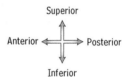

Superior

Anterior ⟵⟶ Posterior

Inferior

F sagittal T2-weighted magnetic resonance image (MRI) of the cervical
and upper thoracic spine. Note the posterior defect due to the
basivertebral veins (12), which is a normal finding

Magnetic resonance imaging (MRI) is the investigation of choice for
assessing the spinal cord and bone marrow. The signal characteristics
vary with age and the type of marrow present. In the spine red marrow
converts to fatty marrow over time in an organised and predictable
fashion. The MR appearance of discs varies according to their water
content with normal discs returning low signal on T1 and high signal on
T2-weighted imaging.

Orbit and Eye

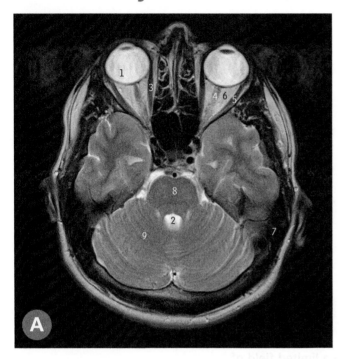

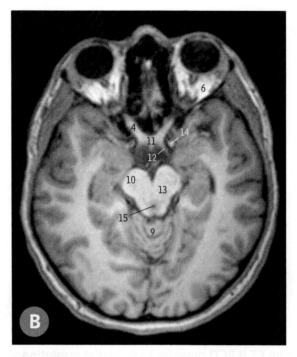

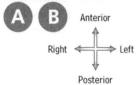

A T2-weighted axial magnetic resonance image (MRI) through the mid-orbit

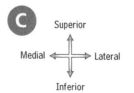

A **B** Anterior
Right ⟷ Left
Posterior

B T2-weighted axial magnetic resonance image (MRI). Note the optic nerves (4) which cross at the optic chiasma (11) and the optic tracts (12) which run posteriorly towards the occipital lobe of the brain

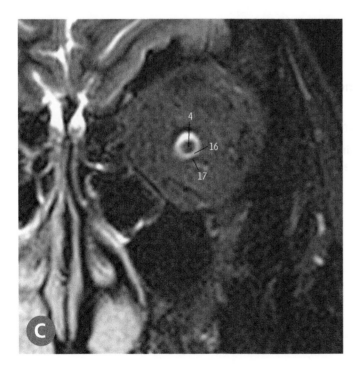

C Superior
Medial ⟷ Lateral
Inferior

1   Globe of eyeball
2   Fourth ventricle
3   Medial rectus
4   Optic nerve II
5   Lateral rectus
6   Retro-orbital fat
7   Petrous part of temporal bone
8   Pons
9   Cerebellum
10 Cerebral peduncle
11 Optic chiasma
12 Optic tract
13 Midbrain
14 Internal carotid artery
15 Cerebral aqueduct
16 Cerebrospinal fluid (CSF)
17 Dural sheath

C T2-weighted coronal magnetic resonance image (MRI). Note the optic nerve I (4) surrounded by a dural sheath (17) and cerebrospinal fluid (CSF) (16) occupying the subarachnoid space

The visual pathway extends from the globes of the eyeballs anteriorly to the occipital cortex posteriorly. The optic nerve (4) is surrounded by meninges containing an extension of the subarachnoid space. Magnetic resonance imaging accurately differentiates bone, fat, muscle and nervous tissue and is very useful in imaging the orbit and visual pathways.

Ear *middle and inner*

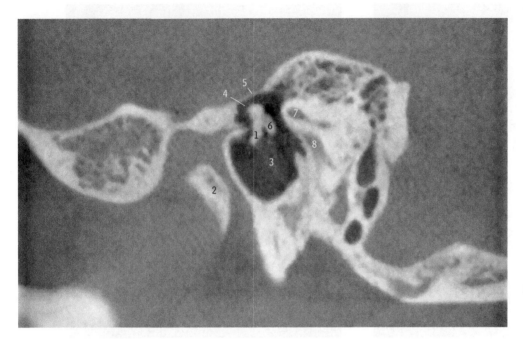

1 Malleus
2 Condyle of mandible
3 Tympanic membrane
4 Epitympanic recess
5 Tegmen tympani
6 Incus
7 Semicircular canal
8 Facial nerve VII

Superior
Anterior ⟵⟶ Posterior
Inferior

Cone beam CT (CBCT) provides high spatial resolution within a limited field of view, which is useful when assessing the structures within the temporal bone, such as the ossicular chain, bony labyrinth, cochlear anatomy and the facial nerve

High-resolution CT provides excellent characterization of the middle and inner ear structures.

The middle ear consists of the tympanic cavity and the antrum.

The inner ear consists of an osseous labyrinth which contains the vestibule, cochlea, semicircular canals, vestibular and cochlear aqueduct.

Brain *main arteries of head and neck*

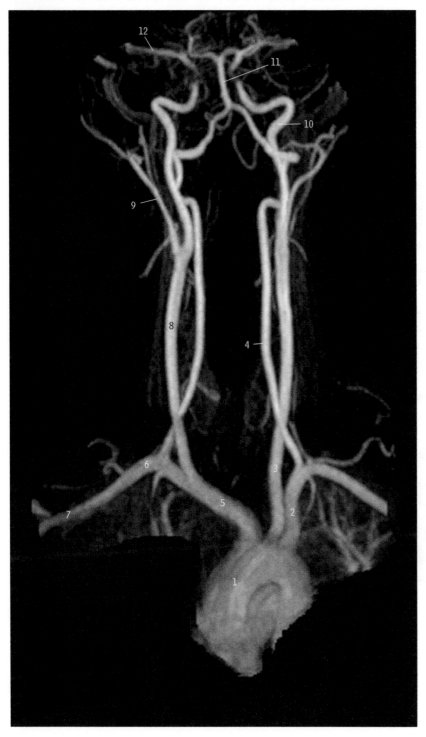

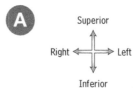

1 Ascending aorta
2 Left subclavian artery
3 Left common carotid artery
4 Left vertebral artery
5 Brachiocephalic artery
6 Right subclavian artery
7 Right axillary artery
8 Right common carotid artery
9 Right external carotid artery
10 Left internal carotid artery
11 Basilar artery
12 Middle cerebral artery

There have been considerable improvements in vascular imaging techniques in recent years. Magnetic resonance angiography provides an alternative to conventional angiography (MRA), eliminating the need for intervention, iodinated contrast media and ionizing radiation. Time of flight angiography (TOF) is an MRI technique to visualize flow within vessels, without the need to administer contrast. In A the aortic arch (1) is seen along with the arterial supply to the head and neck.

Ⓐ magnetic resonance (MR) time of flight (TOF) image of the carotid and vertebral arteries

Brain *Circle of Willis*

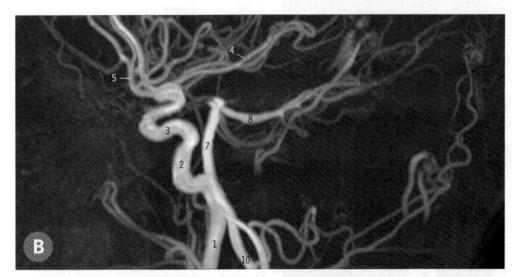

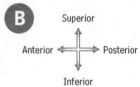

B Superior

Anterior ⟷ Posterior

Inferior

B sagittal magnetic resonance (MR) time of flight (TOF) image of the circle of Willis arising from the carotids and basilar arteries

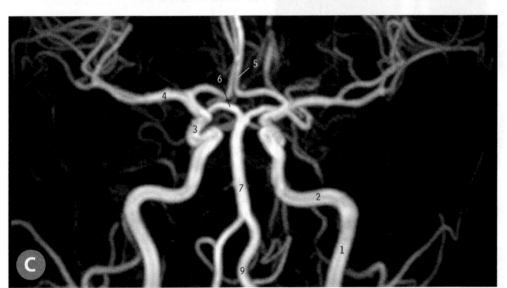

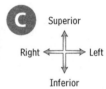

C Superior

Right ⟷ Left

Inferior

C magnetic resonance (MR) time of flight (TOF) image of the circle of Willis

1 Cervical part ⎫
2 Petrous part ⎬ of internal carotid artery
3 Cavernous part ⎭
4 Middle cerebral artery
5 Anterior cerebral artery
6 Posterior communicating artery
7 Basilar artery
8 Posterior cerebral artery
9 Left vertebral artery
10 Vertebral artery

Brain *carotid arteriogram and internal carotid arteriogram*

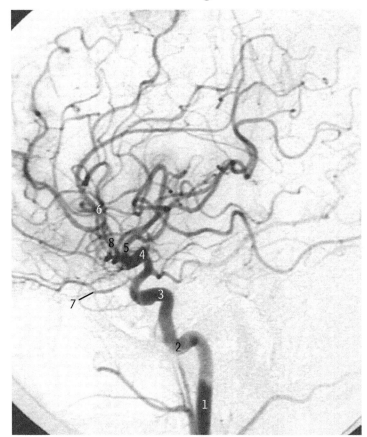

Digital subtraction arteriography (DSA) is a technique that allows unwanted background material to be reduced, thus emphasising the image of the blood vessels. In the lateral view (A) the upper (cervical) part of the internal carotid artery (1) in the neck can be visualised entering the carotid canal in the petrous part of the temporal bone, within which it takes a right-angled turn forwards and medially (2). It then curves upwards along the carotid groove of the sphenoid bone (3) within the cavernous sinus and emerges as the cerebral part (4) which divides into the anterior and middle cerebral arteries (5 and 6). Note the ophthalmic artery (7) passing forwards into the orbit.

1 Cervical ⎫
2 Petrous ⎬ part of internal carotid artery
3 Cavernous ⎪
4 Cerebral ⎭
5 Anterior cerebral artery
6 Branches of middle cerebral artery
7 Ophthalmic artery
8 Middle cerebral artery

(A) lateral projection of a digitally subtracted arterial phase of a carotid arteriogram

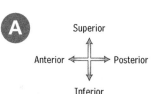

In the anteroposterior view B the characteristic T-shaped division of the internal carotid artery into anterior and middle cerebral branches (2 and 11) is clearly seen.

1 Angular branches of middle cerebral artery
2 Anterior cerebral artery
3 Anterior temporal branches of middle cerebral artery
4 Branches (in insula) of middle cerebral artery
5 Callosomarginal artery
6 Cavernous portion ⎫ of internal carotid artery
7 Cervical portion ⎭
8 Frontopolar artery
9 Genu of middle cerebral artery
10 Lenticulostriate arteries
11 Middle cerebral artery
12 Orbitofrontal branch of pericallosal artery
13 Pericallosal artery
14 Petrous portion of internal carotid artery
15 Posterior parietal branches of middle cerebral artery
16 Recurrent artery of Heubner
17 Sylvian point

(B) anteroposterior view

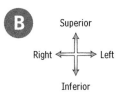

Brain *vertebral arteriograms*

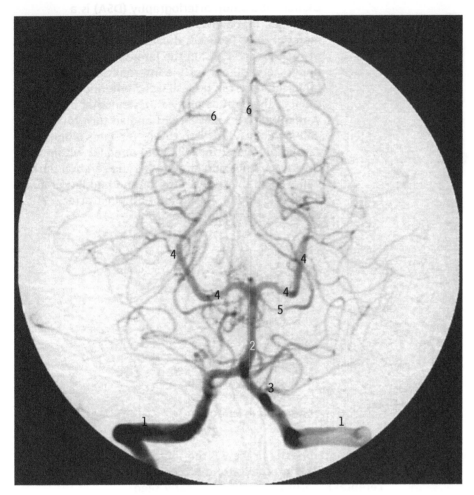

1 Vertebral artery
2 Basilar artery
3 Posterior inferior cerebellar artery
4 Posterior cerebral artery
5 Superior cerebellar artery
6 Occipital and calcarine branches of posterior cerebral artery

A

Superior

Right ←→ Left

Inferior

A **(digitally subtracted arterial phase of vertebral arteriogram) anterior view of both sides**

In A each vertebral artery is first labelled (1) after emerging from the foramen in the transverse processes of the atlas and taking a right-angled turn medially to lie on the posterior arch of the atlas.

After entering the foramen magnum (where both vessels are here unusually tortuous) they unite to form the basilar artery (2) after giving off the posterior inferior cerebellar arteries (3).

The basilar artery divides at its upper end into the posterior cerebrals (4) after giving off the superior cerebellar arteries (5).

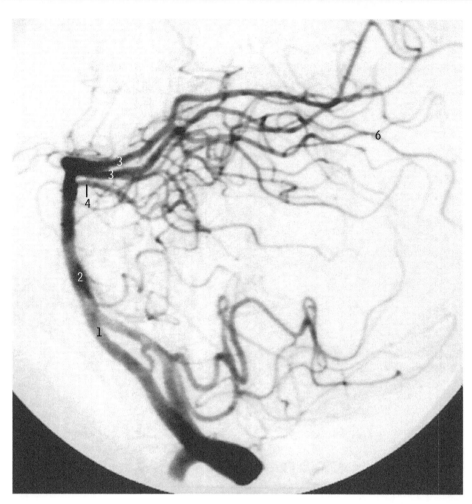

1 Vertebral artery
2 Basilar artery
3 Posterior cerebral artery
4 Superior cerebellar artery

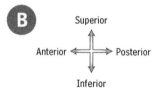

B **(digitally subtracted arterial phase of a vertebral arteriogram) lateral view, left side, from the left**

Superior

Anterior ⟵⟶ Posterior

Inferior

The lateral view B emphasises the mass of vessels converging on the cerebellum and the posterior direction of the posterior cerebral artery (3).

Brain *venous sinuses*

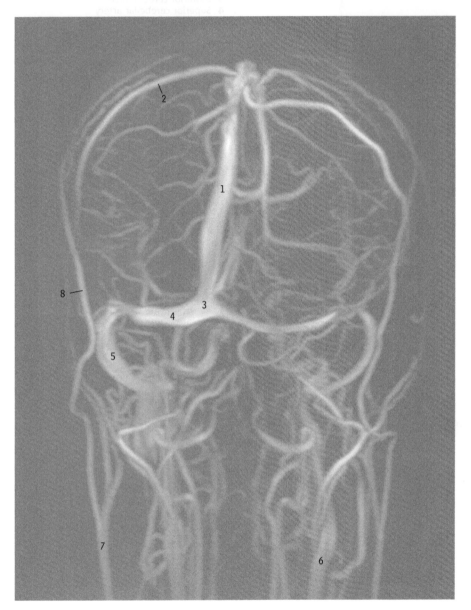

1   Superior sagittal sinus
2   Superior cerebral vein
3   Confluence of the sinuses
4   Transverse sinus
5   Sigmoid sinus
6   Internal jugular vein
7   External jugular vein
8   Superficial temporal vein

A

Superior

Right ⟵⟶ Left

Inferior

A imaging of the intracerebral venous sinuses using maximum intensity projection (MIP) magnetic resonance (MR)

High-resolution contrast enhanced magnetic resonance imaging (MRI) is effective at evaluation of the cerebral veins and sinuses. The intracranial venous system may exhibit a wide range of normal variations, most commonly the right transverse sinus being dominant.

In A the superior sagittal sinus (1) can be traced backwards to the confluence of the sinuses (3) where it runs laterally to become a transverse sinus (usually the right, 4). The other transverse sinus is continuous with the straight sinus, into which drain the inferior sagittal sinus and the great cerebral vein. The transverse sinus turns down to become the sigmoid sinus (5) which leaves the jugular foramen to enter the neck as the internal jugular vein (6).

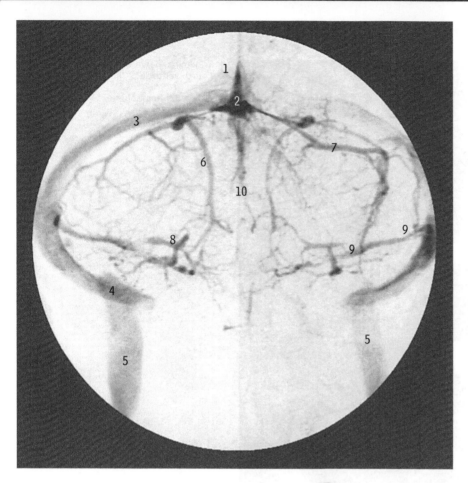

1 Superior sagittal sinus
2 Straight sinus
3 Transverse sinus
4 Sigmoid sinus
5 Internal jugular vein
6 Inferior ⎫
7 Superior ⎬ hemispheric vein
8 Petrosal vein
9 Superior petrosal sinus
10 Inferior vermian vein
11 Confluence of sinuses
12 Great cerebral vein
13 Superior cerebral veins

In B the superior sagittal sinus (1) continues laterally as the right transverse sinus. Other contributory venous systems are also marked in A and B, such as the inferior and superior hemispheric veins (11 and 12) and the inferior vermian vein (15). The petrosal vein (13) and the superior petrosal sinus (14) can also be seen.

B anteroposterior view

B

Superior
Right ⬌ Left
Inferior

C

Superior
Anterior ⬌ Posterior
Inferior

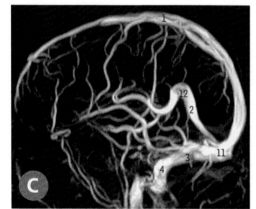

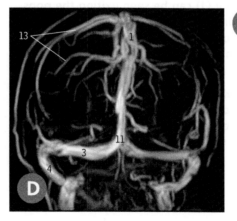

D

Superior
Right ⬌ Left
Inferior

C D phase contrast magnetic resonance (MR) venograms taken at 3.0T in lateral (C), frontal (D) and superior

Brain *cerebellarpontine angle*

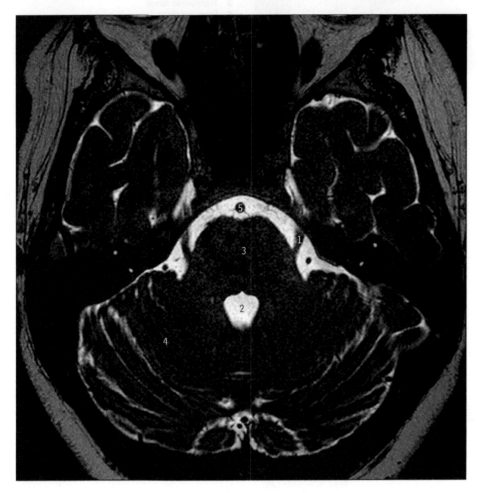

1 Trigeminal nerve V
2 Fourth ventricle
3 Pons
4 Cerebellar hemisphere
5 Basilar artery

Anterior

Right ⟷ Left

Posterior

Magnetic resonance imaging (MRI) is best suited for evaluation of the brainstem, cranial nerves and the fluid-filled spaces of the inner ear

In this axial view, trigeminal nerve V (1) can be seen exiting the pons (3) anteriorly to cross the prepontine cistern to enter Meckel's cave to form the trigeminal ganglion from which it divides into three divisions forming the ophthalmic nerve V^1, the maxillary nerve V^2 and the mandibular nerve V^3.

The internal auditory meatus lies within the petrous temporal bone with the facial (VII) and vestibulocochlear (VIII) cranial nerves running through it. The facial nerve runs posterior to the cochlea to the geniculate ganglion where it then decends and exits the skull through the stylomastoid foramen.

Brain *internal structures*

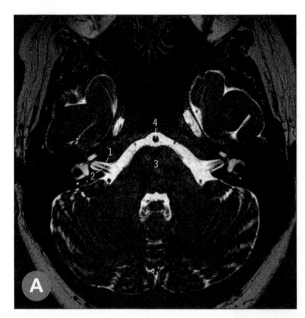

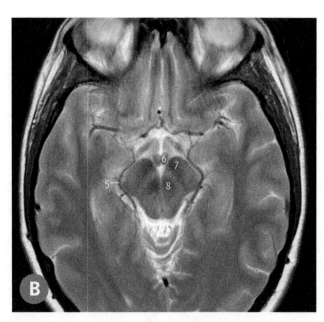

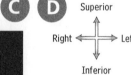

A axial heavily T2-weighted magnetic resonance imaging (MRI) demonstrates the facial nerve VII (1) and the vestibulocochlear nerve VIII (2) as they leave the pons (3) and travel into the internal auditory meatus

A B Anterior

Right ⟷ Left

Posterior

B axial T2-weighted magnetic resonance image (MRI) at the level of the midbrain

C D Superior

Right ⟷ Left

Inferior

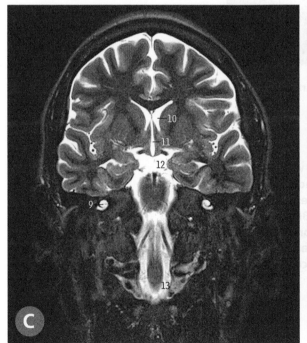

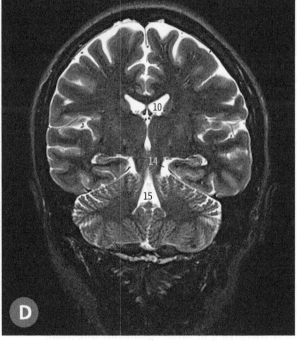

C D coronal T2-weighted magnetic resonance images (MRIs) of the ventricles and basal cisterns.

The internal auditory meatus lies within the petrous temporal bone with the facial nerve VII (1) and vestibulocochlear nerve VIII (2) running through it.

The facial nerve VII runs posterior to the cochlea (9) to the geniculate ganglion where it then descends and exits through the cranium via the stylomastoid foramen.

1 Facial nerve VII	9 Cochlea
2 Vestibulocochlear nerve VIII	10 Lateral ventricle
3 Pons	11 Third ventricle
4 Basilar artery	12 Suprasellar cistern
5 Posterior cerebral artery	13 Cerebellomedullary cistern
6 Mammillary body	14 Quadrigeminal cistern
7 Substantia nigra	15 Fourth venticle
8 Red nuclei	

Brain *internal structures*

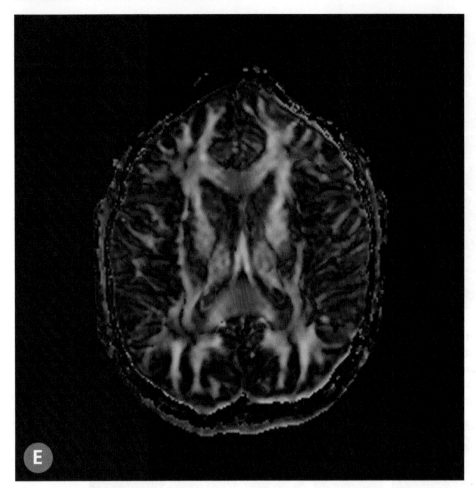

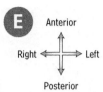

E magnetic resonance (MR) diffusion tractography map showing the major white matter pathways in the brain

The white matter tracts within the brain are not identifiable by conventional CT or MRI methods. Within cerebral white matter, water molecules diffuse more freely along the direction of axonal bundles than across them. This directional dependence of diffusivity is termed anisotropy. Diffusion Tensor Imaging (DTI) tractography allows 3D visualisation of white matter tracts by using anisotropic diffusion to estimate the axonal organisation of the brain. For example, it can determine the location of the corticospinal tract or the thalamocortical tracts. Fiber tractography is a 3D reconstruction technique to demonstrate data collected by DTI in colour form.

Red, for fibres crossing from left to right;

Green, for fibres traversing in anteroposterior direction;

Blue, for fibres going from superior to inferior.

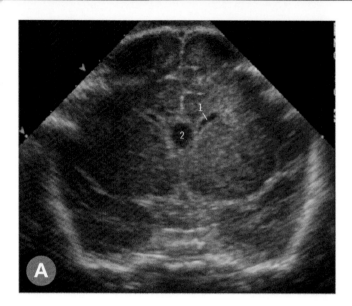

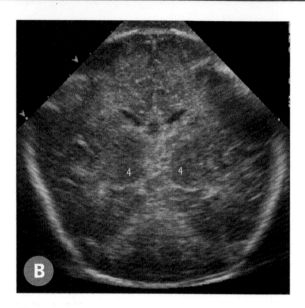

A coronal ultrasound. The cerebrospinal fluid (CSF) in the lateral ventricles (1) is anechoic and appears as a dark image. Note the cavum septum pellucidum (2) (present in almost 100% of neonates and disappears by 8 weeks in 80%)

B coronal ultrasound, angling posteriorly

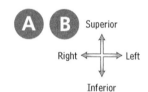

A **B** Superior

Right ⟷ Left

Inferior

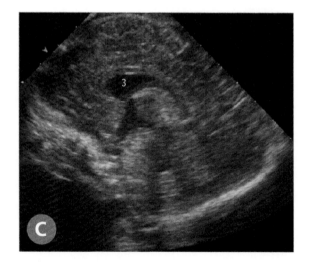

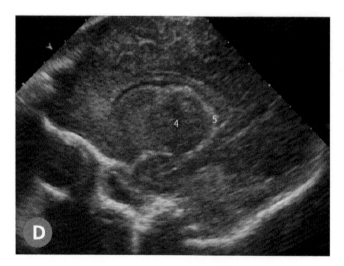

C sagittal ultrasound in the midline. The fourth ventricle lies in front of the cerebellar vermis

1 Anterior horn of lateral ventricles
2 Cavum septum pellucidum
3 Third ventricle
4 Thalamus
5 Choroid plexus

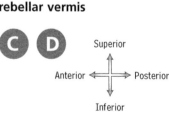

C **D** Superior

Anterior ⟷ Posterior

Inferior

D parasagittal ultrasound. The caudate nucleus lies below the floor of the frontal horn of the lateral ventricle; the thalamus (4) lies behind and below it. The occipital horn of the lateral ventricle is filled with choroid plexus (5)

Ultrasound is a useful clinical technique to assess the neonatal brain and scans are taken in a coronal and sagittal plane. The anterior fontanelle (which normally closes at 18 months) provides an acoustic window.

Appendices

Appendix I *Dental anaesthesia*

In dental practice, anaesthesia of teeth and gingivae can be achieved either by infiltration or regional nerve block. In *infiltration anaesthesia*, the anaesthetic solution is injected into the area concerned, and the anaesthetic agent diffuses through the tissues to anaesthetise local nerve fibres. In *regional nerve block* the injection is placed to affect the nerve(s) supplying the area, which may be at some distance from the operative site.

The bone of the alveolar part of the maxilla, especially that of the buccal (outer) surface, is relatively porous, and anaesthetic solution that penetrates to the region of the apex of a tooth (where the root canal opens and the nerve enters the pulp) will effectively anaesthetise the tooth and surrounding gingiva. Infiltration anaesthesia of the buccal aspect of the jaw is usually effective for all the upper teeth and will allow painless instrumentation, but painless extraction will require anaesthesia of the palatal (inner) aspect as well. Aspiration should precede all injections to avoid intravascular deposition.

For the teeth of the lower jaw, infiltration anaesthesia is less effective, commonly reserved only for the incisors. The other mandibular teeth are embedded in bone that is denser and does not easily allow sufficient penetration of standard anaesthetic solution; for these teeth, a block of the inferior alveolar nerve is most often required. Again for tooth extraction it is necessary to block the lingual and buccal nerves as well in order to anaesthetise the adjacent soft tissues.

The notes that follow describe the anatomical background to the above two common methods of dental anaesthesia, together with some other nerve blocks that may be required.

It is essential that before any injection of local anaesthetic, an attempt is made to aspirate blood into the syringe. A positive aspiration indicates that the needle has inadvertently entered a blood vessel. Direct intravascular injection results not only in failure of the local anaesthetic to work but may cause a variety of cardiovascular effects depending on the agent used.

Inferior alveolar and lingual nerve block

After branching off from the mandibular nerve just below the foramen ovale, the inferior alveolar and lingual nerves pass down between the lateral and medial pterygoid muscles (see page 140, A and B). The inferior alveolar nerve enters the mandibular foramen (with the companion artery behind it), lying at this level immediately lateral to the medial pterygoid muscle and to the sphenomandibular ligament which is attached to the lingula and overlaps the opening of the foramen. Within the mandible the nerve supplies the pulps of all the teeth of its own side and part of the periodontal ligament, and through its mental branch it innervates the lower lip and skin of the chin. The lingual nerve emerges from between the two pterygoid muscles about 1 cm in front of and medial to the inferior alveolar nerve. Running downwards across the medial pterygoid, it enters the mouth by passing under the lower

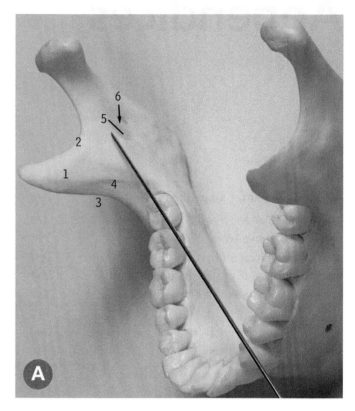

A mandible, obliquely from the left, in front and above, with a needle showing the line of approach to the right mandibular foramen

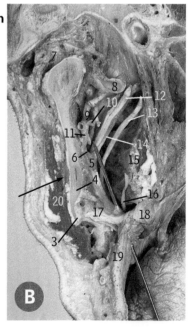

B horizontal section of the right infratemporal fossa, from above, to show the path of the needle

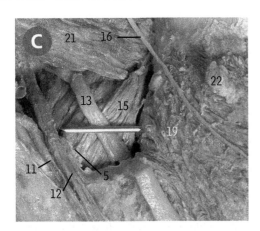

1 Coronoid process
2 Mandibular notch (sigmoid notch)
3 Coronoid notch (external oblique ridge)
4 Internal oblique ridge
5 Lingula
6 Mandibular foramen
7 Parotid gland
8 Styloid process
9 Maxillary artery
10 Inferior alveolar vein
11 Inferior alveolar artery
12 Inferior alveolar nerve
13 Lingual nerve
14 Sphenomandibular ligament
15 Medial pterygoid
16 Buccal nerve
17 Temporalis insertion
18 Pterygomandibular raphe
19 Buccinator
20 Masseter
21 Lateral pterygoid
22 Parotid duct

C **right infratemporal fossa, from the right, with part of the mandible and fat removed, with the needle tip adjacent to the inferior alveolar nerve**

border of the inferior constrictor of the pharynx, lying in contact with the periosteum of the mandible below and behind the third molar tooth. It is the sensory nerve to the anterior part of the tongue, the floor of the mouth and the lingual aspect of the mandible, including the gingivae. It also contributes to the innervation of the periodontal ligament.

Inferior alveolar nerve block, which invariably includes lingual nerve block, is achieved by introducing the anaesthetic solution through the lateral side of the mouth into the fat of the pterygomandibular space—the region between the ramus of the mandible laterally and the medial pterygoid medially.

Through the open mouth the anterior border of the ramus of the mandible (the external oblique ridge) and the ridge of mucous membrane overlying the pterygomandibular raphe are identified. For right-sided anaesthesia this is done by the operator laying the index finger of the left hand on the occlusal surfaces of the molar teeth and moving it backwards to feel first the external oblique ridge (a rather sharp border) and then, slightly behind and more medially, the internal oblique ridge (usually a rather rounded margin). More medially still and with the mouth opened wide, the pterygomandibular raphe is stretched (between its attachments to the pterygoid hamulus of the medial pterygoid plate and the posterior end of the mylohyoid line) to form a ridge in the overlying mucous membrane which can be seen and palpated. With the barrel of the syringe lying over the opposite premolar teeth, the needle is inserted into the mucous membrane 1 cm above the occlusal surface of the third molar tooth and immediately lateral to the ridge over the raphe, i.e. between the ridge medially and the internal oblique line laterally. The needle then pierces the buccinator and about 0.5 cm deeper lies lateral to the lingual nerve, where a small injection is made. After insertion for a further 1 cm the needle tip lies just above the lingula where the main injection is made.

In A a long needle has been used to indicate that the line of approach to the right mandibular foramen (6) is from the left premolar region. This line takes the needle almost parallel to the slope of the ramus between the internal oblique line (4) and the mandibular foramen; the foramen is 1 cm behind the oblique line. The needle tip lies just above the opening of the mandibular foramen.

The section in B is about 1 cm above the mandibular foramen. The fat of the pterygomandibular space has been removed to show the needle tip lying above the mandibular foramen (6), with the inferior alveolar nerve (12) entering it.

The arrow shows the direction of view of the dissection in C, with the needle traversing the pterygomandibular space after piercing the buccinator (19).

If the needle tip is too far lateral it may enter the temporalis muscle insertion (B17) or come into contact with the internal oblique ridge of the mandible (B4).

If the needle is too far medial it may enter the medial pterygoid muscle (B15) and so lie medial to the sphenomandibular ligament (B14) instead of lateral to it. With the needle tip correctly lateral to the ligament, the ligament and the lingual make a kind of funnel directing the anaesthetic solution into the foramen.

If the needle passes too far back it may enter the parotid gland (B7) and part or all of the facial nerve may be paralysed. Even correctly placed injections may sometimes percolate through the inferior orbital fissure and cause transient visual disturbances by affecting the nerve supply of the extra-ocular muscles.

Long buccal nerve block

The long buccal nerve is a branch of the mandibular division of the trigeminal nerve and arises high in the infratemporal fossa from where it passes between the two heads of lateral pterygoid inferiorly and anteriorly where it is medially related to the coronoid notch. It reaches the anterior border of the ascending ramus of the mandible at a similar occlusal level to the lower third molar and crosses the ramus laterally and downwards to the buccal sulcus in the retromolar area. Here it branches out piercing the buccinator supplying the buccal gingivae and the vestibular mucosa forwards to the second premolar. Other fibres continue anteriorly to innervate the skin of the cheek.

When performing extractions or surgery to the molar region, the long buccal nerve must be blocked in addition to the inferior alveolar and lingual nerves. Alternatively, a local buccal infiltration may be used adjacent to the surgical area.

The mucosa is punctured just above the buccal fold of the mucosa in the retromolar area. Using a self-aspiring syringe, the needle is guided horizontally under the mucosa in a posterior direction towards the mandibular ramus where the nerve crosses the external oblique ridge distobuccal to the third molar; 0.5 ml of solution is deposited submucosally.

Mandibular buccal infiltration

Although very dense, some local anaesthetic agents, such as articaine hydrochloride 4%, are able to penetrate through the cortex of the mandible to anaesthetise the inferior alveolar nerve within the bony canal. This results in sufficient anaesthesia for extraction of posterior molars and, only rarely is a 'rescue' inferior alveolar nerve block required. There is some controversy over the use of high strength anaesthetic agents in some countries.

Using a short needle local anaesthetic solution is deposited in the buccal sulcus with further infiltration in the lingual tissues. Care must be taken when infiltrating lingually so as not to directly injure the lingual nerve. Anaesthesia is usually evident within the first 3–5 minutes following the infiltration.

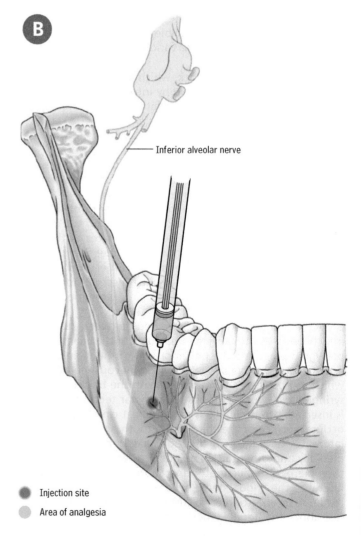

A

Long buccal nerve

Long buccal block

Nerve to mylohyoid

Direct ID block

Lingual nerve

Injection sites

B

Inferior alveolar nerve

Injection site

Area of analgesia

A needle positions for long buccal and inferior alveolar nerve blocks

B needle position for buccal infiltration

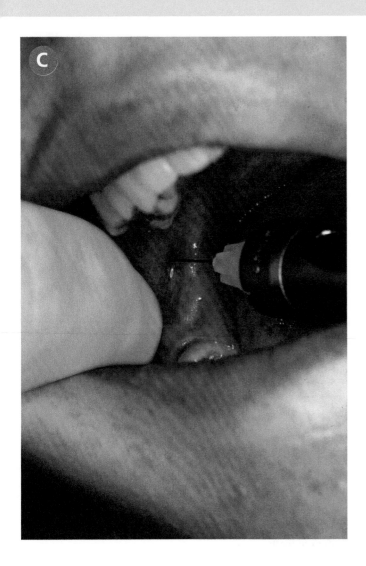

C position of needle and palpating finger in the inferior alveolar nerve block

Infiltration anaesthesia of the upper teeth

For infiltration anaesthesia on the buccal aspect of the jaw, the needle is inserted into or just below the buccal fold (where the mucous membrane is reflected from the jaw to the cheek) opposite the appropriate tooth. The tip of the needle is directed upwards to the level where the apex of the tooth is considered to lie.

For infiltration of the upper teeth on the palatal aspect, the needle is inserted midway between the gingival margin and the midline of the palate opposite the appropriate tooth. As a submucosa is present in this region, anaesthetic solution can be readily accommodated.

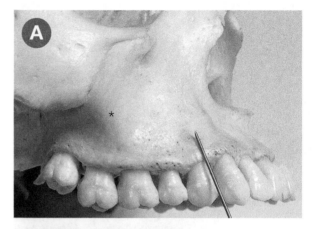

Ⓐ **right maxilla and position of needle for anaesthesia of the first premolar tooth**

Ⓑ **coronal section of maxilla and cheek through the first premolar tooth with buccal and palatal needle placement**

Ⓒ **diagram of injection site and area of anaesthesia (lateral view)**

Ⓓ **diagram of injection site and area of anaesthesia (anterior view)**

Ⓔ **position of needle in buccal sulcus**

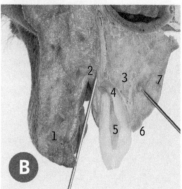

In A the needle is being advanced to the level of the apex of the first premolar, the position for depositing the anaesthetic solution for anaesthesia of this tooth. The asterisk indicates the lower part of the root of the zygomatic process (see note opposite page).

In the coronal section in B the needle on the buccal side is shown penetrating the mucous membrane (2), with the tip lying against the periosteum at the level of the apex of the tooth. Note the presence of a submucosa here. The needle on the palatal side is being inserted midway between the gingival margin (6) and the midline.

1 Lip
2 Buccal fold of mucous membrane
3 Alveolar process of maxilla
4 Apex of tooth
5 Pulp cavity
6 Gingival margin
7 Mucoperiosteum of hard palate

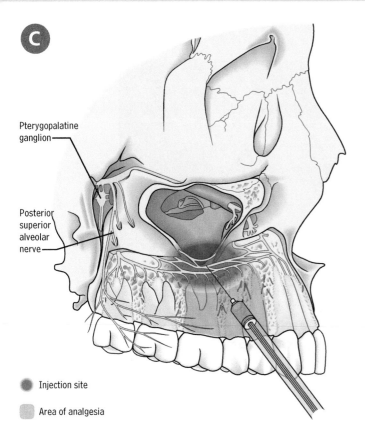

Pterygopalatine ganglion

Posterior superior alveolar nerve

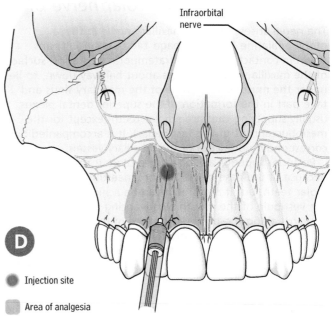

Infraorbital nerve

● Injection site

▨ Area of analgesia

● Injection site

▨ Area of analgesia

The needle must not penetrate the periosteum and strip it off the bone; this causes pain at the time and residual pain when the anaesthesia has worn off.

The bone of the zygomatic process of the maxilla is denser than that of the alveolar process bearing the teeth, and if the root of the zygomatic process (indicated by the asterisk in A) extends lower than usual it may not allow effective penetration in the region of the first and second molar roots. Further injections may be needed.

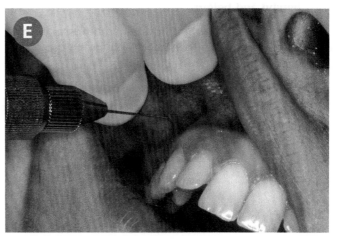

Posterior superior alveolar nerve block

The nerve arises from the maxillary nerve in the pterygopalatine fossa (see page 140, A and B). It runs down in contact with the infratemporal (posterior) surface of the maxilla which it pierces about halfway down, to lie under the mucous membrane of the maxillary sinus and take part in the formation of the superior dental plexus, usually supplying the three molar teeth (except for the mesiobuccal root of the first molar). It is accompanied by corresponding branches of the maxillary vessels.

Posterior superior alveolar nerve block is rarely necessary because of the ease of infiltration anaesthesia of the molar teeth, but if required it can be achieved through the vestibule of the mouth by advancing the needle upwards along the posterior surface of the maxilla.

The needle is inserted through the buccal fold level with the second upper molar tooth, in a direction upwards and backwards at an angle of 45° to the vertical and occlusal planes. The needle is advanced for 2 cm, keeping as close as possible to the maxillary periosteum (10). At this level the tip should be in the region where the nerve enters the bone.

F right infratemporal region and maxilla, from behind and below

G dissection of the right infratemporal fossa, with needle piercing buccinator (17) to lie on the posterior surface of the maxilla

H diagram of position of needle and area of anaesthesia (lateral view)

I position of needle in posterior buccal sulcus

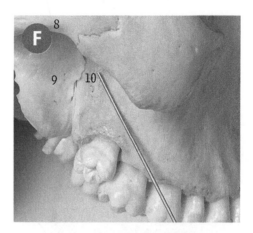

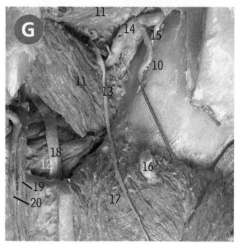

 8 Zygomatic arch
 9 Lateral pterygoid plate
10 Posterior surface of maxilla
11 Lateral pterygoid
12 Medial pterygoid
13 Buccal nerve
14 Maxillary artery
15 Posterior superior alveolar nerve and vessels
16 Parotid duct
17 Buccinator
18 Lingual nerve
19 Inferior alveolar nerve
20 Inferior alveolar artery

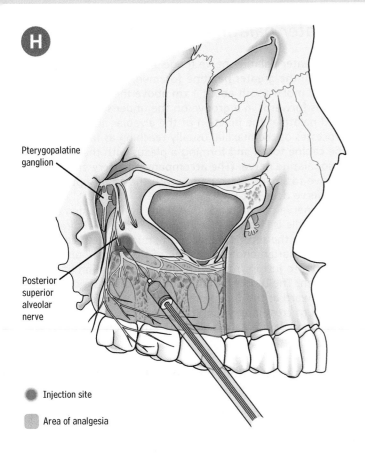

H

Pterygopalatine
ganglion

Posterior
superior
alveolar
nerve

● Injection site

▮ Area of analgesia

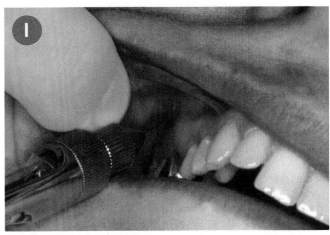

I

If the needle is not kept close to the maxilla, the lateral pterygoid muscle or the pterygoid venous plexus may be entered.

If vessels in the pterygoid venous plexus are damaged by the passage of the needle, a painful haematoma (bruise) will ensue, with limitation of jaw opening due to reflex pterygoid muscle spasm.

Nasopalatine nerve block

The nasopalatine nerve runs downwards and forwards under the mucous membrane of the nasal septum, and passes through the incisive foramen and incisive fossa to enter the roof of the mouth (see page 167, C). It supplies the hard palate and palatal alveolus in the region of the incisor and canine teeth of its own side and the teeth themselves.

The nerve can be blocked as it emerges from the incisive fossa (A1). The injection is made in an upward and slightly medial direction just lateral to the midline above the gingival margin. The incisor teeth of the nerve's own side and possibly the canine will be affected. For procedures involving the adjacent bone of the maxilla, the needle can be pushed up into the incisive canal (B) for 1 cm in a line parallel with the long axis of the central incisor tooth. However, this procedure results in intense pain until the anaesthetic takes effect.

In A the needle is in the normal position for tooth anaesthesia, and in B the needle is being advanced up the incisive canal (1) for more extensive anaesthesia.

Ⓐ upper jaw, from below, with needle tip adjacent to the incisive fossa

Ⓑ upper jaw, from below, with needle advanced into the incisive canal

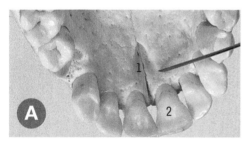

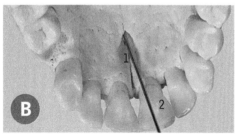

The site of insertion of the needle into the mucoperiosteum is made slightly lateral to the mid-line (A), because the mid-line tissue over the incisive fossa is very sensitive, so that the initial injection more laterally is less painful.

There is no submucosa in this region, the oral mucosa being tightly bound down to the underlying periosteum (mucoperiosteum). Only a small amount of anaesthetic solution is required and only a small amount can be accommodated. If too much is injected too rapidly, the mucosa may be forcibly stripped off the bone, causing considerable postoperative pain.

Greater palatine nerve block

The greater palatine nerve (page 161, D29) emerges through the greater palatine foramen, at the level of the second molar tooth about 1 cm above the gingival margin. It runs forwards in a groove on the under surface of the hard palate at the junction of the alveolar and palatine processes of the maxilla, usually reaching as far forward as the canine tooth and forming a plexus with the nasopalatine nerve. (The accompanying artery enters the incisive fossa and foramen to reach the nasal septum, but the nerve does not.)

The nerve can be blocked in front of its foramen (C5). The needle is inserted in an upward and lateral direction—level with the second molar tooth, midway between the gingival margin and the midline of the palate—and directed to just in front of the expected position of the foramen. The block should produce anaesthesia of teeth as far forward as the first premolar; the canine is in the region of cross-innervation between the greater palatine and nasopalatine nerves, and the effects on this tooth are variable.

Ⓒ hard palate, from the left and below, with needle tip in front of the right greater palatine foramen

Ⓓ dissection of palatal mucoperiosteum to show the greater palatine nerve

In C the needle tip lies in the desired position in front of the greater palatine foramen (5) where, as seen in D, it is adjacent to the greater palatine nerve (7).

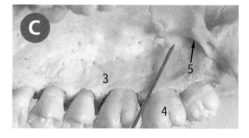

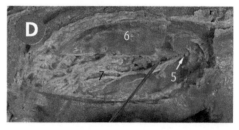

Injection too far back may affect the lesser palatine nerves supplying the tonsillar area and soft palate; this is often an unpleasant sensation.

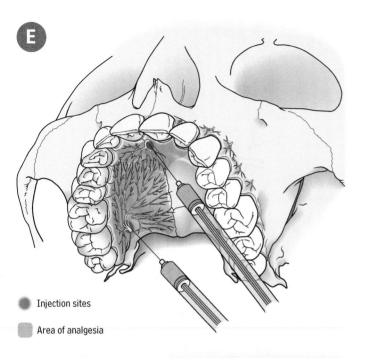

E

Injection sites

Area of analgesia

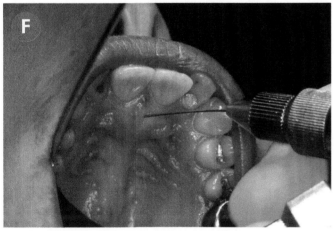

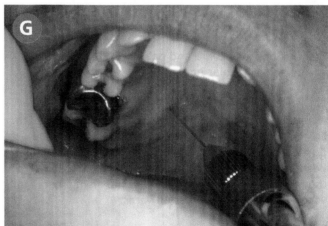

1 Incisive fossa leading to incisive canal
2 Central incisor tooth
3 Alveolar process of maxilla
4 Second molar tooth
5 Greater palatine foramen
6 Mucoperiosteum
7 Greater palatine nerve

Mental and incisive nerve block

The mental nerve supplies the skin of the lower lip and chin and the adjacent mucous membrane and gingiva. The incisive nerve supplies the first premolar, canine and incisor teeth and gingiva. In mental and incisive nerve block, the object is to deposit anaesthetic so that it flows into the mental foramen, thus affecting the mental nerve that emerges from the foramen and runs upwards, and the incisive nerve that continues forwards within the mandible. Since the opening of the mental foramen faces upwards and backwards, the needle must approach it from above and behind so that the tip can enter the opening.

Through the open mouth and with the angle of the mouth retracted, the needle is inserted through the mucous membrane in the depth of the sulcus between the mandible and cheek in the line of the second premolar tooth. After a small mucosal injection, the needle is advanced into the opening of the foramen.

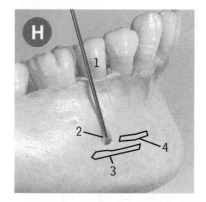

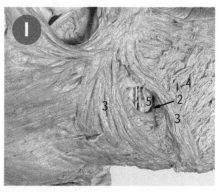

H   right mental foramen

I   dissection

J   diagram of injection site and position of needle for the mental block

K   position of needle and palpating finger in the inferior alveolar nerve block

1 Second premolar tooth
2 Mental foramen
3 Depressor anguli oris
4 Depressor labii inferioris
5 Mental nerve and vessels

In H the tip of the needle has been advanced vertically from above, in the line of the second premolar tooth, to lie at the opening of the mental foramen (2). In the dissection in I the fibres of depressor anguli oris (3) have been separated to show the needle tip at the opening of the mental foramen (2), from which the mental nerve and vessels (5) emerge and pass upwards.

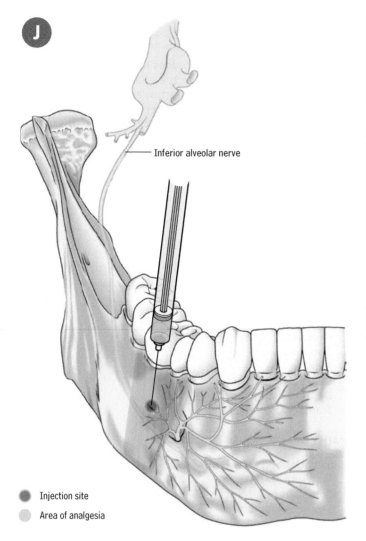

Inferior alveolar nerve

● Injection site
○ Area of analgesia

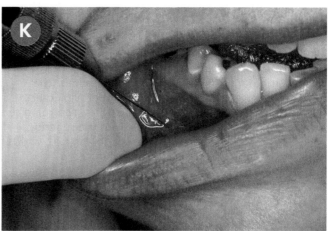

The attachment of depressor labii inferioris (H4) lies in front of the mental foramen (H2), and that of depressor anguli oris (H3) below it. Injected solution may enter these muscles if the needle tip is not at the opening of the foramen.

As this injection results in profound numbness of the lower lip, it is important to warn the patient of the risk of biting the lip until the anaesthetic has completely worn off.

Appendix II *Reference lists*

The following lists are included to provide 'at-a-glance' reference to muscle groups, branches of nerves and arteries, tributaries of veins, and to lymph nodes. The nerves and vessels have been grouped to provide quick identification of parent trunks and branches, according to the indentation of the listed names. Thus the superior laryngeal artery is a branch of the superior thyroid, which in turn is a branch of the external carotid.

An arrow indicates a continuity with a change of name, not a branching.

The inclusion of items here does not necessarily imply that they are all illustrated in the atlas. Many of the smaller vessels and nerves in particular are not shown but have been included to provide a record of generally accepted terms as far as the anatomy of the head and neck is concerned.

A list of skull foramina with the structures that pass through them is also included but some students may find that the simplified list of the more important items on page 19 is sufficient for their purpose.

Muscles

MUSCLES OF THE HEAD

Muscles of the scalp
Epicranius
　Occipitofrontalis
　　Occipital belly
　　Frontal belly
　Temporoparietalis

Muscles of the auricle
Extrinsic
　Auricularis anterior
　Auricularis superior
　Auricularis posterior
Intrinsic
　Helicis major and minor
　Tragicus
　Antitragicus
　Transversus auriculae
　Obliquus auriculae

Muscles of the nose
Procerus
Nasalis
　Transverse part (compressor naris)
　Alar part (dilator naris)
Depressor septi

Muscles of the eyelids
Orbicularis oculi
　Orbital part
　　Depressor supercilii
　Palpebral part
　Lacrimal part
Corrugator supercilii
Levator palpebrae superioris (see Muscles of the orbit)

Muscles of mastication
Temporalis
Masseter
Lateral pterygoid
Medial pterygoid

Muscles of the mouth
Levator labii superioris
Levator labii superioris alaeque nasi
Zygomaticus major
Zygomaticus minor
Levator anguli oris
Buccinator
Orbicularis oris
Risorius
Mentalis
Depressor labii inferioris
Depressor anguli oris
Transversus menti

MUSCLES OF THE NECK

Superficial and lateral muscles
Platysma
Trapezius (see Muscles of the upper limb)
Sternocleidomastoid

Anterior vertebral muscles
Longus colli
Longus capitis
Rectus capitis anterior
Rectus capitis lateralis

Lateral vertebral muscles
Scalenus anterior
Scalenus medius
Scalenus posterior

Suprahyoid muscles
Digastric
Stylohyoid
Mylohyoid
Geniohyoid

Infrahyoid muscles
Sternohyoid
Sternothyroid
Thyrohyoid
Omohyoid

MUSCLE GROUPS IN HEAD AND NECK

Muscles of the pharynx
Superior constrictor
Middle constrictor
Inferior constrictor
Stylopharyngeus
Palatopharyngeus
Salpingopharyngeus

Muscles of the palate
Palatoglossus
Palatopharyngeus
Tensor veli palatini
Levator veli palatini
Musculus uvulae

Muscles of the larynx
Cricothyroid
Posterior crico-arytenoid
Lateral crico-arytenoid
Transverse arytenoid
Oblique arytenoid
Aryepiglottic
Thyro-arytenoid and vocalis
Thyro-epiglottic
(Superior thyro-arytenoid)

Muscles of the tongue
Extrinsic
  Genioglossus
  Hyoglossus and chondroglossus
  Styloglossus
  Palatoglossus
Intrinsic
  Superior longitudinal
  Inferior longitudinal
  Transverse
  Vertical

Muscles of the orbit
Levator palpebrae superioris
Orbitalis

Muscles of the eyeball
Superior rectus
Inferior rectus
Medial rectus
Lateral rectus
Superior oblique
Inferior oblique

MUSCLES OF THE TRUNK

Suboccipital muscles
Rectus capitis posterior major
Rectus capitis posterior minor
Obliquus capitis inferior
Obliquus capitis superior

Deep muscles of the back
Splenius capitis
Splenius cervicis
Erector spinae
  Iliocostalis cervicis
  Iliocostalis thoracis
  Iliocostalis lumborum
  Longissimus capitis
  Longissimus cervicis
  Longissimus thoracis
  Spinalis capitis
  Spinalis cervicis
  Spinalis thoracis
Transversospinalis
  Semispinalis capitis
  Semispinalis cervicis
  Semispinalis thoracis
  Multifidus
  Rotatores
Interspinal
Intertransverse

MUSCLES OF THE UPPER LIMB

Connecting limb and vertebral column
Trapezius
Latissimus dorsi
Levator scapulae
Rhomboid major
Rhomboid minor

Connecting limb and thoracic wall
Pectoralis major
Pectoralis minor
Subclavius
Serratus anterior

Scapular muscles
Deltoid
Subscapularis
Supraspinatus
Infraspinatus
Teres minor
Teres major

Nerves

CRANIAL NERVES AND BRANCHES

I   Olfactory (from olfactory mucous membrane)

II   Optic (from retina)

III Oculomotor
Superior branch (to superior rectus and levator palpebrae superioris)
Inferior branch (to medial rectus, inferior rectus and inferior oblique)
Oculomotor root to ciliary ganglion

IV   Trochlear (to superior oblique)

V   Trigeminal
Sensory root
  Trigeminal ganglion
Motor root (joining mandibular nerve)
Ophthalmic
  Tentorial
  Lacrimal
    Communicating branch with zygomatic
  Frontal
    Supra-orbital
    Supratrochlear
  Nasociliary → anterior ethmoidal → external nasal
        Communicating branch with ciliary ganglion
        Long ciliary
        Posterior ethmoidal
        Anterior ethmoidal
          Lateral and medial internal nasal
          External nasal
        Infratrochlear
        Palpebral
Maxillary → infra-orbital
  Meningeal
  Ganglionic branches to pterygopalatine ganglion
    Orbital
    Nasal (lateral and medial posterior superior nasal and nasopalatine)
    Pharyngeal
  Greater palatine
    Posterior inferior nasal
  Lesser palatine
  Zygomatic
    Zygomaticotemporal
    Zygomaticofacial
  Infra-orbital
    Superior alveolar
      Posterior, middle and anterior superior alveolar
        Superior dental plexus
          Superior dental
          Superior gingival
    Inferior palpebral
    External nasal
    Internal nasal
    Superior labial

Mandibular
  Meningeal
  Masseteric
  Deep temporal
  Nerve to lateral pterygoid
  Nerve to medial pterygoid
    Nerve to tensor veli palatini and tensor tympani via otic ganglion
  Buccal
  Auriculotemporal
    Nerve to external acoustic meatus
    Tympanic membrane
    Communicating branches with facial nerve
    Anterior auricular
    Superficial temporal
  Lingual
    Faucial
    Communicating branches with hypoglossal nerve
    Communicating branches with chorda tympani
    Sublingual
    Lingual
    Ganglionic branches to submandibular ganglion
  Inferior alveolar
    Mylohyoid
    Inferior dental plexus
      Inferior dental
      Inferior gingival
    Mental
      Mental
      Inferior labial

VI   Abducent (to lateral rectus)

VII Facial
Greater petrosal
Nerve to stapedius
Chorda tympani
Communicating branch with tympanic plexus
Communicating branch with vagus nerve
Posterior auricular
  Occipital (to occipital belly of occipitofrontalis)
  Auricular (to auricular muscles)
  To digastric (posterior belly)
  To stylohyoid
  Communicating branch with glossopharyngeal nerve
Parotid plexus

Temporal	to frontal belly of occipitofrontalis, muscles of facial expression and platysma
Zygomatic	
Buccal	
Marginal mandibular	
Cervical	

VIII Vestibulocochlear
Cochlear (from coils of cochlea)
Vestibular (from utricle, saccule and ampullae of
semicircular canals)

IX   Glossopharyngeal
Tympanic
Tubal
Caroticotympanic
Lesser petrosal
Carotid sinus
Pharyngeal
Muscular (to stylopharyngeus)
Tonsillar
Lingual

X   Vagus
Meningeal
Auricular
Pharyngeal (to muscles of pharynx and soft palate
except stylopharyngeus and tensor veli palatini)
Superior cervical cardiac
Carotid body
Superior laryngeal
Internal laryngeal
External laryngeal (to cricothyroid)
Inferior cervical cardiac
Recurrent laryngeal
Tracheal
Oesophageal
Inferior laryngeal (to muscles of larynx except
cricothyroid)
Thoracic cardiac
Bronchial
Oesophageal plexus
Anterior vagal trunk
Gastric
Hepatic
Posterior vagal trunk
Coeliac
Gastric

XI   Accessory
Trunk of accessory
Internal ramus (cranial or vagal part, from cranial
roots, to muscles of palate, except tensor veli
palatini, and larynx via fibres joining vagus nerve)
External ramus (spinal part, from cervical roots, to
sternocleidomastoid and trapezius)

XII Hypoglossal
Lingual (to muscles of tongue except palatoglossus)
Muscular (derived from cervical nerves and including
upper root of ansa cervicalis, to geniohyoid,
thyrohyoid, sternohyoid, sternothyroid and superior
belly of omohyoid. See cervical plexus, page 282).

SOME HEAD AND NECK NERVE SUPPLIES

All the muscles of	Supplied by	Except	Supplied by
Pharynx	Pharyngeal plexus*	Stylo-pharyngeus	Glosso-pharyngeal nerve
Palate	Pharyngeal plexus	Tensor veli palatini	Nerve to medial pterygoid
Larynx	Recurrent laryngeal nerve	Crico-thyroid	External laryngeal nerve
Tongue	Hypoglossal nerve	Palato-glossus	Pharyngeal plexus
Facial expression (including buccinator)	Facial nerve		
Mastication	Mandibular nerve		

*The cricopharyngeus part of the inferior constrictor may
sometimes be supplied by the recurrent or external laryngeal
branches of the vagus nerve.

Nerves

CERVICAL PLEXUS AND BRANCHES
Lesser occipital C2
Great auricular C2, 3
Transverse cervical C2, 3
Supraclavicular C3, 4
Phrenic (to diaphragm) C3, 4, 5
Communicating (with vagus and hypoglossal nerves and
   superior cervical sympathetic ganglion)
Muscular (to rectus capitis lateralis, rectus capitis anterior,
   longus capitis and longus colli, and by lower root of
   ansa cervicalis to sternohyoid, sternothyroid and inferior
   belly of omohyoid) C1, 2, 3

BRACHIAL PLEXUS AND BRANCHES

Supraclavicular branches
From the roots
   To scalenes and longus colli C5, 6, 7, 8
   To join phrenic nerve C5
   Dorsal scapular (to rhomboids) C5
   Long thoracic (to serratus anterior) C5, 6, 7
From the upper trunk
   Nerve to subclavius C5, 6
   Suprascapular (to supraspinatus and infraspinatus)
      C5, 6

Infraclavicular branches
From the lateral cord
   Lateral pectoral (to pectoralis major and minor)
      C5, 6, 7
   Musculocutaneous C5, 6, 7
   Lateral root of the median C(5), 6, 7
From the medial cord
   Medial pectoral (to pectoralis major and minor) C8, T1
   Medial root of the median C8, T1
   Medial cutaneous of arm C8, T1
   Medial cutaneous of forearm C8, T1
   Ulnar C(7), 8, T1
From the posterior cord
   Upper subscapular (to subscapularis) C5, 6
   Thoracodorsal (to latissimus dorsi) C6, 7, 8
   Lower subscapular (to subscapularis and teres major)
      C5, 6
   Axillary C5, 6
   Radial C5, 6, 7, 8, T1

Lymphatic system

THORACIC DUCT AND RIGHT LYMPHATIC DUCT

Thoracic duct
   Left jugular trunk
   Left subclavian trunk
   Left bronchomediastinal trunk

Right lymphatic duct
   Right jugular trunk
   Right subclavian trunk
   Right bronchomediastinal trunk

Cisterna chyli
   Left lumbar trunk
   Right lumbar trunk
   Intestinal trunks

LYMPH NODES OF THE HEAD AND NECK

Deep cervical
   Superior (including jugulodigastric)
   Inferior (including jugulo-omohyoid)

Draining superficial tissues in the head
   Occipital
   Retro-auricular (mastoid)
   Parotid
   Buccal (facial)

Draining superficial tissues in the neck
   Submandibular
   Submental
   Anterior cervical
   Superficial cervical

Draining deep tissues in the neck
   Retropharyngeal
   Paratracheal
   Lingual
   Infrahyoid
   Prelaryngeal
   Pretracheal

Arteries

AORTA AND BRANCHES

Ascending aorta → arch of aorta → thoracic aorta → abdominal aorta

Ascending aorta

Right coronary
    Marginal
    Posterior interventricular
Left coronary
    Circumflex
    Anterior interventricular

Arch of aorta

Brachiocephalic trunk
    Right common carotid
      Right internal carotid
    Right external carotid
    Right subclavian → axillary → brachial
    Thyroidea ima (occasional)
Left common carotid
    Left internal carotid
    Left external carotid
Left subclavian → axillary → brachial

SUBCLAVIAN ARTERY AND BRANCHES

Subclavian → axillary → brachial
Vertebral
  Prevertebral part
  Transversarial (cervical) part
    Spinal (radicular)
    Muscular
  Atlantic part
  Intracranial part
    Anterior and posterior meningeal
    Anterior spinal
    Posterior inferior cerebellar
      Choroidal of fourth ventricle
      To cerebellar tonsil
      Medial and lateral medullary
      Posterior spinal
Basilar (from union of both vertebrals)
  Anterior inferior cerebellar
  Labyrinthine
  Pontine
  Mesencephalic
  Superior cerebellar
  Posterior cerebral
    Precommunicating part
      Posteromedial central
    Postcommunicating part
      Posterolateral central
      Thalamic
      Medial and lateral posterior choroidal
      Peduncular
    Terminal (cortical) part
      Lateral occipital
        Anterior, middle and posterior temporal
      Medial occipital
        Dorsal corpus callosal
        Parietal
        Calcarine
        Occipitotemporal
Thyrocervical trunk
  Inferior thyroid
    Inferior laryngeal
    Glandular
    Pharyngeal
    Oesophageal
    Tracheal
    Ascending cervical
      Spinal
    Superficial (transverse) cervical
    Suprascapular
      Acromial
  Internal thoracic
  Costocervical trunk
    Deep cervical
    Superior intercostal
      First posterior intercostal
      Second posterior intercostal
        Dorsal
        Spinal
  Dorsal scapular

CAROTID ARTERIES AND BRANCHES

Internal carotid
  Cervical part
    Carotid sinus
  Petrous part
    Caroticotympanic
    Pterygoid canal
  Cavernous part
    Basal and marginal tentorial
    Meningeal
    To trigeminal and trochlear
    Cavernous sinus
    Inferior hypophysial
  Cerebral part
    Superior hypophysial
    Ophthalmic
      Central of retina
      Lacrimal
      Anastomotic branch with middle meningeal
      Lateral palpebral
    Short and long posterior ciliary
    Muscular
      Anterior ciliary
    Anterior and posterior conjunctival
    Episcleral
    Supra-orbital
    Posterior ethmoidal
    Anterior ethmoidal
      Anterior meningeal
    Medial palpebral
    Supratrochlear
    Dorsal nasal
  Anterior cerebral
    Precommunicating part
      Anteromedial central (thalamostriate)
      Short central
      Long central (recurrent)
      Anterior communicating
    Postcommunicating part (pericallosal)
      Medial frontobasal (orbitofrontal)
      Callosomarginal
        Anteromedial frontal
        Intermediomedial frontal
        Posteromedial frontal
        Cingular
      Paracentral
      Precuneal
      Parieto-occipital

  Middle cerebral
    Sphenoidal part
      Anterolateral central (thalamostriate)
        Medial and lateral (striate)
    Insular part
      Insular
      Lateral frontobasal (orbitofrontal)
      Anterior, intermediate and posterior temporal
    Terminal (cortical) part
      To central sulcus
      To precentral sulcus
      To postcentral sulcus
      Anterior and posterior parietal
      To angular gyrus
  Anterior choroidal
    Choroidal of lateral ventricle
    Choroidal of third ventricle
    To anterior perforated substance
    To optic tract
    To lateral geniculate body
    To internal capsule
    To globus pallidus
    To tail of caudate nucleus
    To tuber cinereum
    To hypothalamic nuclei
    To substantia nigra
    To red nucleus
    To amygdaloid body
  Posterior communicating (joining posterior cerebral)
    Chiasmatic
    To oculomotor nerve
    Thalamic
    Hypothalamic
    To tail of caudate nucleus

External carotid
  Superior thyroid
    Infrahyoid
    Sternocleidomastoid
    Superior laryngeal
      Cricothyroid
  Ascending pharyngeal
    Posterior meningeal
    Pharyngeal
    Inferior tympanic
  Lingual
    Suprahyoid
    Sublingual
    Dorsal lingual
    Deep lingual
  Facial
    Ascending palatine
    Tonsillar
    Submental
    Glandular
    Inferior labial
    Superior labial
    Angular
  Occipital
    Mastoid
    Auricular
    Sternocleidomastoid
    Meningeal
    Occipital
    Descending
  Posterior auricular
    Stylomastoid
    Posterior tympanic
      Mastoid
      Stapedial
    Auricular
    Occipital
  Superficial temporal
    Parotid
    Transverse facial
    Anterior auricular
    Zygomatico-orbital
    Middle temporal
    Frontal
    Parietal

  Maxillary
    Deep auricular
    Anterior tympanic
    Inferior alveolar
      Dental
      Mylohyoid
      Mental
    Middle meningeal
      Accessory meningeal
      Petrosal
      Superior tympanic
      Frontal
      Parietal
      Orbital
      Anastomotic branch with lacrimal
    Masseteric
    Deep temporal
    Pterygoid
    Buccal
    Posterior superior alveolar
      Dental
    Infra-orbital
      Anterior superior alveolar
        Dental
    Pterygoid canal
    Descending palatine
      Greater palatine
      Lesser palatine
    Sphenopalatine
      Posterior, lateral and septal nasal

Veins

TRIBUTARIES OF MAJOR VEINS

Superior vena cava
Left brachiocephalic
Left internal jugular
Left subclavian
Left vertebral
Left supreme (first posterior) intercostal
Left superior intercostal (2-4)
Inferior thyroid
Thymic
Pericardial
Right brachiocephalic
Right internal jugular
Right subclavian
Right vertebral
Right supreme (first posterior) intercostal
Azygos

Internal jugular
Inferior petrosal sinus
Pharyngeal
Lingual
Facial
Superior thyroid
Middle thyroid

External jugular
Posterior auricular
Posterior branch of retromandibular
Occipital
Posterior external jugular
Suprascapular
Transverse of neck
Anterior jugular

Retromandibular
Superficial temporal
Maxillary
Transverse facial
Pterygoid plexus
Middle meningeal
Greater palatine
Sphenopalatine
Buccal
Dental
Deep facial
Inferior ophthalmic
Anterior branch to join facial
Posterior branch to external jugular

Facial
Supratrochlear
Supra-orbital
Superior ophthalmic
Palpebral
External nasal
Labial
Deep facial
Submental
Submandibular
Tonsillar
External palatine (paratonsillar)

DURAL VENOUS SINUSES

Posterosuperior group
Superior sagittal
Inferior sagittal
Straight
Transverse
Sigmoid
Petrosquamous
Occipital

Antero-inferior group
Cavernous
Intercavernous
Inferior petrosal
Superior petrosal
Sphenoparietal
Basilar
Middle meningeal veins

EMISSARY VEINS

The most common are found in the
Parietal foramen
Mastoid foramen
Foramen lacerum
Foramen ovale
Venous (emissary sphenoidal) foramen
Carotid canal
Hypoglossal canal
Condylar canal

CEREBRAL VEINS
Superficial cerebral veins
Superior cerebral
Superficial middle cerebral
Superior anastomotic
Inferior anastomotic
Inferior cerebral
Deep cerebral veins
Great cerebral
Internal cerebral
Thalamostriate
Choroidal
Basal
Anterior cerebral
Deep middle cerebral
Striate

Skull foramina

INSIDE THE SKULL

MIDDLE CRANIAL FOSSA

Optic canal: in the sphenoid between the body and the two roots of the lesser wing
Optic nerve
Ophthalmic artery

Superior orbital fissure: in the sphenoid between the body and the greater and lesser wings, with a fragment of the frontal bone at the lateral extremity
Oculomotor, trochlear and abducent nerves
Lacrimal, frontal and nasociliary nerves
Filaments from the internal carotid (sympathetic) plexus
Orbital branch of the middle meningeal artery
Recurrent branch of the lacrimal artery
Superior ophthalmic vein

Foramen rotundum: in the greater wing of the sphenoid
Maxillary nerve

Foramen ovale: in the greater wing of the sphenoid
Mandibular nerve
Lesser petrosal nerve (usually)
Accessory meningeal artery
Emissary veins (from cavernous sinus to pterygoid plexus)

Foramen spinosum: in the greater wing of the sphenoid
Middle meningeal vessels
Meningeal branch of the mandibular nerve

Venous (emissary sphenoidal) foramen: in 40% of skulls, in the greater wing of the sphenoid medial to the foramen ovale
Emissary vein (from the cavernous sinus to the pterygoid plexus)

Petrosal (innominate) foramen: occasional, in the greater wing of the sphenoid, medial to the foramen spinosum
Lesser petrosal nerve (if not through foramen ovale)

Foramen lacerum: between the sphenoid, apex of the petrous temporal and the basilar part of the occipital
Internal carotid artery (entering from behind and emerging above)
Greater petrosal nerve (entering from above and behind, and leaving anteriorly as nerve of pterygoid canal)
Nerve of pterygoid canal (leaving through anterior wall)
A meningeal branch of the ascending pharyngeal artery
Emissary veins (from the cavernous sinus to the pterygoid plexus)

Hiatus for the greater petrosal nerve: in the tegmen tympani of the petrous temporal, in front of the arcuate eminence
Greater petrosal nerve
Petrosal branch of the middle meningeal artery

Hiatus for the lesser petrosal nerve: in the tegmen tympani of the petrous temporal, about 3 mm in front of the hiatus for the greater petrosal nerve
Lesser petrosal nerve

ANTERIOR CRANIAL FOSSA

Foramina in the cribriform plate of the ethmoid
Olfactory nerve filaments
Anterior ethmoidal nerve and vessels

Foramen caecum: between the frontal crest of the frontal bone and the ethmoid in front of the crista galli
Emissary vein (between nose and superior sagittal sinus)

POSTERIOR CRANIAL FOSSA

Internal acoustic meatus: in the posterior surface of the petrous temporal
Facial nerve
Vestibulocochlear nerve
Labyrinthine artery

Aqueduct of the vestibule: in the petrous temporal about 1 cm behind the internal acoustic meatus
Endolymphatic duct and sac
A branch from the meningeal branch of the occipital artery
A vein (from the labyrinth and vestibule to the sigmoid sinus)

Jugular foramen: between the jugular fossa of the petrous temporal and the occipital bone
Glossopharyngeal, vagus and accessory nerves
Meningeal branches of the vagus nerve
Inferior petrosal sinus
Internal jugular vein
A meningeal branch of the occipital artery

Hypoglossal canal: in the occipital bone above the anterior part of the condyle
Hypoglossal nerve and its (recurrent) meningeal branch
A meningeal branch of the ascending pharyngeal artery
Emissary vein (from the basilar plexus to the internal jugular vein)

Condylar canal: occasional, from the lower part of the sigmoid groove in the lateral part of the occipital bone to the condylar fossa on the external surface of the occipital bone behind the condyle
Emissary vein (from the sigmoid sinus to occipital veins)
A meningeal branch of the occipital artery

Mastoid foramen: in the petrous temporal near the posterior margin of the lower part of the sigmoid groove, passing backwards to open behind the mastoid process
Emissary vein (from the sigmoid sinus to occipital veins)
A meningeal branch of the occipital artery

Foramen magnum: in the occipital bone
Apical ligament of the odontoid process of the axis
Tectorial membrane
Medulla oblongata and meninges (including first digitations of denticulate ligament)
Spinal parts of the accessory nerves
Meningeal branches of upper cervical nerves
Vertebral arteries
Anterior spinal artery
Posterior spinal arteries

Skull foramina

IN THE BASE OF THE SKULL EXTERNALLY

Foramen lacerum
Foramen ovale
Foramen spinosum
Jugular foramen   } see *INSIDE THE SKULL*
Hypoglossal canal
Condylar canal
Mastoid foramen
Foramen magnum

Inferior orbital fissure—see IN THE ORBIT

Lateral incisive foramen: opens into the incisive fossa, in the midline at the front of the hard palate
Nasopalatine nerve
Greater palatine vessels

Greater palatine foramen: between the maxilla and the palatine bone at the lateral border of the hard palate behind the palatomaxillary fissure
Greater palatine nerve and vessels

Lesser palatine foramina: two or three, in the inferior and medial aspects of the pyramidal process of the palatine bone
Lesser palatine nerves and vessels

Palatovaginal canal: between lower surface of the vaginal process of the root of the medial pterygoid plate and the upper surface of the sphenoidal process of the palatine bone
Pharyngeal branch of the pterygopalatine ganglion
Pharyngeal branch of the maxillary artery

Vomerovaginal canal: occasional, medial to the palatovaginal canal, between the upper surface of the vaginal process of the root of the medial pterygoid plate and the lower surface of the ala of the vomer
Pharyngeal branch of the sphenopalatine artery

Petrosquamous fissure: between the squamous temporal and the tegmen tympani
Petrosquamous vein

Petrotympanic fissure: between the tympanic part of the temporal bone and the tegmen tympani
Chorda tympani
Anterior ligament of the malleus
Anterior tympanic branch of the maxillary artery

Cochlear canaliculus: in the petrous temporal, at the apex of a notch in front of the medial part of the jugular fossa
Perilymphatic duct
Emissary vein (from the cochlea to the internal jugular vein or inferior petrosal sinus)

Carotid canal: in the inferior surface of the petrous temporal
Internal carotid artery
Internal carotid (sympathetic) plexus
Internal carotid venous plexus (from the cavernous sinus to the internal jugular vein)

Tympanic canaliculus: in the inferior surface of the petrous temporal, on the ridge of bone between the carotid canal and the jugular fossa
Tympanic branch of the glossopharyngeal nerve
Inferior tympanic branch of the ascending pharyngeal artery

Mastoid canaliculus: in the inferior surface of the petrous temporal, on the lateral wall of the jugular fossa
Auricular branch of the vagus nerve

Stylomastoid foramen: between the styloid and mastoid processes of the temporal bone
Facial nerve
Stylomastoid branch of the posterior auricular artery

IN THE ORBIT

Superior orbital fissure
Optic canal } see *INSIDE THE SKULL*

Frontal notch or foramen: in the supra-orbital margin of the frontal bone one fingerbreadth from the mid-line
Supratrochlear nerve and vessels

Supra-orbital notch or foramen: in the supra-orbital margin of the frontal bone two fingerbreadths from the mid-line
Supra-orbital nerve and vessels

Anterior ethmoidal foramen: in the medial wall of the orbit between the orbital part of the frontal bone and the ethmoid labyrinth
Anterior ethmoidal nerve and vessels

Posterior ethmoidal foramen: occasional, 1-2 cm behind the anterior ethmoidal foramen
Posterior ethmoidal nerve and vessels

Zygomatico-orbital foramen: in the orbital surface of the zygomatic bone
Zygomatic branch of the maxillary nerve

Nasolacrimal canal: at the front, lower, medial corner of the orbit formed by the lacrimal bone and maxilla
Nasolacrimal duct

Inferior orbital fissure: towards the back of the orbit, between the maxilla and the greater wing of the sphenoid
Maxillary nerve
Zygomatic nerve
Orbital branches of the pterygopalatine ganglion
Infra-orbital vessels
Inferior ophthalmic veins

Infra-orbital canal: in the orbital surface of the maxilla
Infra-orbital nerve and vessels

MISCELLANEOUS

Infra-orbital foramen: the anterior opening of the infra-orbital canal, in the maxilla below the infra-orbital margin
Infra-orbital nerve and vessels

Mental foramen: on the outer surface of the body of the mandible below the second premolar tooth or slightly more anteriorly
Mental nerve and vessels

Mandibular foramen: on the inner surface of the ramus of the mandible, overlapped anteriorly and medially by the lingula
Inferior alveolar nerve and vessels

Foramina in the infratemporal (posterior) surface of the maxilla
Posterior superior alveolar nerves and vessels

Pterygomaxillary fissure: between the lateral pterygoid plate and the infratemporal (posterior) surface of the maxilla, and continuous above with the posterior end of the inferior orbital fissure
Maxillary artery (entering pterygopalatine fossa)
Maxillary nerve (entering inferior orbital fissure)
Sphenopalatine veins

Sphenopalatine foramen: at the upper end of the perpendicular plate of the palatine between its orbital and sphenoidal processes and (above) the body of the sphenoid; in the medial wall of the pterygopalatine fossa (viewed laterally through the pterygomaxillary fissure) and lateral wall of the nasal cavity (viewed medially)
Nasopalatine and posterior superior nasal nerves
Sphenopalatine vessels

Foramina in the perpendicular plate of the palatine
Posterior inferior nasal nerves

Pterygoid canal: at the root of the pterygoid process of the sphenoid in line with the medial pterygoid plate, leading from the anterior wall of the foramen lacerum to the posterior wall of the pterygopalatine fossa (and only clearly seen in a disarticulated sphenoid)
Nerve of the pterygoid canal
Artery of the pterygoid canal

Musculotubular canal: at the lateral side of the apex of the petrous temporal, at the junction of the petrous and squamous parts, and divided by a bony septum into upper and lower semicanals
Tensor tympani (upper semicanal)
Auditory tube (lower semicanal)

Parietal foramen: in the parietal bone near the posterosuperior (occipital) angle
Emissary vein (from the superior sagittal sinus to the scalp)

Index

Page numbers followed by "*f*" indicate figures, "*t*" indicate tables, "*b*" indicate boxes, and "*e*" indicate online content.

Printed and bound by CPI Group (UK) Ltd, Croydon, CR0 4YY

03/10/2024

01040303-0005